PATIEN DATA COLLECTION, AND COMMUNICATION

A POCKET GUIDE FOR NURSES

CALLIE SCHLICHT

Clinical Assistant Professor
Marquette University
Milwaukee, Wisconsin

JONES & BARTLETT
LEARNING

World Headquarters
Jones & Bartlett Learning
5 Wall Street
Burlington, MA 01803
978-443-5000
info@jblearning.com
www.jblearning.com

Jones & Bartlett Learning books and products are available through most bookstores and online booksellers. To contact Jones & Bartlett Learning directly, call 800-832-0034, fax 978-443-8000, or visit our website, www.jblearning.com.

> Substantial discounts on bulk quantities of Jones & Bartlett Learning publications are available to corporations, professional associations, and other qualified organizations. For details and specific discount information, contact the special sales department at Jones & Bartlett Learning via the above contact information or send an email to specialsales@jblearning.com.

Copyright © 2019 by Jones & Bartlett Learning, LLC, an Ascend Learning Company

All rights reserved. No part of the material protected by this copyright may be reproduced or utilized in any form, electronic or mechanical, including photocopying, recording, or by any information storage and retrieval system, without written permission from the copyright owner.

The content, statements, views, and opinions herein are the sole expression of the respective authors and not that of Jones & Bartlett Learning, LLC. Reference herein to any specific commercial product, process, or service by trade name, trademark, manufacturer, or otherwise does not constitute or imply its endorsement or recommendation by Jones & Bartlett Learning, LLC and such reference shall not be used for advertising or product endorsement purposes. All trademarks displayed are the trademarks of the parties noted herein. *Patient Evaluation, Data Collection, and Communication: A Pocket Guide for Nurses* is an independent publication and has not been authorized, sponsored, or otherwise approved by the owners of the trademarks or service marks referenced in this product.

There may be images in this book that feature models; these models do not necessarily endorse, represent, or participate in the activities represented in the images. Any screenshots in this product are for educational and instructive purposes only. Any individuals and scenarios featured in the case studies throughout this product may be real or fictitious, but are used for instructional purposes only.

The authors, editor, and publisher have made every effort to provide accurate information. However, they are not responsible for errors, omissions, or for any outcomes related to the use of the contents of this book and take no responsibility for the use of the products and procedures described. Treatments and side effects described in this book may not be applicable to all people; likewise, some people may require a dose or experience a side effect that is not described herein. Drugs and medical devices are discussed that may have limited availability controlled by the Food and Drug Administration (FDA) for use only in a research study or clinical trial. Research, clinical practice, and government regulations often change the accepted standard in this field. When consideration is being given to use of any drug in the clinical setting, the health care provider or reader is responsible for determining FDA status of the drug, reading the package insert, and reviewing prescribing information for the most up-to-date recommendations on dose, precautions, and contraindications, and determining the appropriate usage for the product. This is especially important in the case of drugs that are new or seldom used.

Production Credits

VP, Product Management: David D. Cella
Director of Product Management: Amanda Martin
Product Manager: Teresa Reilly
Product Assistant: Christina Freitas
Production Manager: Carolyn Rogers Pershouse
Vendor Manager: Molly Hogue
Marketing Communications Manager: Katie Hennessy
Product Fulfillment Manager: Wendy Kilborn
Composition: S4Carlisle Publishing Services

Project Management: S4Carlisle Publishing Services
Cover Design: Kristin E. Parker
Director of Rights & Media: Joanna Gallant
Rights & Media Specialist: John Rusk
Media Development Editor: Troy Liston
Cover Image (Title Page, Part Opener, Chapter Opener): © a-r-t-i-s-t/ DigitalVision Vectors/Getty
Printing and Binding: Sheridan Books
Cover Printing: Sheridan Books

Library of Congress Cataloging-in-Publication Data
Names: Schlicht, Callie J., author.
Title: Patient evaluation, data collection, and communication : a pocket guide for nurses / Callie J. Schlicht.
Description: Burlington, Massachusetts : Jones & Bartlett Learning, [2019] | Includes bibliographical references and index.
Identifiers: LCCN 2018024081 | ISBN 9781284130416 (pbk. : alk. paper)
Subjects: | MESH: Nursing Assessment | Communication | Nurse-Patient Relations | Handbooks
Classification: LCC RT48 | NLM WY 49 | DDC 616.07/5--dc23 LC record available at https://lccn.loc.gov/2018024081

6048

Printed in the United States of America
22 21 20 19 18   10 9 8 7 6 5 4 3 2 1

Contents

Contents

Contents

Contents

Contents

Contents

Contents

Chapter 19: Hemoptysis   339

Chapter 20: Hyperglycemia   355

Chapter 21: Hypertension   367

Contents

Chapter 22: Hypoglycemia   389

Chapter 23: Hypotension   403

Chapter 24: Insomnia   427

Contents

Chapter 25: Nausea and Vomiting   443

Chapter 26: Palpitations   471

Chapter 27: Pressure Injury   491

Contents

Contents

Acknowledgments

To my husband, Aaron . . . your support and unwavering love for me is why I am what I am. I will love you as long as the stars are above you.

To my sweet baby, Theo, the heart warrior, my angel. . . We love you and miss you, every second, of every day.

To my family, friends, colleagues, and the CICU staff at Children's Hospital of Wisconsin. . . thank you for being my factious doctors, nurses, and patients throughout this book.

To my editors and reviewers. . . thank you for all of your support, flexibility, and time throughout this insane process.

To my students. . . this book is for you. "To know even one life has breathed easier because you have lived. This is to have succeeded." ~Ralph Waldo Emerson

BE THE DIFFERENCE.

Callie Schlicht

Reviewers

Janet J. Adams, MSN, RT (ARRT), RN-ONC
Instructor
Southeast Missouri State University
Cape Girardeau, MO

Linda Ann Aubrey, MSN, CMSRN
Nursing Instructor
Delaware Technical Community College, Owens Campus
Georgetown, DE

Susan D. Beck, PhD-C, RN
Assistant Professor
Bloomsburg University
Bloomsburg, PA

Eva M. Bell, DNP, APRN, FNP-BC, PMHNP-BC
Assistant Professor
Texas A&M University, Corpus Christi
Corpus Christi, TX

Jeri L. Brandt, PhD, RN
Professor of Nursing
Nebraska Wesleyan University
Lincoln, NE

Donna J. Brauer, PhD
Professor Emerita
Minnesota State University
Mankato, MN

Reviewers

Gloria Browning, PhD, MSN, RN, HN-BC
Nursing Professor
University of Tennessee
Knoxville, TN

Karen Camargo, PhD, RN
Assistant Professor
MCPHS University
Boston, MA
University of Houston, Victoria
Victoria, TX

Ann S. Cleary, DN, RN, NP-C, CNE
Associate Professor Nursing
Long Island University Brooklyn Campus
Brooklyn, NY

Barbara E. Connell, RN, MSN
Program Director
Southwestern Community College
Sylva, NC

Rachel W. Cozort, RN, PhD, CNE
Associate Professor
Pfeiffer University
Misenheimer, NC

Jena Cruciani, MSN, APRN
Nurse Practitioner
Thoracic Surgery
Aurora Medical Group
Milwaukee, WI

Jennifer L. Bailey DeJong, PhD, FNP-BC, CNE, IBCLC
Associate Professor of Nursing
Concordia College
Moorhead, MN

Reviewers

Jacqueline Sayre Dorsey, RN, MS, ANP
Associate Professor in Nursing
Monroe Community College
Rochester, NY

Diane Dressler, MSN, RN
Clinical Assistant Professor
College of Nursing
Marquette University
Milwaukee, WI

Aida L. Egues, DNP, RN, APHN-BC, CNE
Associate Professor
The City University of New York
New York City, NY

Gloria J. Green, PhD, RN
Chairperson
Department of Nursing
Southeast Missouri State University
Cape Girardeau, MO

Stephanie Grode, MSN, RN, CNE
Associate Professor of Nursing
Community College of Beaver County
Monaca, PA

Susan Hanna, MSN, APRN, PMHNP-BC, HN-BC
Nursing Instructor
Maurine Church Coburn School of Nursing
Monterey Peninsula College
Monterey, CA

Kimberley S. Hawkins, PhD, APRN, FNP-C, CHSE
Associate Professor
Bellarmine University
Louisville, KY

Reviewers

Tametra L. Jones, DNP
Professor
Maryville University
St. Louis, MO

Cathy Koetting, DNP, APRN, CPNP, PMHS, FNP-C
Assistant Professor
Saint Louis University School of Nursing
St. Louis, MO

Brandy H. Larmon, MSN-RN, EdD
Associate Professor
Mississippi University for Women
Columbus, MS

Cheryl Leiningen, DNP, RN, APN-C
Professor
Monmouth University
West Long Branch, NJ

Sherri Lindsey, MSN Ed., MSA, RN
Nursing Fundamentals Coordinator
College of Southern Nevada
Henderson, NV

Shirley MacNeill, MSN, RN, CNE
Department Chair, Allied Health
Program Director Upward Mobility LVN to ADN Program
Lamar State College, Port Arthur
Port Arthur, TX

Rhonda R. Martin, PhD, RN
Associate Professor
University of Tulsa
Tulsa, OK

Barbara McGraw, MSN, RN, CNE
Nursing Instructor
Central Community College
Grand Island, NE

J. Jean Mitchell, PhD
Professor
Northwest Florida State College
Niceville, FL
University of Florida
Gainesville, FL

Mina Mirhoseini, MD
Surgical Resident
Vanderbilt University Medical Center
Nashville, TN

Kathleen S. Murtgah, RN, MSN, CAN
Assistant Professor
St. Elizabeth School of Nursing
University of Saint Francis
Fort Wayne, IL

Michael Potnek, BSN, RN
College of Nursing
Marquette University
Milwaukee, WI

Elizabeth Pratt, MSN, RNC-OB, CNE
Associate Professor in Nursing
SUNY Delhi
Delhi, NY

Carmen Presti, DNP, ARNP-BC
Assistant Professor
University of Miami School of Nursing and Health Studies
Coral Gables, FL

Reviewers

Veronica Rankin, MSN, RN-BC, NP-C, CNL, CMSRN
Adjunct Professor and Clinical Nurse Leader Program Coordinator
Queens University of Charlotte
Charlotte, NC

Janet M. Reed, RN, MSN
Nursing Lecturer
Kent State University at Stark
North Canton, OH

L. Jane Rosati, EdD, MSN, RN, ANEF
Professor
School of Nursing
Daytona State College
Daytona Beach, FL

Mckenzie Saunders, BSN, RN
Post Anesthesia Care Unit
SSM Health St. Mary's Hospital
Madison, WI

Theresa Schnable, MSN, RN
College of Nursing
Marquette University
Milwaukee, WI

Brooke Schultz, DNP, APRN
Epilepsy Nurse Practitioner
Spectrum Health
Grand Rapids, MI

Nancy Steffen, MSN, RN, CNE
Nursing Instructor
Century College
White Bear Lake, MN

Reviewers

Nerina J. Stepanovsky, PhD, MSN, CTRN
Adjunct Professor
St. Petersburg College
St. Petersburg, FL

Beryl Stetson, RNBC, MSN, CNE, LCCE, CLC
Professor of Nursing
Chairperson in Health Science Education Department
Raritan Valley Community College
Branchburg, NJ

Becky White, MSN, RN
Assistant Professor
Blessing Rieman College of Nursing and Health Sciences
Quincy, IL

Polly Gerber Zimmermann, RN, MS, MBA, CEN, FAEN
Assistant Professor of Nursing
Ivy Tech Community College of Indiana
Indianapolis, IN

Disclaimer

The information in this book is to be used as a resource only and should not be used as a substitute for an institution's protocols and/or professional provider diagnosis and treatment. The author does not endorse any specific test, treatment, procedure, or intervention. Readers should be aware that best practice is changing continuously, and it is their responsibility to be up to date with new research, changes in practice, and treatment. All appropriate safety measures need to be taken with each patient situation. To the fullest extent of the law, neither the author, publisher, nor the contributors/reviewers, assume any liability for any injury and/or damage to persons or property arising out of or related to any use of the material contained in this book.

CHAPTER 1

Introduction

Intimidating Conversations

You are working the night shift and it is 3 a.m. Your patient has just put on the call light and is complaining of shortness of breath. You freeze. You think to yourself, "This can't be happening. She was fine an hour ago. I've only been a nurse a few weeks. What is wrong with my patient? What should I do first? Did I do something wrong to cause this? Should I ask for help? Oh man, the doctor is going to be so mad at me when I call; they're definitely sleeping. What am I going to say first? What are they going to want to know?"

Does this situation sound familiar to you? As a new nurse, you may not feel confident in your ability to handle this situation and can become nervous about the upcoming conversation with the provider. You are not alone.

Differences in Communication Styles

Typically, nurses and providers communicate differently. As you are reading this guide, this statement should not come as a surprise. Nurses tend to be more narrative and descriptive, whereas providers prefer a bulleted, to-the-point description of a patient's condition. In so many situations, time is of the essence, and while attempting to be expedient, information can be lost in the process. Differences in communication styles can lead to strained interprofessional relationships, causing nurses to avoid contact with providers, and conversely, providers dreading their phone calls. It is a frustrating situation, but can be especially difficult for newer nurses, because they often lack confidence and may be unprepared to collect essential data about an acute clinical situation.

Ineffective communication among medical professionals is a leading contributor to adverse medical events, errors, and patient death. It can also lead to increased length of hospital stay, diminished nurse and provider job satisfaction, and higher health care costs. Improving patient safety is a top priority, and a key component to addressing this issue is improving communication among caregivers.

How Do We Fix This?

The World Health Organization, The Joint Commission, and the Institute for Healthcare Improvement recommend using the SBAR communication tool to create a common language among all caregivers. SBAR can be used by anyone, but it is most widely used and initiated by nurses.

SBAR stands for:

Situation: Why are you calling the provider?

Background: What background information is pertinent to the situation?

Assessment: What do you think is wrong with the patient?

Recommendation: What is your recommendation regarding the patient's care, or what do you need from the provider?

SBAR was originally created by the United States military and was then adopted and developed by Kaiser Permanente to encourage standardized communication in the medical environment. It can be used in a variety of settings, including inpatient, rehabilitation, and long-term care. Studies examining the effectiveness of SBAR have found that it improves the perception of communication between nurses and providers; creates a safer environment; and reduces medical errors, incident reports, re-hospitalizations, and unexpected deaths. Using SBAR can reduce anxiety and allow the nurse to better prepare for the conversation with the provider and, accordingly, help to eliminate unnecessary or incomplete narration. The use of SBAR allows the nurse to deliver a thorough, concise report, which gives the provider enough information to ask additional meaningful and deliberate questions in order to develop a comprehensive plan of care. SBAR requires the nurse to critically think and use their clinical judgment in order to be a part of the decision-making process.

Why Aren't We Doing This Already?

Even though the use of SBAR has been shown to be effective, it is not always utilized in actual patient care settings unless required by the employer. Nursing programs are beginning to embed SBAR communication techniques into their curriculum, but it is not consistent nationwide. Another obstacle to the wider use of this communication tool is that there are many variations of SBAR; the most up-to-date variation is ISBARR, which adds *Introduction* and *Read Back Order* components. Giving the provider a professional introduction and reading back the given orders have been found to be simple, yet critical, strategies to improve communication within the standard SBAR model.

The ISBARR examples currently available may vary by author and do not usually provide specific descriptions for different clinical situations. While the concept of ISBARR is simple and easy to understand, the undertaking of the assessment that provides the content to complete the report may be challenging for a new nurse. Because utilizing ISBARR effectively takes experience and skill, novice nurses can have difficultly recognizing a patient's decline, formulating an action plan, and collecting the pertinent data needed to make the ISBARR report complete. *I-S-A-V-E-P-L-A-N* is an acronym that can be used to fill in the different components of the ISBARR tool.

I-S-A-V-E-P-L-A-N stands for:

Introduction: Introduce yourself and the patient.

Sign/Symptom: What is the main sign/symptom you are concerned about?

Associated Signs/Symptoms: What other associated signs/symptoms is the patient experiencing?

Vitals: What is the most recent set of vital signs (and trends if applicable)?

Exam: What are the pertinent physical exam findings you have assessed?

Past Medical History: What past medical history elements may be related to the sign/symptom?

Labs and Medication: What labs and medication may be affecting the current situation?

Assessment: What do you think is wrong with the patient?

Nursing Recommendations, Interventions, and Read Back: What nursing interventions have you implemented so far? What interventions are you recommending for the situation? What other interventions does the provider want done? Any orders given by the provider should be read back to the provider to verify.

I-S-A-V-E-P-L-A-N can be used to ensure that you are gathering all the pertinent data regarding the patient's issue before calling the provider. It was developed by the author from *The Guidelines for SBAR Use* by Kaiser Permanente. The complete ISBARR template is described below.

How Do You Use the Rest of This Book?

The next 29 chapters provide common clinical signs/symptoms that you might encounter as a nurse. You may not need to use all the information from the chapter for the ISBARR, and it will not replace clinical judgment or your institution's policies, but you will know the information if the provider asks, and it will help prompt questions during the conversation.

The chapters are meant to guide you through the complaint, ensure that you are collecting comprehensive information that the provider may need, and organize it utilizing the ISBARR format. Each chapter has the following: a brief overview of the sign/symptom; a description of differentials for the sign/symptom; questions you should ask your patient, family member, witness, or yourself; the physical exams that should be completed; and the past medical history (including medications and labs) that should be assessed. The chapters also provide evidence-based nursing interventions that can be initiated before (or while) you call the provider and plan-of-care recommendations to discuss with the provider.

As a reference, an example of an ISBARR conversation is given for the sign/symptom at the end of each chapter, along with

ISBARR Template

I **Introduction**	**Introduce Yourself and the Patient** • Patient name/room number/location • Brief HPI if the provider is not familiar with the patient • CODE status (if applicable)
S **Situation**	**Sign/Symptom You Are Concerned About** • Brief description of the sign/symptom you are concerned about and why you are calling **Associated Signs/Symptoms** • All associated signs/symptoms the patient is experiencing

B
Background
	Vitals
	• Blood pressure (orthostatic if applicable), pulse, respiratory rate, O_2 sat, and temperature
	Exam
	• Pertinent physical exam findings
	Past Medical History
	• Past medical history that may be related to the sign/symptom
	Labs and Medications
	• Recent labs that may be related to the sign/symptom
	  • Date/time the lab was done
	  • Trends of the lab (if available)
	• Medications that may be contributing or used to treat the sign/symptom
	• Know the times they were last taken

A **Assessment**	**Assessment** • What do you think is wrong with the patient, or what are you concerned about? • Let the provider know if you are unsure what is wrong.

ISBARR Template	
R **Recommendation** **R** **Read Back**	**Nurse's Recommendations, Interventions, and Read Back** • What nursing interventions have already been done or are in progress • Give order recommendations to the provider (if appropriate) • Make the provider aware if you want them to assess the patient STAT • Ask what other orders the provider wants • Read back orders and ask the provider to put the orders in the electronic medical record (if available)

a brief overview of select common or emergent differentials (for the sign/symptom) and how they may present. It is the provider's job to determine the diagnosis and plan of care; however, it is important that the nurse is able to develop an idea of what may be causing the patient's issue. It is also important to remember that nothing in medicine is exact and that presentations of each disease can vary with every patient.

References

Arora, V., Auerbach, A. D., & Sokol, H. N. (2017). Patient handoffs. In J. A. Melin (Ed.), *UpToDate*. Retrieved from https://www.uptodate.com/contents/patient-handoffs

Ashcraft, A. S., & Owen, D. C. (2014). From nursing home to acute care: Signs, symptoms, and strategies used to prevent transfer. *Geriatric Nursing, 35,* 316–320.

Beckett, C. D., & Kipnis, G. (2009). Collaborative communication: Integrating SBAR to improve quality/patient safety. *Journal for Healthcare Quality, 31*(5), 19–28.

Blom, L., Petersson, P., Hagell, P., & Westergren, A. (2015). The situation, background, assessment and recommendation (SBAR) model for communication between health care professionals: A clinical intervention pilot study. *International Journal of Caring Sciences, 8*(3), 530–535.

Boaro, N., Fancott, C., Baker, R., Velji, K., & Andreoli, A. (2010). Using SBAR to improve communication in interprofessional rehabilitation teams. *Journal of Interprofessional Care, 24*(1), 111–114. doi: 10.3109/13561820902881601

Compton, J., Copeland, K., Flanders, S., Cassity, C., Spetman, M., Xiao, Y., & Kennerly, D. (2012). Implementing SBAR across a large multihospital health system. *The Joint Commission Journal on Quality and Patient Safety, 38*(6), 261–268.

Cornell, P., Townsend-Gervis, M., Yates, L., & Vandaman, J. M. (2014). Impact of SBAR on nurse shift reports and staff rounding. *MEDSURG Nursing, 23*(5), 334–342.

Crawford, C. L., Omery, A., & Seago, J. A. (2012). The challenges of nurse-physician communication. *Journal of Nursing Administration, 42*(12), 548–550. doi: 10.1097/NNA.0b013e318274b4c0

De Meester, K., Verspuy, M., Monsieurs, K. G., & Bogaert, P. V. (2013). SBAR improves nurse–physician communication and reduces unexpected death: A pre- and post-intervention study. *Resuscitation, 84*, 1192–1196.

Enlow, M., & Guhde, J. (2010). Incorporating interprofessional communication skills (ISBARR) into an undergraduate nursing curriculum. *Nurse Educator, 35*(4), 176–180. doi: 10.1097/NNE.0b013e3181e339ac

Hart, P. L., Brannan, J. D., Long, J. M., Brooks, B. K., Maguire, M. B., Robley, L. R., & Kill, S. R. (2015). Using combined teaching modalities to enhance nursing students' recognition and response to clinical deterioration. *Nursing Education Perspectives, 36*(3), 194–196.

Institute for Healthcare Improvement. (2014). *SBAR: Situation-background-assessment recommendation.* Retrieved from http://www.ihi.org/Topics/SBARCommunicationTechnique/Pages/default.aspx

Institute of Medicine. (1999). *To err is human: Building a safer health system.* Retrieved from https://iom.nationalacademies.org/~/media/Files/Report%20Files/1999/To-Err-is-Human/To%20Err%20is%20Human%201999%20%20report%20brief.pdf

Joffe, E., Turley, J. P., Hwang, K. O., Johnson, T. R., Johnson, C. W., & Bernstam, E. V. (2013). Evaluation of a problem-specific SBAR tool to improve after-hours nurse-physician phone communication: A randomized trial. *The Joint Commission Journal on Quality and Patient Safety, 39*(11), 495–501.

The Joint Commission. (2012a). *Improving patient and worker safety: Opportunities for synergy, collaboration and innovation.* Retrieved from http://www.jointcommission.org/assets/1/18/TJC-ImprovingPatientAndWorkerSafety-Monograph.pdf

The Joint Commission. (2012b). *Transitions of care: The need for a more effective approach to continuing patient care. Hot topics in health care.* Retrieved from http://www.jointcommission.org/assets/1/18/Hot_Topics _Transitions_of_Care.pdf

Kaiser Permanente. (n.d.). *Guidelines for communication with physician using the SBAR process.* Retrieved from http://bcpsqc.ca/documents/2012/12/SQAN -Teamwork-Communication-SBAR-Guidelines-Kaiser-Permanente.pdf

Kostiuk, S. (2015). Can learning in ISBARR framework help to address nursing students' perceived anxiety and confidence levels associated with handover reports? *Journal of Nursing Education, 54*(10), 583–587. doi:10.3928/01484834-20150916-07

Lancaster, R. J., Westphal, J., & Jambunathan, J. (2015). Using SBAR to promote clinical judgment in undergraduate nursing students. *Journal of Nursing Education, 54*(3), 31–34.

Narayan, M. C. (2013). Using SBAR communications in efforts to prevent patient rehospitalizations. *Home Healthcare Nurse, 31*(9), 504–515.

Nasarwanji, M. F., Badir, A., & Gurses, A. P. (2016). Standardizing hand-off communication. *Journal of Nursing Care Quality, 31*(3), 238–244. doi:10.1097/NCQ.0000000000000174

Randmaa, M., Martensson G., Swenne, C. L., & Engstrom, M. (2014). SBAR improves communication and safety climate and decreases incident reports due to communication errors in an anesthetic clinic: A prospective intervention study. *BMJ Open, 4*(1), 1–8. doi:10.1136 /bmjopen-2013-004268

Renz, S. M., Boltz, M. P., Wagner, L. M., Capezuti, E. A., & Lawrence, T. E. (2013). Examining the feasibility and utility of an SBAR protocol in long-term care. *Geriatric Nursing, 34,* 295–301.

Scotten, M., LaVerne-Manos, E., Malicoat, A., & Paolo, A. M. (2015). Minding the gap: Interprofessional communication during inpatient and post discharge chasm care. *Patient Education and Counseling, 98,* 895–900.

Townsend-Gervis, M., Cornell, P., & Vardaman, J. M. (2014). Interdisciplinary rounds and structured communication reduce re-admissions and improve some patient outcomes. *Western Journal of Nursing Research, 36*(7), 917–928. doi: 10.1177/0193945914527521

WHO Collaborating Centre for Patient Safety Solutions. (2007). *Communication during patient hand-overs.* Retrieved from http://www.who .int/patientsafety/solutions/patientsafety/PS-Solution3.pdf

CHAPTER 2

Abdominal Pain

Abdominal pain is a common complaint in primary care and emergency room settings. It is important to evaluate every complaint of abdominal pain with a thorough history and objective evaluation before calling the provider. Acute abdominal pain has a large spectrum of causes ranging from self-limiting conditions, such as gas pain, to surgical emergencies like appendicitis. The differential diagnoses encompass GI, GU, cardiac, respiratory, and musculoskeletal problems. To complicate things further, presentations can be different depending on the patient's age, sex, and comorbidities. The first step by the nurse is to determine if the abdominal pain is suspicious for an emergent issue. Surgical abdominal pain emergencies include incarcerated hernias, ectopic pregnancy, intestinal obstruction, appendicitis, bowel perforation, internal GI bleeding, and abdominal aortic aneurysms. If any of these are suspected, the provider needs to be called immediately and a surgical consult may be indicated. Most individuals with abdominal pain have a nonsurgical issue but will eventually require a workup that includes laboratory and imaging diagnostics. It is the nurse's priority to clearly identify the location, severity, and other descriptive characteristics of the pain, manage the patient's acute pain and hydration status, and evaluate their past medical history and medication in order to help the provider determine the cause and course of action. In this chapter, nursing intervention considerations and plan of care recommendations should reflect whatever the suspected cause is.

Differential Diagnosis Considerations

Common: appendicitis, cholecystitis, constipation, diverticulitis, dysmenorrhea, ectopic pregnancy, esophagitis, food/lactose intolerance, gas pain, gastritis, gastroenteritis, GERD, *Helicobacter pylori* infection, (incarcerated) hernia, IBD,

IBS, (post-surgical) ileus, intestinal obstruction, ovarian cyst rupture, pancreatitis, PID, PUD, pyelonephritis, urinary retention, urolithiasis, uterine fibroids, UTI

Consider: AAA rupture, anaphylaxis, celiac disease, cirrhosis, DKA, endometriosis, gastroparesis, GI/GU malignancy, hepatitis, herpes zoster, internal GI bleeding, intra-abdominal abscess, ischemic bowel disease, mesenteric infarction, MI, PE, pericarditis, peritonitis, pneumonia, salpingitis, sickle cell crisis, splenic rupture, TB, testicular torsion

Questions to Ask the Patient/Family/Witness/Yourself

- When did the abdominal pain start? Did it start gradually or suddenly?
- What were you doing before/when the symptoms started?
- Where is the pain exactly? Can you point to it?
- Is the pain constant, or does it come and go? If intermittent, how long does it last? How often is it happening per hour/day?
- Can you describe the pain (pressure, sharp, cramping, dull, achy, ripping, burning, heavy)?
- What makes the pain better (bowel/bladder elimination, certain positions, eating, medication, rest)?
- What triggers the pain or makes it worse (activity, bearing down, bowel/bladder elimination, breathing, certain positions, changing positions, coughing, eating, psychological stress, sexual intercourse, touching)?
- Does the pain radiate to the back, chest, or flank?
- How severe is the pain? Can you rate it on a scale from 0 to 10? Is it waxing and waning in severity? Does it wake you from your sleep?
- When was your last bowel movement? What did it look like (consistency, amount, color)?
- Are you able to pass gas?

- How is your appetite? Are you able to keep down food and/or fluids?
- Do you have a history of lactose intolerance? If so, have you recently ingested any milk, cheese, yogurt, ice cream, or other dairy products?
- Do you have a history of abdominal pain? If so, does this feel similar? What have you done or used to treat it?
- Have you had any recent: GI/GU illness? dietary changes or eaten anything out of the ordinary? exposure to GI infection, contaminated drinking water, or been around anyone who is sick? GI/GU surgery? trauma to the abdomen, back, chest, flank, or pelvis? travel outside of the United States?
- Have you had any recent invasive interventions, such as a urinary catheter?
- When was your last menstrual period? (if applicable)
- Have you taken any NSAIDs (ASA, ibuprofen, naproxen)?
- Have you taken any new prescribed or over-the-counter medications? Have there been any recent changes to your current medications?
- What are you allergic to? Have you been exposed to a known allergen?
- Do you drink alcohol? How many drinks do you have per day/week? What kind and amount of alcohol do you drink? When was your last drink? (if applicable)

Associated Signs/Symptoms: PAIN: pain anywhere else; GENERAL: chills, fever, fatigue, weight changes; CARDIO-VASCULAR: chest pain/tightness, palpitations; RESPIRATORY: cough, painful breathing/coughing, dyspnea; GASTROINTESTI-NAL: bloating, constipation, diarrhea, heartburn, nausea, signs of GI bleeding, swallowing difficulties, vomiting; GENITOURI-NARY: dysuria, hematuria, incontinence, penile/vaginal discharge, testicular pain, urinary frequency, urgency, or retention, vaginal bleeding; NEUROLOGICAL: dizziness; ENDOCRINE: poly-dipsia, polyphagia, polyuria

Recommended Assessments

- Vital signs
- Temperature
- Weight and nutritional status
- I/O
- Pain scale
  - Tolerable pain level
- General
  - Level of consciousness and orientation
  - Inspect: signs of acute distress, acute illness, affect, restlessness
- Skin
  - Inspect: diaphoresis, dryness, ecchymosis, jaundice, pallor, surgical site (if applicable)
  - Palpate: temperature, turgor
- Mouth
  - Inspect: mucous membrane moisture level
- Cardiovascular
  - Auscultate: heart sounds, rate, rhythm
- Respiratory
  - Inspect: respiratory effort, depth, use of accessory muscles
  - Auscultate: lung sounds
- Gastrointestinal
  - Inspect: distention, pulsation, scarring
  - Auscultate: bowel sounds, bruits
  - Palpate: guarding, hernias, masses, organomegaly, (rebound) tenderness
- Rectal (if applicable)
  - Palpate: stool impaction, masses, tenderness
- Genitourinary
  - Inspect: external drainage, erythema, lesions, swelling
  - Palpate: bladder distention, CVAT
- Extremities
  - Inspect: IV site (if applicable)

Past Medical History Considerations
- Allergies

Puts the patient at risk for differential considerations
- Abdominal/GYN surgery
- Alcohol abuse/use
- Bleeding/clotting disorders
- Cholelithiasis
- Diabetes
- Diverticulosis
- Immobilization
- Nicotine use
- Ovarian cysts
- Radiation therapy to the abdomen/pelvis
- Sickle cell anemia

Reoccurrence/exacerbation should be considered
- Anaphylaxis
- Diverticulitis
- GI bleed
- *H. pylori* infection
- Hernia
- Intestinal obstruction
- MI
- Ovarian cyst rupture
- Urolithiasis
- UTI

Chronic conditions that can cause abdominal pain
- AAA
- Angina
- Celiac disease
- Cirrhosis
- Constipation
- Dysmenorrhea
- Endometriosis

- GERD
- GI/GU malignancy
- Hepatitis
- IBD
- IBS
- Lactose intolerance
- Pancreatitis
- PUD
- Urinary retention
- Uterine fibroids

Medication Evaluation
Has GI tract inflammation as a side effect
- Ascorbic acid
- Bisphosphonates
- Chemotherapy
- Iron supplements
- NSAIDs
- Potassium supplements

Used to treat common differential considerations
- Antibiotics → various GI/GU infections
- Antispasmodics → diarrhea, IBS, acute pain
- Opioids → acute pain
- PPIs, H2 antagonists, antacids → upper GI tract inflammation
- Laxatives, enemas, stool softeners, suppositories → constipation

Lab Evaluation and Trends
- BMP/CMP
- CBC

Nursing Intervention Considerations
- Call for help or rapid response/code team if vital signs are unstable or there are signs of urgent distress

- Maintain a patent airway
  - Apply oxygen if hypoxic
- Verify patent IV if IVF or IV medication treatment is anticipated
  - Flush according to facility protocol; watch for swelling, erythema, pain, and other signs of infiltration
- Medications (if ordered or protocol allows)
  - Hold suspected causative medication until discussion with the provider
  - Hold all oral medication if NPO status is anticipated
  - PRN anti-emetic for nausea, IV/IM if vomiting
  - PRN pain medication
  - PRN stool softener, laxative, enema, suppository if constipated
- Diet
  - NPO if procedure or surgery is anticipated
  - NPO if intestinal obstruction is suspected
  - Offer bland, simple foods that the patient can tolerate
  - Avoid foods that trigger symptoms
- Positioning
  - Supine or side lying position with knees flexed to chest to take tension off the abdominal wall if the patient has active abdominal pain
  - Side lying position if there is a decrease in LOC or the patient is vomiting
  - Reposition every 2–4 hours or establish an individualized turning schedule
- Collect
  - Urine sample if there are signs/symptoms of UTI, ectopic pregnancy, or hematuria
  - Stool sample for diarrhea or signs of GI bleeding
- Monitor
  - Stay with the patient until stable
  - Pain levels
  - Vital signs and trends
  - Temperature trends
  - I/O

- Bowel sounds
- Weight trends
- Agitation levels
- Orientation status changes
- Skin assessment every 8–24 hours
- Signs of dehydration such as lethargy, decreased skin turgor, dry mucous membranes, tachycardia, and (orthostatic) hypotension
- Signs and symptoms of sepsis such as fever, chills, hypotension, altered mental status, hypoxia, cool clammy skin, dyspnea, oliguria, tachycardia, and tachypnea
- Signs and symptoms of GI bleeding such as fatigue, dizziness, dyspnea, melena, hematochezia, hematemesis, pallor, ecchymosis, altered mental status, hypotension, tachycardia, and tachypnea
- Stool output color, consistency, frequency, and volume
- Emesis output color, consistency, frequency, and volume
- Urine output color, frequency, and volume
- Safety
  - Perform a fall risk assessment and implement the appropriate strategies
- Environment
  - Provide a calm, quiet environment and reduce stimulation
  - Provide distractions
  - Avoid bothersome odors in the room
  - Maintain a comfortable room temperature
  - Offer aromatherapy and/or music therapy (if appropriate)
  - Utilize a fan (if appropriate)
- Supportive care
  - Maintain effective communication between yourself, patient, and family
  - Provide emotional support and reassurance to the patient and family
  - Maintain a calm manner during patient interactions
  - Discuss plan of care with the patient and decide reasonable goals together

- Notify the patient and family of changes in the plan of care
- Promote skin care and integrity
- Offer heat or ice therapy
- **Educational topics (as applicable to the patient):**
  - General information regarding the patient's abdominal pain and differential considerations
  - Procedure and intervention explanation and justification
  - Explanation regarding referrals and specialist who may see them for this issue
  - New medication education including reason, side effects, and administration needs
  - Medication changes
  - Pain scale and pain goals
  - Relaxation techniques and breathing exercises
  - Cough and deep breathing techniques
  - Trigger avoidance
  - Skin care
  - Proper positioning and turning schedule
  - BRAT diet, clear liquid diet, NPO diet
  - Avoidance of food/fluid that trigger symptoms
  - Alcohol cessation and support
  - Smoking cessation
  - Safety needs and fall risk
  - When to notify the nurse or provider
  - Signs and symptoms of GI/GU infection
  - Signs and symptoms of GI bleeding
  - Constipation prevention
  - Dehydration prevention
  - Pressure injury prevention

ISBARR Recommendation Considerations

- Ask the provider to come assess the patient STAT if they are unstable or showing signs of emergent differential considerations

- Transfer to the ICU if hemodynamically unstable, advanced medication management is required, or closer monitoring is needed
- Medication
  - Discontinue/change suspected causative medication
  - Hold oral medications if the patient is unable to tolerate or NPO
  - Discuss changing medication routes with the provider (and pharmacy) if the patient is NPO
  - Add PPI, H2 antagonist, or antacid for dyspepsia, heartburn, or other signs/symptoms of GERD
  - Add PRN anti-emetic for nausea
  - Add PRN and/or scheduled pain medication
  - Add PRN and/or scheduled enema, fiber supplement, stool softener, laxative, or suppository for constipation
- IV fluid needs if oral intake is poor, there are signs of dehydration, and the patient is NPO or hypotensive
- ECG if cardiac etiology is suspected
- Imaging (depending on the suspected cause)
  - Abdominal CT scan or US, HIDA scan, KUB, chest X-ray
- Labs (depending on the suspected cause)
  - Amylase, lipase
  - BMP/CMP
  - CBC
  - Hcg (urine or serum)
  - *H. pylori* breath/stool/serum
  - Occult stool
  - Stool culture
  - Urinalysis
  - Urine culture
- Safety
  - Fall risk protocol
- Monitoring needs
  - Daily weights
  - Strict I/O

- Vital signs including frequency and parameters to call the provider
- Change diet to (depending on the suspected cause)
  - NPO
  - BRAT or bland
  - Clear liquid
- Referrals
  - General surgeon
- Ask if the provider wants anything else done
- Read back orders; ask that they enter all orders into the electronic medical record

ISBARR Template	
I **Introduction**	**Introduce Yourself and the Patient** • "Hello, Dr. Thompson, this is Marlowe Walder. I am the nurse for patient Cora Dilling in Room 109. I know you are not familiar with her; she is a 60-year-old patient of Dr. Bergstrom, admitted two days ago after her left knee replacement."
S **Situation**	**Sign/Symptom You Are Concerned About** • "Mrs. Dilling started complaining of acute generalized abdominal pain about three hours ago. She describes it as sharp and cramping. It has been getting worse. Now she rates it at a constant 10/10. Moving around makes the pain worse." **Associated Signs/Symptoms** • "She is also having intermittent nausea for the past hour. She vomited one time 10 minutes ago. It appeared to be regurgitated food. There was no blood. She has not had an appetite today and didn't eat lunch. She is also feeling very bloated and unable to pass gas. Her last bowel movement was four days ago."

ISBARR Template	
B **Background**	**Vitals** • "Blood pressure is 166/89, heart rate is 102, respirations are 18, and oral temperature is 98.3." **Exam** • "She appears to be in pain. I noticed she is diaphoretic, her abdomen is firmer, distended and tender throughout with guarding." **Past Medical History** • "She has a history of chronic constipation secondary to the use of narcotics for her knee pain." **Labs and Medications** • "She took one Vicodin at 1200 for her knee pain. The day shift nurse gave her one dose of Miralax at 1030 with no results yet. She did not have lab work done this morning."
A **Assessment**	**Assessment** • "I am concerned about an intestinal obstruction."
R **Recommendations** **R** **Read Back**	**Nurse's Recommendations, Interventions, and Read Back** • "I currently have her at NPO. Can we give her something IV for pain? Did you want any updated lab work or a KUB? Should I continue the patient at NPO? Do you want any IV fluids started? Do you want anything else done at this time?" • "Just to verify your orders, Dr. Thompson, you would like a STAT KUB, call with the results when they are available. Start 1–2 mg IV push morphine every two to four hours as needed for pain, and normal saline at 100mL per hour? You would also like me to hold all PO meds for now and keep the patient NPO?"

Disclaimer: This dialogue is factitious and any resemblance to actual persons, living or dead, or actual events is purely coincidental.

In order to avoid order discrepancies, it is recommended that all orders be entered by the provider in the electronic medical record.

Select Differential Diagnosis Presentations

Abdominal Aortic Aneurysm Rupture

Overview: abnormal dilation of the abdominal aorta leads to vessel rupture

Patient may complain of: severe abdominal/back pain, palpitations, nausea, vomiting, dizziness

Objective findings: signs of acute distress, altered mental status, diaphoresis, tachycardia, hypotension, pulsating abdominal mass, abdominal bruit

PMH considerations/risk factors: hx of CAD, HTN, heart failure, diabetes, connective tissue disorders, trauma to the abdomen, nicotine use, family hx of AAA, male gender, older age

Diagnostics: abdominal US/CT/MRI

Appendicitis

Overview: inflammation of the appendix

Patient may complain of: chills, fever, fatigue, umbilical abdominal pain (initially), RLQ abdominal pain, anorexia, nausea, vomiting, diarrhea

Objective findings: signs of acute distress/illness, lethargy, low-grade fever, RLQ tenderness with guarding, positive McBurney's point tenderness, and positive psoas and obturator sign

PMH considerations/risk factors: hx of IBD, previous GI surgery, younger age (<30 years)

Diagnostics: CBC, abdominal CT

Cholecystitis

Overview: inflammation of the gallbladder

Patient may complain of: fever, chills, fatigue, RUQ/epigastric pain, right shoulder pain, nausea, vomiting, anorexia, dyspepsia

Objective findings: signs of acute distress/illness, lethargy, fever, diaphoresis, jaundice, tachycardia, RUQ/epigastric tenderness with guarding, positive Murphy's sign, palpable gallbladder

PMH considerations/risk factors: hx of cholelithiasis, obesity, female gender

Diagnostics: CBC, CMP, abdominal CT/US, HIDA scan

Diabetic Ketoacidosis

Overview: lack of insulin leads to extreme hyperglycemia and the production of ketones, causing the blood to be more acidic

Patient may complain of: fatigue, generalized abdominal pain, nausea, vomiting, dyspnea, polyuria, polyphagia, polydipsia

Objective findings: altered mental status, lethargy, acetone breath, decreased skin turgor, dry mucous membranes, tachycardia, hypotension, tachypnea

PMH considerations/risk factors: hx of type 1 diabetes, medication non-compliance, substance abuse, recent major illness or stress

Diagnostics: anion gap, BMP/CMP, ABG, hemoglobin A1C, urine ketones

Diverticulitis

Overview: inflammation of diverticulum

Patient may complain of: fever, chills, LLQ abdominal pain (typically), constipation/diarrhea, nausea, vomiting

Objective findings: signs of acute distress/illness, fever, palpable abdominal mass, LLQ tenderness with guarding

PMH considerations/risk factors: hx of IBD, IBS, diverticulosis, GI cancer, obesity, nicotine use, older age

Diagnostics: CBC, occult stool, abdomen CT/US

Dysmenorrhea

Overview: painful pelvic cramping during menstruation

Patient may complain of: fatigue, pelvic pain and cramping, nausea, vomiting, headache

Objective findings: irritability, lethargy, vague diffuse pelvic tenderness without guarding, vaginal bleeding; exam is typically unremarkable

PMH considerations/risk factors: hx of dysmenorrhea, early menarche, irregular or heavy menstrual cycles, uterine fibroids, nicotine use, younger age (<30 years)

Diagnostics: clinical diagnosis; workup to rule out more emergent causes may be indicated

Ectopic Pregnancy

Overview: fertilized egg implants outside of the uterus, typically in the fallopian tubes

Patient may complain of: chills, fever, breast tenderness, severe lower abdominal pain, nausea, vomiting, irregular vaginal bleeding, dizziness

Objective findings: signs of acute distress/illness, fever, hypotension, tachycardia, lower abdominal tenderness, vaginal bleeding

PMH considerations/risk factors: hx of infertility, IUD, previous GYN surgeries

Diagnostics: urine or serum Hcg, pelvic US, pelvic exam

Esophagitis (various types)

Overview: inflammation of the esophagus

Patient may complain of: painful swallowing, dysphagia, chest pain, heartburn, upper abdominal/epigastric pain, dyspepsia, nausea, vomiting, signs of GI bleeding, dry coughing

Objective findings: oral herpes or thrush (depending on etiology), poor dentition, cough; exam is typically unremarkable

PMH considerations/risk factors: hx of esophagitis, GERD, hiatal hernia, cancer, immunosuppression, allergic diseases (food allergies, asthma, eczema), obesity, radiation therapy of the head, neck, and chest, alcohol abuse/use, nicotine use, NSAID use

Diagnostics: endoscopy with biopsy

Gastritis

Overview: inflammation of the stomach

Patient may complain of: anorexia, nausea, vomiting, dyspepsia, epigastric pain, signs of GI bleeding

Objective findings: nonspecific epigastric tenderness; exam is typically unremarkable

PMH considerations/risk factors: hx of PUD, *H. pylori* infection, NSAID use, alcohol abuse/use, recent travel outside of the United States, older age

Diagnostics: *H. pylori* serum/breath/stool test, endoscopy with biopsy

Gastroenteritis

Overview: broad term for infection (typically viral) of the stomach and intestines

Patient may complain of: chills, fever, fatigue, anorexia, nausea, vomiting, diarrhea, generalized abdominal pain, dyspepsia

Objective findings: fever, lethargy, decreased skin turgor, dry mucous membranes, generalized abdominal tenderness without guarding

PMH considerations/risk factors: recent ingestion of undercooked food/contaminated water, hx of immunosuppression, recent antibiotic use, older age

Diagnostics: clinical diagnosis; stool cultures may be considered if symptoms are severe or prolonged

Gastroesophageal Reflux Disease

Overview: abnormal reflux of acid from the stomach back into the esophagus

Patient may complain of: sore throat, sour taste in mouth, dysphagia, chest pain, or heartburn that may be worse lying flat or after meals, nausea, dyspepsia, epigastric pain, chronic coughing, insomnia

Objective findings: epigastric tenderness; exam is typically unremarkable

PMH considerations/risk factors: hx of GERD, hiatal hernia, obesity, diabetes, pregnancy, nicotine use, alcohol abuse/use

Diagnostics: clinical diagnosis

Helicobacter pylori Infection

Overview: gram-negative bacterial infection in the stomach that disrupts the gastric mucosal lining making it vulnerable to peptic damage

Patient may complain of: abdominal pain, bloating, nausea, anorexia, dyspepsia, signs of GI bleeding

Objective findings: nonspecific epigastric tenderness; exam is typically unremarkable

PMH considerations/risk factors: hx of PUD, immunosuppression, recent travel outside of the United States, low socioeconomic status, ingestion of contaminated drinking water, NSAID use

Diagnostics: H. pylori serum/breath/stool testing, endoscopy with biopsy

Hernia (abdominal)

Overview: bulging of intestines through a weakened abdominal wall

Patient may complain of: abnormal abdominal bulging with or without pain

Objective findings: visualization of the hernia in abdominal or groin (inguinal) area, should be able to palpate/reduce without any pain; incarcerated hernia will be erythematous, tender, and unable to reduce

PMH considerations/risk factors: hx of obesity, constipation, pregnancy, heavy lifting, previous hernia repair, trauma to the abdomen/pelvis/groin

Diagnostics: clinical diagnosis

Inflammatory Bowel Disease

Overview: chronic inflammation of all or different parts of the gastrointestinal tract

Patient may complain of: chills, fever, fatigue, weight loss, anorexia, abdominal pain/cramping, nausea, vomiting, dyspepsia, constipation/diarrhea, change in bowel habits, signs of GI bleeding

Objective findings: signs of acute distress/illness, lethargy, fever, signs of malnourishment, diaphoresis, pallor, tachycardia, abdominal tenderness, hematochezia

PMH considerations/risk factors: hx of Crohn's disease or ulcerative colitis, food intolerance/allergies, bleeding/clotting disorders, NSAID use, recent travel outside of the United States, nicotine use, family hx of IBS, younger age

Diagnostics: occult stool, CRP, CBC, endoscopy with biopsy

Intestinal Obstruction

Overview: inability of digestive material to move through the gastrointestinal tract normally

Patient may complain of: abdominal pain, anorexia, nausea, vomiting, inability to pass gas, constipation/diarrhea

Objective findings: signs of acute distress/illness, decreased skin turgor, dry mucous membranes, tachycardia, abdominal distention and tenderness, hypoactive or absent bowel sounds, fecal impaction (rectal exam)

PMH considerations/risk factors: hx of hernia, GI cancer, IBD, previous GI surgery, radiation therapy to the abdomen, opioid use

Diagnostics: KUB, abdominal CT

Irritable Bowel Syndrome

Overview: recurrent benign intestinal pain syndrome with associated bowel habit changes

Patient may complain of: abdominal pain and cramping, constipation/diarrhea, bloating, dyspepsia, heartburn, nausea, sensation of incomplete bowel movements

Objective findings: irritable, mild abdominal bloating and generalized tenderness; exam is typically unremarkable

PMH considerations/risk factors: hx of IBS, IBD, depression, or anxiety, family hx of IBS, female gender, younger age

Diagnostics: may not require any diagnostic testing; colonoscopy with biopsy, stool cultures, and CRP may be considered initially

Myocardial Infarction

Overview: decreased or no blood flow through the coronary arteries causing cardiac muscle death

Patient may complain of: fatigue, chest pain not improved with rest, radiation of the pain to the left arm/neck/jaw, palpitations, dyspnea, activity intolerance, abdominal pain, nausea, dizziness, anxiety, feelings of impending doom; symptoms have longer duration than stable angina

Objective findings: signs of acute distress, lethargy, irritability, altered mental status, diaphoresis, cool clammy skin, hypertension/hypotension, tachycardia/bradycardia, arrhythmia, murmur, ST elevations, pathologic Q waves, weak pulses, sluggish capillary refill, tachypnea

PMH considerations/risk factors: hx of MI, CAD, HTN, heart failure, hyperlipidemia, diabetes, cardiac valve disorders, sedentary lifestyle, NSAID use, nicotine use, substance abuse, family hx of heart disease, older age

Diagnostics: cardiac enzymes, ECG, stress test, coronary angiography

Ovarian Cyst Rupture

Overview: rupture of a fluid filled sac on the ovary

Patient may complain of: generalized weakness, nausea, vomiting, sudden onset of unilateral pelvic pain typically after sexual intercourse, vaginal bleeding

Objective findings: signs of acute distress, irritability, unilateral abdominal/pelvic tenderness; tachycardia, hypotension, positive Cullen's sign (abdominal ecchymosis) if there is intraabdominal bleeding

PMH considerations/risk factors: hx of ovarian cysts or PCOS, fertility treatments, nicotine use, family hx of ovarian cancer, younger age (<40 years)

Diagnostics: clinical diagnosis; pelvic US, pelvic exam may be considered

Pancreatitis

Overview: inflammation of the pancreas

Patient may complain of: fatigue, chills, fever, epigastric/upper abdominal pain, radiation of the pain to the back, worse with movement, nausea, vomiting, dyspepsia, diarrhea

Objective findings: signs of acute distress/illness, lethargy, fever, diaphoresis, pallor, jaundice, tachycardia, hypotension, upper abdominal/epigastric tenderness, abdominal distention, positive Cullen's sign or Grey Turner sign (abdominal ecchymosis)

PMH considerations/risk factors: hx of chronic pancreatitis, hypertriglyceridemia, cholelithiasis, GI cancer, recent GI surgery or trauma to the abdomen, nicotine use, alcohol abuse/use

Diagnostics: amylase, lipase, abdominal CT/US

Pelvic Inflammatory Disease

Overview: broad term for inflammation and infection of the female reproductive organs

Patient may complain of: chills, fever, pelvic/abdominal pain, back pain, vaginal discharge, abnormal vaginal bleeding, pain with sexual intercourse, urinary frequency

Objective findings: signs of acute distress/illness, fever, abdominal/pelvic tenderness with guarding, mucopurulent vaginal discharge, cervical motion tenderness

PMH considerations/risk factors: multiple sexual partners, hx of STDs, nicotine use, younger age

Diagnostics: pelvic exam, STD testing, serum or urine Hcg, pelvic US

Peptic Ulcer Disease

Overview: ulcers that develop in the lining of a stomach and/or duodenum

Patient may complain of: chest pain, dyspepsia, epigastric pain, heartburn, pain relief with food or antacids, nausea, signs of GI bleeding

Objective findings: nonspecific epigastric tenderness; exam is typically unremarkable

PMH considerations/risk factors: hx of PUD, *H. pylori* infection, NSAID use, recent travel outside of the United States, nicotine use, alcohol abuse/use

Diagnostics: CBC, *H. pylori* serum/breath/stool testing, occult stool, endoscopy with biopsy

Pulmonary Embolism

Overview: a blood clot in the pulmonary vasculature

Patient may complain of: chills, fever, chest pain, pain with deep breaths, palpitations, activity intolerance, dyspnea, coughing, hemoptysis, abdominal pain, dizziness

Objective findings: signs of acute distress, fever, pallor, cyanosis, diaphoresis, tachycardia, hypotension, S3/S4 heart sounds, tachypnea, hypoxia, cough, signs of DVT

PMH considerations/risk factors: hx of DVT, PE or CVA, bleeding/clotting disorder, cancer, pregnancy, HRT/birth control use, IV drug use, recent surgery, immobility, nicotine use

Diagnostics: D-dimer, chest CT, V/Q scan, chest X-ray

Pyelonephritis

Overview: bacterial infection of the kidney

Patient may complain of: fever, chills, nausea, vomiting, abdominal/back/flank pain, increased urinary frequency, retention, and urgency, dysuria, hematuria, urine odor, confusion (elderly)

Objective findings: signs of acute distress/illness, altered mental status (elderly), fever, tachycardia, CVAT, abdominal tenderness, bladder distention

PMH considerations: hx of frequent UTIs, diabetes, urolithiasis, urinary retention, immunosuppression, pregnancy, poor fluid intake, immobility, recent catheter use or GU surgery, female gender

Diagnostics: CBC, urinalysis, urine culture, renal US

Urolithiasis

Overview: calculi that form in the urinary tract

Patient may complain of: severe flank/back pain, may radiate to the abdomen, nausea, vomiting, urinary urgency, retention and frequency, dysuria, hematuria

Objective findings: signs of acute distress/illness, irritability, fidgeting, CVAT, abdominal tenderness

PMH considerations/risk factors: hx of urolithiasis, short bowel syndrome, malnutrition, diabetes, gout, obesity, dehydration, bariatric surgery, family hx of urolithiasis, female gender

Diagnostics: urinalysis, KUB, renal US

Urinary Tract Infection

Overview: broad term for infection of the urinary tract including the urethra, bladder, ureters, and kidneys

Patient may complain of: fever, chills, abdominal/back/flank/pelvic pain, nausea, vomiting, dysuria, increased urinary frequency, retention and urgency, hematuria, incontinence, urine odor, confusion (elderly)

Objective findings: fever, altered mental status (elderly), pelvic tenderness, bladder distention; exam is typically unremarkable

PMH considerations/risk factors: hx of frequent UTIs, diabetes, interstitial cystitis, urinary retention, immunosuppression, dehydration, pregnancy, incontinence, recent catheter use, GU surgery or sexual activity, immobility, female gender

Diagnostics: urinalysis, urine culture

References

American College of Gastroenterology. (n.d.). *Common Gastrointestinal Problems: A consumer health guide.* Retrieved from http://s3.gi.org/patients/cgp/pdf/abdomi.pdf

American Medical Directors Association. (2010). *Know-it-all before you call: Data collection system.* Columbia, MD: Author.

Brown, H. F., & Kelso, L. (2014). Abdominal pain: An approach to a challenging diagnosis. *AACN Advanced Critical Care, 25*(3), 266–278.

Bulechek, G. M., Butcher, H. K., Dochterman, J. M., & Wagner, C. (2013). *Nursing intervention classification (NIC).* St. Louis, MO: Elsevier Mosby.

Cartwright, S. L., & Knudson, M. P. (2015). Diagnostic imaging of acute abdominal pain in adults. *American Family Physician, 91*(7), 452–460.

Desai, S. P. (2009). *Clinician's guide to laboratory medicine* (3rd ed.). Houston, TX: MD2B.

Epee-Bekima, M., & Overton, C. (2013). Diagnosis and treatment of ectopic pregnancy. *The Practitioner, 257*(1759), 15–17.

Fritz, D., & Weilitz, P. B. (2016). Abdominal assessment. *Home Healthcare Now, 34*(3), 151–155.

Gans, S. L., Pols, M. A., Stoker, J., & Boermeester, M. A. (2015). Guidelines for the diagnostic pathway in patients with acute abdominal pain. *Digestive Surgery, 32*(1), 23–31.

Gulanick, M., & Myers, J. L. (2017). *Nursing care plans: Diagnosis, interventions, & outcomes* (9th ed.). St. Louis, MO: Elsevier.

Hale, A., & Hovey, M. J. (2014). *Fluid, electrolyte and acid-base imbalances.* Philadelphia, PA: F.A. Davis Company.

Jarvis, C. (2015). *Physical examination & health assessment.* St. Louis, MO: Elsevier.

Kruszka, P. S., & Kruszka, S. J. (2010). Evaluation of acute pelvic pain in women. *American Family Physician, 82*(2), 141–147.

LeBlond, R. F., Brown, D. D., Suneja, M., & Szot, J. F. (2015). *DeGowin's diagnostic examination* (10th ed.). New York, NY: McGraw-Hill.

Macaluso, C. R., & McNamara, R. M. (2012). Evaluation and management of acute abdominal pain in the emergency department. *International Journal of General Medicine, 5,* 789–797.

Mayumi, T., Yoshida, M., Tazuma, S., Furukawa, A., Nishii, O., Shigematsu, K., . . . Hirata, K. (2016). Practice guidelines for primary care of acute abdomen 2015. *Journal of Hepato-Biliary-Pancreatic Sciences, 23,* 3–36.

McCance, K. L., Huether, S. E., Brashers, V. L., & Rote, N. S. (2014). *Pathophysiology: The biologic basis for disease in adults and children* (7th ed.). St. Louis, MO: Elsevier

Norton, C., Czuber-Dochan, W., Artom, M., Sweeney, L., & Hart, A. (2017). Systematic review: Interventions for abdominal pain management in inflammatory bowel disease. *Alimentary Pharmacology & Therapeutics, 46,* 115–125.

Papadakis, M. A., & McPhee, S. J. (2017). *Current medical diagnosis and treatment* (56th ed.). New York, NY: McGraw-Hill.

Penner, R. M. & Fishman, M. B. (2017). Evaluation of the adult with abdominal pain. In D. J. Sullivan (Ed.), *UpToDate*. Retrieved from https://www.uptodate.com/contents/evaluation-of-the-adult-with-abdominal-pain

Penner, R. M. & Fishman, M. B. (2018). Causes of abdominal pain in adults. In D. J. Sullivan (Ed.), *UpToDate*. Retrieved from https://www.uptodate.com/contents/causes-of-abdominal-pain-in-adults

Quinlan, J. D. (2014). Acute pancreatitis. *American Family Physician, 90*(9), 632–639.

Raftery, A. T., Lim, E., & Ostor, A. J. (2014). *Differential diagnosis* (4th ed.). London, UK: Elsevier.

Saccomano, S. J., & Ferrara, L. R. (2013). Evaluation of acute abdominal pain. *The Nurse Practitioner, 38*(11), 46–53.

Seller, R. H., & Symons, A. B. (2012). *Differential diagnosis of common complaints* (6th ed.). Philadelphia, PA: Elsevier.

Thompson, J. (2017). Improving clinical care for patients with irritable bowel syndrome. *British Journal of Nursing, 26*(2), 76–80.

Uphold, C. R., & Graham, M. V. (2013). *Clinical guidelines in family practice* (5th ed.). Gainesville, FL: Barmarrae Books.

Yaghmai, V., Rosen, M. P., Lalani, T., Baker, M. E., Blake, M. A., Cash, B. D., . . . Yee, J. (2012). *ACR appropriateness criteria: Acute (nonlocalized) abdominal pain and fever or suspected abdominal abscess.* Retrieved from https://www.guideline.gov/summaries/summary/37926/acr-appropriateness-criteria--acute-nonlocalized-abdominal-pain-and-fever-or-suspected-abdominal-abscess

Zalon, M. (2014). Mild, moderate and severe pain in patients recovering from major abdominal surgery. *Pain Management Nursing, 15*(2), 1–12.

CHAPTER 3

Anaphylaxis

Anaphylaxis is a life-threatening hypersensitivity reaction that causes widespread vasodilation and increased vascular permeability leading to hypotension, impaired tissue perfusion, and altered cell metabolism. Signs and symptoms of anaphylaxis are acute and include angioedema, flushing, GI irritability, hypotension, respiratory distress, and urticarial rash. If suspected, it needs to be dealt with **immediately**. Anaphylaxis can be defined as three possible presentations:

1. Acute skin symptoms (angioedema, flushing, pruritus, urticarial rash) **plus** respiratory distress and/or hypotension
2. Involvement of **two** organ systems (as described next) after exposure to a **likely** allergen
   a. Skin symptoms (angioedema, flushing, pruritus, urticarial rash)
   b. Respiratory distress (dyspnea, wheezing, hypoxia)
   c. Hypotension (SBP <90)
   d. GI irritability (abdominal pain, vomiting)
3. Hypotension (SBP <90) after exposure to a **known** allergen

Symptoms can begin within seconds to hours after an exposure. Not all patients will fit the preceding definition(s) of anaphylaxis, and because it can be unpredictable, careful monitoring of any of these symptoms is needed. Food, medication, exercise, blood transfusions, contrast dye, latex, immunizations, venom, and biological agents can all cause anaphylaxis; however, some anaphylactic reactions are idiopathic in nature. Priorities for the nurse include maintaining the patient's airway, breathing and circulation, ending exposure to the suspected causative agent, calling for urgent help, and administering epinephrine. Once the patient is stable, it will also be important for the nurse to give education on allergen avoidance and the use of an EpiPen®. If the causal allergen is unknown, a referral to an allergist may be required for further testing.

Differential Diagnosis Considerations

Consider: anxiety, asthma exacerbation, carcinoid syndrome, chronic urticaria, COPD exacerbation, dehydration, epiglottitis, hereditary angioedema, hyperventilation, mastocytosis, menopausal flushing, MI, PE, red man syndrome, sepsis, shock, syncope, thyroid tumor, vasovagal reflex

Questions to Ask the Patient/Family/Witness/Yourself

- What are you allergic to? Have you been exposed to a known allergen?
- When did your symptoms start?
- What were you doing before/when the symptoms started?
- Do you have a history of anaphylaxis? If so, did you use an EpiPen®?

If the allergen is unknown

- Have you eaten any peanuts, shellfish, milk, eggs, or tree nuts recently or before the symptoms started?
- Have you had any recent dietary changes or eaten anything out of the ordinary? vigorous exercise? insect bite/sting? immunizations? contrast dye? exposure to latex?
- Have you had any recent invasive interventions such as a blood transfusion?
- Have you taken any new prescribed or over-the-counter medications? Have there been any recent changes to your current medication?
- Does anyone in your family have a history of anaphylaxis or severe allergic reactions?

Associated Signs/Symptoms: PAIN: pain anywhere; GENERAL: fatigue; EENT: swelling of the lips/mouth/throat, hoarseness, rhinorrhea; CARDIOVASCULAR: chest pain/tightness, palpitations; RESPIRATORY: cough, dyspnea, wheezing; GASTROINTESTINAL: diarrhea, nausea, swallowing difficulties, vomiting; NEUROLOGICAL: dizziness, (pre)syncope; SKIN: flushing, pruritus, rash; PSYCHOLOGICAL: anxiety, confusion, feelings of impending doom

Recommended Assessments

- Vital signs
- Temperature
- Pain scale (if applicable)
  - Tolerable pain level
- General
  - Level of consciousness and orientation
  - Inspect: signs of acute distress, affect, restlessness
  - Speech changes due to breathlessness or hoarseness
- Skin
  - Inspect: cyanosis, diaphoresis, pallor, urticarial rash
  - Palpate: temperature
- Eyes
  - Inspect: lid swelling
- Mouth
  - Inspect: swelling or erythema of the lips, posterior pharynx and/or tongue
- Head/face/neck
  - Palpate: swelling, tenderness
- Cardiovascular
  - Auscultate: heart sounds, rate, rhythm
- Respiratory
  - Inspect: respiratory effort, depth, pattern, use of accessory muscles
  - Auscultate: lung sounds, stridor
- Gastrointestinal
  - Auscultate: bowel sounds
  - Palpate: (rebound) tenderness
- Extremities
  - Inspect: IV site
  - Palpate: capillary refill, pulses

Past Medical History Considerations

- Allergies

Puts the patient at risk for differential considerations

- CAD
- Drug abuse/use
- Eczema
- HTN
- Nicotine use
- Obesity

Reoccurrence/exacerbation should be considered

- Anaphylaxis
- Asthma
- COPD
- MI
- PE

Chronic conditions that can mimic signs and symptoms of anaphylaxis

- Anxiety
- Asthma
- Chronic urticaria
- COPD
- Hereditary angioedema
- Menopausal flushing

Medication Evaluation

Most common causative/exacerbating medication

- ACE inhibitors
- Anesthetics
- Antibiotics
- Biologic/immunosuppressive agents
- Chemotherapy

- Contrast dye
- Neuromuscular blockers
- NSAIDs
- Opioids

May effect response to epinephrine because of antagonistic effects
- Alpha-adrenergic blockers
- Beta blockers

Lab Evaluation and Trends
- Baseline tryptase level

Nursing Intervention Considerations
- **Remove/stop suspected causative agent immediately**
- Call for help or rapid response/code team immediately. Ideally, a provider should be present to give STAT orders.
- Maintain a patent airway
  - Apply high-flow oxygen and wean as appropriate
  - Encourage slow relaxed deep breathing if hyperventilating
  - Suction as needed
  - Call respiratory therapy for signs of respiratory distress
- Verify patent IV if IVF or IV medication treatment is anticipated
  - Flush according to facility protocol; watch for swelling, erythema, pain, and other signs of infiltration
  - Large bore IV is preferred
- Medications (if ordered or protocol allows)
  - Hold suspected causative medication until discussion with the provider
  - Epinephrine 1:1,000 IM (1mg/1mL) in outer thigh STAT (max single dose of 0.5mg)
  - Rapid or bolus IV fluids per rapid response orders
  - PRN bronchodilator treatment per respiratory therapy if the patient is coughing or short of breath

- Diet
  - NPO until discussion with the provider
- Activity
  - Keep the patient in bed until discussion with the provider
- Positioning
  - Lay supine with feet elevated if the patient is hypotensive
  - HOB raised to comfort for respiratory distress
  - Side lying position if there is a decrease in LOC or the patient is vomiting
- Monitor
  - Stay with the patient until stable
  - Vital signs and trends
  - Oxygen saturation/pulse oximetry
  - Temperature trends
  - Telemetry/cardiac monitor
  - Orientation status changes
  - Agitation levels
  - Peripheral pulses
  - Skin assessment every 8–24 hours
  - Signs of decreased cardiac output, such as weak pulses, cool skin, altered mental status, hypotension, oliguria, and mottling
  - Signs of respiratory distress, such as cyanosis, tachypnea, hypoxia, use of accessory muscles, diaphoresis, and adventitious lung sounds
- Safety
  - Perform a fall risk assessment and implement the appropriate strategies
- Environment
  - Maintain a well-lit environment
  - Avoid overstimulation
  - Maintain a comfortable room temperature
  - Utilize a fan (if appropriate)

- Supportive care
  - Maintain effective communication between yourself, patient, and family
  - Provide emotional support and reassurance to the patient and family
  - Maintain a calm manner during patient interactions
  - Discuss plan of care with the patient and decide reasonable goals together
  - Notify the patient and family of changes in the plan of care
  - Provide light clothing and bed linen
  - Promote skin care and integrity
  - **Educational topics (as applicable to the patient):**
    - General information regarding the patient's anaphylaxis and differential diagnosis considerations
    - Procedure and intervention explanation and justification
    - Explanation regarding referrals and specialist who may see them for this issue
    - New medication education including reason, side effects, and administration needs
    - Medication changes
    - Relaxation techniques and breathing exercises
    - Oxygen therapy and maintenance
    - Trigger and allergen avoidance
    - Telemetry
    - Skin care
    - Safety needs and fall risk
    - NPO diet
    - When to notify the nurse or provider
    - Signs and symptoms of cardiac emergencies
    - Signs and symptoms of respiratory emergencies
    - Signs and symptoms of anaphylaxis
    - Home anaphylaxis management
    - Pressure injury prevention

ISBARR Recommendation Considerations

- Ask the provider to come assess the patient STAT
- Transfer to the ICU if hemodynamically unstable, advanced medication management is required, or closer monitoring is needed
- Medication
  - Discontinue/change suspected causative medication
  - Hold oral medications if the patient is unable to tolerate or NPO
  - Discuss changing medication routes with the provider (and pharmacy) if the patient is NPO
  - Add antihistamines
  - Add corticosteroids
  - Add glucagon if the patient is on a beta blocker and not responding to epinephrine
  - Add PRN and/or scheduled bronchodilator nebulizer treatments per respiratory therapy for coughing, dyspnea, or other signs of respiratory distress
- IV fluid needs if oral intake is poor, there are signs of dehydration, and the patient is NPO or hypotensive. Rapid infusion or bolus rates should be discussed.
- Labs
  - ABG
  - Plasma histamine
  - Tryptase
- Safety
  - Activity-level changes
  - Fall risk protocol
- Monitoring needs
  - Continuous O_2 monitoring
  - Telemetry/continuous cardiac monitoring
  - Vital signs including frequency and parameters to call the provider

- Change diet to
  - NPO
  - Avoidance of suspected food allergen (if applicable)
- Referrals
  - Allergist

ISBARR Template	
I **Introduction**	**Introduce Yourself and the Patient** • "Hello, Dr. Brown, this is Andrea Chiroff. I am the nurse for your patient Aaron Schlicht in Room 402. He was admitted for pneumonia this morning."
S **Situation**	**Sign/Symptom You Are Concerned About** • "Mr. Schlicht developed respiratory distress and hypotension 10 minutes after his IV Zosyn dose was started." **Associated Signs/Symptoms** • "He was feeling short of breath and was wheezing. He also felt like his tongue and the back of his throat were swollen."
B **Background**	**Vitals** • "Respirations were 32, O_2 sat was 87% on room air, and blood pressure was 82/40." **Exam** • "When I examined him, his lips and tongue were moderately swollen, he was tachypnic and wheezing throughout all of his lung fields." **Past Medical History** • "He denies a history of angioedema, anaphylaxis, or known drug allergies," **Labs and Medications** • "and has not taken any other medications today or eaten any suspicious foods."
A **Assessment**	**Assessment** • "I was concerned about anaphylaxis."

ISBARR Template	
R Recommendations R Read Back	**Nurse's Recommendations, Interventions, and Read Back** • "I stopped the Zosyn immediately and called the rapid response team. Eight liters of oxygen via mask was placed and his O_2 came up to 95%. We gave 0.5mg of IM epinephrine twice and an albuterol nebulizer treatment was done by respiratory therapy. Normal saline was started at 500 milliliters per hour. Systolic blood pressures remain in the 80s. His dyspnea and tachypnea has improved. I ask that you come see the patient STAT and we transfer him to the ICU for closer monitoring. Would you like a tryptase or plasma histamine drawn? Would you like anything else done at this time?" • "Thank you, Dr. Brown. I would like to read back your orders. You would like a STAT tryptase drawn, discontinue Zosyn, and would like the patient transferred to the ICU. Is that correct?"

Disclaimer: This dialogue is factitious and any resemblance to actual persons, living or dead, or actual events is purely coincidental.

In order to avoid order discrepancies, it is recommended that all orders be entered by the provider in the electronic medical record.

- Ask if the provider wants anything else done
- Read back orders; ask that they enter all orders into the electronic medical record

Select Differential Diagnosis Presentations

Anxiety

Overview: psychiatric disorder that can cause intense fear and worry

Patient may complain of: fatigue, chest pain, palpitations, dyspnea, nausea, vomiting, abdominal pain, constipation/

diarrhea, paresthesias, tremors, headache, insomnia, dizziness, mind racing, feelings of impending doom

Objective findings: signs of acute distress, irritability, inability to focus, diaphoresis, tachycardia, hypertension, tachypnea, muscle tension

PMH considerations/risk factors: hx of anxiety, depression, PTSD, insomnia, substance abuse, physical abuse, recent physical or emotional trauma, family hx of psychiatric diseases

Diagnostics: clinical diagnosis; workup to rule out more emergent causes may be indicated

Asthma Exacerbation

Overview: acute inflammation and swelling of the airway, progressively worsening asthma symptomology

Patient may complain of: activity intolerance, chest pain/tightness, coughing, dyspnea, wheezing, sputum production, insomnia

Objective findings: signs of acute distress, irritability, diaphoresis, cyanosis, breathlessness, hypoxia, tachypnea, cough, sputum, use of accessory muscles, adventitious breath sounds

PMH considerations/risk factors: hx of asthma, allergies, obesity, eczema, recent respiratory illness, nicotine use

Diagnostics: clinical diagnosis; chest X-ray, spirometry, PEF may be considered

COPD Exacerbation

Overview: acute inflammation and swelling of the airway, progressively worsening COPD symptomology

Patient may complain of: worsening fatigue, activity intolerance and sputum production from baseline, chest pain/tightness, coughing, dyspnea, wheezing, hemoptysis, insomnia

Objective findings: signs of acute distress, lethargy, cyanosis, diaphoresis, hypoxia, breathlessness, cough, adventitious breath sounds, sputum, prolonged expirations, use of accessory muscles, barrel chest, digital clubbing

PMH considerations/risk factors: hx of COPD, asthma, allergies, GERD, recent respiratory illness, nicotine use

Diagnostics: clinical diagnosis, chest X-ray, spirometry may be considered

Dehydration

Overview: abnormal loss of extracellular fluid volume

Patient may complain of: fatigue, thirst, dry mouth, constipation, palpitations, oliguria, muscle cramps, dizziness, headache

Objective findings: fever, altered mental status, lethargy, irritability, decreased skin turgor, generalized skin dryness, dry mucous membranes, (orthostatic) hypotension, tachycardia, oliguria

PMH considerations/risk factors: liver or renal disease hx of/failure, recent vomiting and/or diarrhea, GI bleeding, polyuria, diuretic use, burn injury, or intense physical activity

Diagnostics: BMP/CMP, CBC, urine Na, I/O

Myocardial Infarction

Overview: decreased or no blood flow through the coronary arteries causing cardiac muscle death

Patient may complain of: fatigue, chest pain not improved with rest, radiation of the pain to the left arm/neck/jaw, palpitations, dyspnea, activity intolerance, abdominal pain, nausea, dizziness, anxiety, feelings of impending doom; symptoms have longer duration than stable angina

Objective findings: signs of acute distress, lethargy, irritability, altered mental status, diaphoresis, cool clammy skin, hypertension/hypotension, tachycardia/bradycardia, arrhythmia, murmur, ST elevations, pathologic Q waves, weak pulses, sluggish capillary refill, tachypnea

PMH considerations/risk factors: hx of MI, CAD, HTN, heart failure, hyperlipidemia, diabetes, cardiac valve disorders, sedentary lifestyle, NSAID use, nicotine use, substance abuse, family hx of heart disease, older age

Diagnostics: cardiac enzymes, ECG, stress test, coronary angiography

Pulmonary Embolism

Overview: a blood clot in the pulmonary vasculature

Patient may complain of: chills, fever, chest pain, pain with deep breaths, palpitations, activity intolerance, dyspnea, coughing, hemoptysis, abdominal pain

Objective findings: signs of acute distress, fever, pallor, cyanosis, diaphoresis, tachycardia, hypotension, S3/S4 heart sounds, tachypnea, hypoxia, cough, signs of DVT

PMH considerations/risk factors: hx of DVT, PE or CVA, bleeding/clotting disorder, cancer, pregnancy, HRT/birth control use, IV drug use, recent surgery, immobility, nicotine use

Diagnostics: D-dimer, chest CT, V/Q scan, chest X-ray

Sepsis

Overview: severe inflammatory response due to an infection causing organ dysfunction

Patient may complain of: fever, chills, fatigue, generalized weakness, palpitations, (pre)syncope, dyspnea, oliguria; symptoms of whatever infection is suspected (i.e., appendicitis, diverticulitis, cholecystitis, pneumonia, cellulitis, meningitis, UTI)

Objective findings: signs of acute distress/illness, lethargy, fever, altered mental status, cyanosis, cool clammy skin or warm to the touch, tachycardia, hypotension, tachypnea, hypoxia, oliguria; signs of whatever infection is suspected

PMH considerations/risk factors: hx of immunosuppression, diabetes, cancer, recent infection or hospitalization, older/younger age

Diagnostics: blood culture, lactate, CBC, BMP/CMP, PT/INR; workup may also relate to whatever infection is suspected

References

Australian Society of Clinical Immunology and Allergy. (2017). *Advanced acute management of anaphylaxis.* Retrieved from https://www.allergy.org.au/images/stories/pospapers/ASCIA_Guidelines_Acute_Management_Anaphylaxis_2017.pdf

Campbell, R. L., & Kelso, J. M. (2017). Anaphylaxis: Emergency treatment. In A. M. Feldweg (Ed.), *UpToDate.* Retrieved from https://www.uptodate.com/contents/anaphylaxis-emergency-treatment

Campbell, R. L., & Kelso, J. M. (2018). Anaphylaxis: Acute diagnosis. In A. M. Feldweg (Ed.), *UpToDate.* Retrieved from https://www.uptodate.com/contents/anaphylaxis-acute-diagnosis

Chen, C., Cheng, C., Lin, H., Hung, S., Chen, W., & Lin, M. (2012). A comprehensive 4-year survey of adverse drug reactions using a network-based hospital system. *Journal of Clinical Pharmacy & Therapeutics, 37*(6), 647–651. doi:10.1111/j.1365-2710.2012.01359.x

Desai, S. P. (2009). *Clinician's guide to laboratory medicine* (3rd ed.). Houston, TX: MD2B.

Dhami, S., Panesar, S., Roberts, G., Muraro, A., Worm, M., Bilo, M.B., . . . Sheikh, A. (2014). Management of anaphylaxis: A systematic review. *European Journal of Allergy and Clinical Immunology, 69,* 168–175.

Dhami, S., Sheikh, A., Muraro, A., Roberts, G., Halken, S., Fernandez-Rivas, M., . . . Sheikh, A. (2017). Quality indicators for the acute and long-term management of anaphylaxis: A systematic review. *Clinical and Translational Allergy, 7*(15), 1–16.

Gulanick, M., & Myers, J. L. (2017). *Nursing care plans: Diagnosis, interventions, & outcomes* (9th ed.). St. Louis, MO: Elsevier.

Hale, A., & Hovey, M. J. (2014). *Fluid, electrolyte and acid-base imbalances.* Philadelphia, PA: F.A. Davis Company.

Irani, A. M., & Akl, E. G. (2015). Management and prevention of anaphylaxis. *F1000Research, 4*(1492), 1–8.

Jarvis, C. (2015). *Physical examination & health assessment.* St. Louis, MO: Elsevier.

Kelso, J. M. (2018). Anaphylaxis: Confirming the diagnosis and determining the cause(s). In A. M. Feldweg (Ed.), *UpToDate.* Retrieved from https://www.uptodate.com/contents/anaphylaxis-confirming-the-diagnosis-and-determining-the-causes

Kemp, S. F. (2018). Pathophysiology of anaphylaxis. In A. M. Feldweg (Ed.), *UpToDate.* Retrieved from https://www.uptodate.com/contents/pathophysiology-of-anaphylaxis

LeBlond, R. F., Brown, D. D., Suneja, M., & Szot, J. F. (2015). *DeGowin's diagnostic examination* (10th ed.). New York, NY: McGraw-Hill.

Lieberman, P., Nicklas, R. A., Randolph, C., Oppenheimer, J., Bernstein, D., Bernstein, J., . . . Portnoy, J. M. (2015). Anaphylaxis-a practice parameter update 2015. *Annals of Allergy, Asthma & Immunology, 115*(5), 341–384. doi:10.1016/j.anai.2015.07.019

McCance, K. L., Huether, S. E., Brashers, V. L., & Rote, N. S. (2014). *Pathophysiology: The biologic basis for disease in adults and children* (7th ed.). St. Louis, MO: Elsevier.

Muraro, A., Roberts, G., Worm, M., Bilo, M. B., Brockow, K., Fernandez-Rivas, M., . . . Sheikh, A. (2014). Anaphylaxis: Guideline from the European academy of allergy and clinical immunology. *European Journal of Allergy and Clinical Immunology, 69,* 1026–1045.

Nowak, R., Farrar, J. R., Brenner, B. E., Lewis, L., Silverman, R. A., Emerman, C., . . . Wood, J. (2013). Customizing anaphylaxis guidelines for emergency medicine. *The Journal of Emergency Medicine, 45*(2), 299–306.

Papadakis, M. A., & McPhee, S. J. (2017). *Current medical diagnosis and treatment* (56th ed.). New York, NY: McGraw-Hill.

Raftery, A. T., Lim, E., & Ostor, A. J. (2014). *Differential diagnosis* (4th ed.). London, UK: Elsevier.

Ring, J., Beyer, K., Biedermann, T., Bircher, A., Duda, D., Fischer, J., . . . Brockow, K. (2014). Guideline for acute therapy and management of anaphylaxis. *Allergo Journal International, 23,* 96–112.

Ruppert, S. D. (2013). Recognizing and managing acute anaphylaxis. *The Nurse Practitioner, 38*(9), 10–13.

Sampson, H., Muñoz-Furlong, A., Campbell, R., Adkinson, N. F., Bock, S. A., Branum, A., . . . Decker, W. W. (2006). Second symposium on the definition and management of anaphylaxis: Summary report—second national institute of allergy and infectious disease/food allergy and anaphylaxis network symposium. *Annals of Emergency Medicine, 47*(4), 373–380.

Seifert, P. C. (2017). Crisis management of anaphylaxis in the OR. *AORN Journal, 105*(2), 219–227.

Seller, R. H., & Symons, A. B. (2012). *Differential diagnosis of common complaints* (6th ed.). Philadelphia, PA: Elsevier.

Simons, F. E., Ebisawa, M., Sanchez-Borges, M., Thong, B. Y., Worm, M., Tanno, L. K., . . . Sheikh, A. (2015). 2015 update of the evidence base: World allergy organization anaphylaxis guidelines. *World Allergy Journal, 8*(32), 1–16.

Uphold, C. R., & Graham, M. V. (2013). *Clinical guidelines in family practice* (5th ed.). Gainesville, FL: Barmarrae Books.

Wood, J. P. (2016). Anaphylaxis management: Achieving optimal care. *Clinical Advisor, 19*(7), 31–39.

Wood, R. A., Camargo, C. A., Lieberman, P., Sampson, H. A., Schwartz, L. B., Zitt, M., . . . Simons, E. R. (2014). Anaphylaxis in America: The prevalence and characteristics of anaphylaxis in the United States. *Journal of Allergy and Clinical Immunology, 133*(2), 461–467.

Worth, A., & Sheikh, A. (2013). Prevention of anaphylaxis in healthcare settings. *Expert Review of Clinical Immunology, 9*(9), 855–869.

Zilberstein, J., McCurdy, M. T., & Winters, M. E. (2014). Anaphylaxis. *The Journal of Emergency Medicine, 47*(2), 182–187.

CHAPTER 4

Bradycardia

Bradycardia is defined as a heart rate less than 60 beats per minute. A slower heart rate can be a normal finding in healthy individuals, while in others it may cause hypoperfusion of vital organs. It can be due to an underlying arrhythmia, such as an AV block, but may have a reversible etiology like hypoglycemia, electrolyte disturbances, and infection. Bradycardia needs to be determined by two sequential measurements more than 5 minutes apart and confirmed with an ECG.

Once bradycardia has been verified, it is the nurse's priority to maintain and monitor the patient's airway, breathing, circulation, and hemodynamic stability. Signs and symptoms of poor perfusion and instability include altered mental status, hypotension, chest pain, and shock. If the patient is found to be unstable, they will need immediate rapid response attention and may require pharmacological intervention or transcutaneous pacing. If bradycardia persists, and the patient requires a permanent pacemaker, a consult for cardiology or electrophysiology will be required.

Differential Diagnosis Considerations

Common: age, athleticism, AV block, CAD, cardiomyopathy, heart failure, hyperkalemia, hypocalcemia, hypoglycemia, hypokalemia, hypoxia, medication induced, MI, pacemaker malfunction, sick sinus syndrome, vasovagal reflex

Consider: anorexia nervosa, carotid sinus hypersensitivity, familial AV block, hypothermia, hypothyroidism, increased ICP, infectious causes (Chagas disease, legionella, Lyme's disease, malaria, syphilis, typhoid, yellow fever), infiltrative malignancies, junctional escape rhythm, myocarditis, pericarditis, rheumatoid arthritis, seizure, SLE, sleep apnea, ventricular escape rhythm, wandering atrial pacemaker

Questions to Ask the Patient/ Family/Witness/Yourself

- When did the bradycardia/slow heart rate start?
- Is it constant or does it come and go? If intermittent, how long does it last? How often is it happening per hour/day?
- What makes the bradycardia/slow heart rate better (activity, certain positions)?
- What makes the bradycardia/slow heart rate worse (bearing down, medication, rest)?
- Do you have a history of a slow heart rate? If so, what has been done or used to treat it?
- Have you had any recent: illness/infection? exposure to extreme cold temperatures? insect bite/sting? CV surgery? trauma to the chest or /head? travel outside of the United States?
- Have you taken any new prescribed or over-the-counter medications? Have there been any recent changes to your current medication?
- Do you have a pacemaker? If so, when was it placed? Who is the manufacturer?
- How often do you exercise?
- Do you have a family history of slow heart rates or abnormal heart rhythms?

If the patient has a history of HTN

- What medications do you take for your blood pressure?
- Have you been using your blood pressure medications as prescribed? Have you been taking more than what is prescribed?

Associated Signs/Symptoms: PAIN: pain anywhere; GENERAL: fatigue, fever, weakness; CARDIOVASCULAR: chest pain/tightness, edema, palpitations; RESPIRATORY: dyspnea; GASTROINTESTINAL: nausea, diarrhea, vomiting; NEUROLOGICAL: dizziness, headache, (pre)syncope; PSYCHOLOGICAL: confusion

Recommended Assessments

- Vital signs
- Temperature
- I/O
- Pain scale (if applicable)
  - Tolerable pain level
- General
  - Level of consciousness and orientation
  - Inspect: signs of acute distress, acute illness, affect, restlessness
- Skin
  - Inspect: cyanosis, diaphoresis, mottling, pallor
  - Palpate: temperature
- Cardiovascular
  - Auscultate: heart sounds, rate, rhythm
  - Palpate: heaves, thrills
- Respiratory
  - Inspect: chest asymmetry, respiratory effort, depth, pattern, use of accessory muscles
  - Auscultate: lung sounds
- Extremities
  - Inspect: IV site
  - Palpate: capillary refill, edema, pulses

Past Medical History Considerations

Puts the patient at risk for differential considerations

- Cancer
- Cardiac valve disorders
- CKD
- CVA/TIA
- Diabetes
- HTN
- Pacemaker/ICD
- TBI

Reoccurrence/exacerbation should be considered

- MI

Chronic conditions that can cause bradycardia

- Anorexia nervosa
- Arrhythmias (various)
- CAD
- Cardiomyopathy
- Heart failure
- Rheumatoid arthritis
- Sick sinus syndrome
- SLE
- Sleep apnea
- Thyroid disease

Medication Evaluation

Most common causative/exacerbating medication

- ACE inhibitors
- Alpha-1 adrenergic agonist
- Antiarrhythmics
- ARBs
- Beta blockers
- CCBs
- Chemotherapy
- Cimetidine
- Digoxin
- Diuretics
- Ivabradine
- Lithium
- Opioids
- Tricyclic antidepressants

Lab Evaluation and Trends

- Bedside capillary glucose trends
- BMP/CMP
- Cardiac enzymes

Nursing Intervention Considerations

- Call for help or rapid response/code team if vital signs are unstable or there are signs of urgent distress
- Maintain a patent airway
  - Apply oxygen if hypoxic
  - Call respiratory therapy for signs of respiratory distress
- Verify patent IV if IVF or IV medication treatment is anticipated
  - Flush according to facility protocol; watch for swelling, erythema, pain, and other signs of infiltration
- ECG STAT
- Blood sugar if hypoglycemia is suspected
- Medications (if ordered or protocol allows)
  - Hold suspected causative medication until discussion with the provider
  - Atropine 0.5mg IV push, repeat every 3–5 minutes, max dose 3mg (done only during a rapid response and after discussion with the provider has taken place; contraindicated in patients with a heart transplant)
  - If hypoglycemic and has altered mental status or unable to swallow, give 1mg IV/IM/SQ glucagon, and/or 25–50mL IV 50% dextrose, or follow your facility's hypoglycemia protocol (goal is >100)
- Transcutaneous pacing if atropine is ineffective
- Diet
  - NPO if procedure or surgery is anticipated
  - If hypoglycemic, alert, and can swallow, give a fast-acting carbohydrate like a glucose tablet, 4oz of fruit juice, 8oz of milk, 4oz of non-diet soda, hard candy, or teaspoon of

honey/sugar. Repeat until sugar is normalized
(goal is >100).
- Activity
  - Keep the patient in bed until discussion with the
    provider
- Positioning
  - HOB raised to comfort for respiratory distress
  - Lay supine with feet elevated if the patient is hypotensive
  - Reposition every 2–4 hours or establish an individualized
    turning schedule
- Monitor
  - Stay with the patient until stable
  - Vital signs and trends
  - Oxygen saturation/pulse oximetry
  - Temperature trends
  - I/O
  - Telemetry/cardiac monitor
  - Blood sugar trends (if applicable)
  - Orientation status changes
  - Peripheral pulses
  - Skin assessment every 8–24 hours
  - Signs of decreased cardiac output such as weak pulses,
    cool skin, altered mental status, hypotension, oliguria,
    and mottling
  - Signs of respiratory distress such as cyanosis, tachypnea,
    hypoxia, use of accessory muscles, diaphoresis, and
    adventitious lung sounds
- Safety
  - Perform a fall risk assessment and implement the appro-
    priate strategies
- Environment
  - Maintain a well-lit environment
  - Maintain a comfortable room temperature
- Supportive care
  - Maintain effective communication between yourself,
    patient, and family

- Provide emotional support and reassurance to the patient and family
- Maintain a calm manner during patient interactions
- Discuss plan of care with the patient and decide reasonable goals together
- Notify the patient and family of changes in the plan of care
- Avoid vagal maneuvers
- Reorient the patient as needed
- Promote skin care and integrity
- **Educational topics (as applicable to the patient):**
  - General information regarding the patient's bradycardia and differential diagnosis considerations
  - Procedure and intervention explanation and justification
  - Explanation regarding referrals and specialist who may see them for this issue
  - New medication education including reason, side effects, and administration needs
  - Medication changes
  - Oxygen therapy and maintenance
  - Pacemaker needs
  - Telemetry
  - Energy conservation techniques: placing items within reach, sitting to do tasks, taking breaks in between activities, sliding rather than lifting, pushing rather than pulling
  - Proper positioning and turning schedule
  - Skin care
  - Safety needs and fall risk
  - NPO diet
  - When to notify the nurse or provider
  - Signs and symptoms of hypoglycemia
  - Signs and symptoms of cardiac emergencies
  - Signs and symptoms of respiratory emergencies
  - Pressure injury prevention

ISBARR Recommendation Considerations

- Ask the provider to come assess the patient STAT if they are symptomatic or unstable
- Transfer to the ICU if hemodynamically unstable, advanced medication management is required, or closer monitoring is needed
- Medication
  - Discontinue/change suspected causative medication
  - Hold oral medications if the patient is unable to tolerate or NPO
  - Discuss changing medication routes with the provider (and pharmacy) if the patient is NPO
  - Atropine if not already given
- IV fluid needs if oral intake is poor, there are signs of dehydration, and the patient is NPO or hypotensive
- ECG if repeat testing is needed
- Transcutaneous pacing if not already initiated
- Labs (depending on the suspected cause)
  - ABG
  - BMP/CMP
  - BNP
  - Cardiac enzymes
  - Digoxin
  - TSH
- Safety
  - Activity level changes
  - Fall risk protocol
- Monitoring needs
  - Blood sugars including frequency and parameters to call the provider (if applicable)
  - Continuous O_2 monitoring
  - Telemetry/continuous cardiac monitoring
  - Vital signs including frequency and parameters to call the provider
- Change diet to
  - NPO

- Referrals
  - Cardiology or electrophysiology
- Ask if the provider wants anything else done
- Read back orders; ask that they enter all orders into the electronic medical record

ISBARR Template	
I **Introduction**	**Introduce Yourself and the Patient** • "Hello, Dr. Ali, this is Katherine Wallace. I am the nurse for your patient Sheila Helm in Room 305 and understand you are the covering physician for this patient?"
S **Situation**	**Sign/Symptom You Are Concerned About** • "It was noticed during vitals that Mrs. Helm's heart rate was 48. It has ranged from 40 to 55 over the past 30 minutes. From what I know, this bradycardia is new, and she has not had this with any other set of vitals." **Associated Signs/Symptoms** • "Other than her heart rate being low, she denies any other symptoms like chest pain, dizziness, fatigue, or shortness of breath."
B **Background**	**Vitals** • "Her blood pressure is 124/70, respirations are 16, temperature is 98.4, and oxygen on room air is 98%." **Exam** • "Her head to toe is unremarkable. Heart rhythm sounds regular, and her lungs are clear." **Past Medical History** • "She does have a history of hypertension," **Labs and Medications** • "and is currently on amlodipine and metoprolol. Due to higher blood pressures, her metoprolol dose was changed from 25mg BID to 50mg BID yesterday. Her last dose was this morning at 0800."

ISBARR Template	
A Assessments	**Assessment** • "I am concerned the bradycardia is related to her new metoprolol dose."
R Recommendations R Read Back	**Nurse's Recommendations, Interventions, and Read Back** • "I did an ECG, which showed sinus bradycardia. She does not appear to have any heart block, and has no signs of ST elevations. I held her 2,000 metoprolol dose for now. Do you want her on telemetry? Do you want any changes to her medication? Do you want anything else done at this time?" • "Thanks, Dr. Ali, I would just like to read back your orders. You would like me to hold her current metoprolol dose and restart 25mg BID metoprolol dose in the AM, place her on telemetry protocol, and do an ECG and CMP in the AM?"

Disclaimer: This dialogue is factitious and any resemblance to actual persons, living or dead, or actual events is purely coincidental.

In order to avoid order discrepancies, it is recommended that all orders be entered by the provider in the electronic medical record.

Select Differential Diagnosis Presentations

Arrhythmia

Overview: any irregular heart rhythm

Patient may complain of: fatigue, generalized weakness, (pre) syncope, palpitations, chest pain, dyspnea, dizziness, seizures, anxiety

Objective findings: signs of acute distress, lethargy, irritability, diaphoresis, irregular heart rhythm, bradycardia/tachycardia, murmur, hypotension, tachypnea, seizures

PMH considerations/risk factors: hx of arrhythmia, CAD, HTN, heart failure, MI, cardiac valve disorders, diabetes, previous CV surgery, substance abuse, increased psychological stress, nicotine use, family hx of heart disease

Diagnostics. BMP/CMP, CBC, TSH, ECG, ECHO, Holter monitor/loop recorder/event recorder

Heart Failure

Overview: broad term to describe pumping malfunction of the heart

Patient may complain of: fatigue, activity intolerance, chest pain, palpitations, dyspnea, orthopnea, PND, coughing, sputum production, weight gain/loss, anorexia, nausea, nocturia, insomnia

Objective findings: signs of acute distress, lethargy, diaphoresis, cyanosis, JVD, bradycardia/tachycardia, hypertension/hypotension, displaced PMI, murmur, gallop, weak pulses, sluggish capillary refill, digital clubbing, edema, breathlessness, tachypnea, cough, adventitious lung sounds, sputum, hepatomegaly, ascites

PMH considerations/risk factors: hx of heart failure, HTN, CAD, cardiac valve disorders, MI, diabetes, arrhythmias, hyper/hypothyroidism, obesity, nicotine use, substance abuse, family hx of heart disease

Diagnostics: BNP, BMP/CMP, TSH, ECG, I/O, chest X-ray, ECHO, cardiac catheterization

Hyperkalemia

Overview: elevated serum potassium

Patient may complain of: fatigue, palpitations, diarrhea, nausea, vomiting, dyspepsia, muscle weakness and cramps, paresthesias; patient is typically asymptomatic unless severe

Objective findings: lethargy, hypotension, peaked T waves, arrhythmia, weak pulses, hyperactive bowel sounds; exam is typically unremarkable unless severe

PMH considerations/risk factors: hx of arrhythmia, CKD, AKI, Addison's disease, diabetes, burn injury, recent surgery

Diagnostics: serum K, ECG

Hypocalcemia

Overview: low serum calcium

Patient may complain of: fatigue, diarrhea, muscle cramps, paresthesias, seizures, anxiety; patient is typically asymptomatic unless severe

Objective findings: lethargy, altered mental status, irritability, positive Trousseau's and Chvostek's sign, prolonged QT interval, hypotension, bradycardia, tachypnea, hyperactive bowel sounds, hyperactive reflexes; exam is typically unremarkable unless severe

PMH considerations/risk factors: hx of cancer, immobility, malnutrition, hypoparathyroidism, alcohol abuse/use, vitamin D deficiency

Diagnostics: serum Ca, ECG

Hypokalemia

Overview: low serum potassium

Patient may complain of: fatigue, palpitations, nausea, vomiting, constipation, muscle weakness and cramping, seizures, anxiety; patient is typically asymptomatic unless severe

Objective findings: lethargy, irritability, altered mental status, wide QRS, arrhythmia, bradypnea, hypoactive bowel sounds, decreased reflexes; exam is typically unremarkable unless severe

PMH considerations/risk factors: hx of CKD, diabetes, diarrhea, alcohol abuse/use, eating disorders, NPO status, diuretic use

Diagnostics: serum K, ECG

Hypothyroidism

Overview: underactive thyroid gland

Patient may complain of: fatigue, cold intolerance, constipation, weight gain, irregular menstrual cycles, headaches, paresthesias

Objective findings: lethargy, skin dryness, facial swelling, goiter, bradycardia, hypotension, hypoactive bowel sounds, decreased reflexes

PMH considerations/risk factors: hx of thyroid dysfunction, autoimmune diseases, radiation therapy of the head and neck, previous thyroidectomy, female gender

Diagnostics: TSH, T3, free T4, TPO; thyroid US may be considered

Increased Intracranial Pressure

Overview: rise in pressure within the cranial cavity

Patient may complain of: vision changes, nausea, vomiting, headache, confusion, dizziness, seizures

Objective findings: signs of acute distress, altered mental status, GCS changes, sluggish/fixed pupillary response, hypertension, bradycardia, bradypnea

PMH considerations/risk factors: hx of TBI, CVA, CNS infections, hydrocephalus, cancer, seizures, HTN

Diagnostics: ICP monitoring, head CT/MRI

Myocardial Infarction

Overview: decreased or no blood flow through the coronary arteries causing cardiac muscle death

Patient may complain of: fatigue, chest pain not improved with rest, radiation of the pain to the left arm/neck/jaw, palpitations, dyspnea, activity intolerance, abdominal pain, nausea, dizziness, anxiety, feelings of impending doom; symptoms have longer duration than stable angina

Objective findings: signs of acute distress, lethargy, irritability, altered mental status, diaphoresis, cool clammy skin, hypertension/hypotension, tachycardia/bradycardia, arrhythmia, murmur, ST elevations, pathologic Q waves, weak pulses, sluggish capillary refill, tachypnea

PMH considerations/risk factors: hx of MI, CAD, HTN, heart failure, hyperlipidemia, diabetes, cardiac valve disorders, sedentary lifestyle, NSAID use, nicotine use, substance abuse, family hx of heart disease, older age

Diagnostics: cardiac enzymes, ECG, stress test, coronary angiography

References

American Heart Association. (2015). *Adult bradycardia with a pulse algorithm.* Retrieved from https://eccguidelines.heart.org/index.php/figures/page/2/

American Heart Association. (2016). *Bradycardia: Slow heart rate.* Retrieved from http://www.heart.org/HEARTORG/Conditions/Arrhythmia/AboutArrhythmia/Bradycardi a-Slow-Heart-Rate_UCM_302016_Article.jsp#.WEeTxXeZPVo

American Medical Directors Association. (2010). *Know-it-all before you call: Data collection system.* Columbia, MD: Author.

Bulechek, G. M., Butcher, H. K., Dochterman, J. M., & Wagner, C. (2013). *Nursing Intervention Classification (NIC).* St. Louis, MO: Elsevier Mosby.

Chon, S., Kwak, Y. H., Hwang, S., Oh, W. S., & Bae, J. (2013). Severe hyperkalemia can be detected immediately by quantitative electrocardiography and clinical history in patients with symptomatic or extreme bradycardia: A retrospective cross-sectional study. *Journal of Critical Care, 28*(6), 1112.e7–1112.e13. doi:http://0 dx.doi.org.libus.csd.mu.edu/10.1016/j.jcrc.2013.08.013

Deal, N. (2013). Evaluation and management of bradydysrhythmias in the emergency department. *Emergency Medicine Practice, 15*(9), 1–16.

Desai, S.P. (2009). *Clinician's guide to laboratory medicine* (3rd ed.). Houston, TX: MD2B.

Epstein, A. E., DiMarco, J. P., Ellenbogen K. A., Estes, N. A., Freedman, R. A., Gettes, L. S., . . . Varosy, P. D. (2013). 2012 ACCF/AHA/HRS focused update incorporated into the ACCF/AHA/HRS 2008 guidelines for device-based therapy of cardiac rhythm abnormalities: A report of the American college of cardiology foundation/American heart association task force on practice guidelines and the heart rhythm society. *Journal of the American College of Cardiology, 61*(3), 6–75.

Hale, A., & Hovey, M. J. (2014). *Fluid, electrolyte and acid-base imbalances.* Philadelphia, PA: F.A. Davis Company.

Hayes, D. L. (2018). Permanent cardiac pacing: Overview of devices and indications. In B. C. Downey (Ed.), *UpToDate*. Retrieved from https://www .uptodate.com/contents/permanent-cardiac-pacing-overview-of-devices-and -indications

Homoud, M. K. (2017a). Sick sinus syndrome: Clinical manifestations, diagnosis, and evaluation. In B. C. Downey (Ed.), *UpToDate*. Retrieved from https://www.uptodate.com/contents/sick-sinus -syndrome-clinical-manifestations-diagnosis-and-evaluation

Homoud, M. K. (2017b). Sinus bradycardia. In B. C. Downey (Ed.), *UpToDate*. Retrieved from https://www.uptodate.com/contents/sinus -bradycardia

Jarvis, C. (2015). *Physical examination & health assessment*. St. Louis, MO: Elsevier.

LeBlond, R. F., Brown, D. D., Suneja, M., & Szot, J. F. (2015). *DeGowin's diagnostic examination* (10th ed.). New York, NY: McGraw-Hill.

Link, M. S., Berkow, L. C., Kudenchuk, P. J., Halperin, H. R., Hess, E. P., Moitra, V. K., ... Donnino, M. W. (2015). Part 7: Adult advanced cardiovascular life support: 2015 American heart association guidelines update for cardiopulmonary resuscitation and emergency cardiovascular care. *Circulation, 132*, 444–464. doi:10.1161/CIR.0000000000000261

McCance, K. L., Huether, S. E., Brashers, V. L., & Rote, N. S. (2014). *Pathophysiology: The biologic basis for disease in adults and children* (7th ed.). St. Louis, MO: Elsevier.

Nicholson, C. (2014). Advanced cardiac examination: The arterial pulse. *Nursing Standard, 28*(47), 50–59. doi:10.7748/ns.28.47.50.e8664

Papadakis, M. A., & McPhee, S. J. (2017). *Current medical diagnosis and treatment* (56th ed.). New York, NY: McGraw-Hill.

Pozner, C. N. (2018). Advanced cardiac life support (ACLS) in adults. In J. Grayzel (Ed.), *UpToDate*. Retrieved https://www.uptodate.com /contents/advanced-cardiac-life-support-acls-in-adults

Raftery, A. T., Lim, E., & Ostor, A. J. (2014). *Differential diagnosis* (4th ed.). London, UK: Elsevier.

Sauer, W. H. (2017). Etiology of atrioventricular block. In B. C. Downey (Ed.), *UpToDate*. Retrieved from https://www.uptodate.com/contents /etiology-of-atrioventricular-block

Seifert, P. C., Yang, Z., & Reines, H. D. (2016). Crisis management of unstable bradycardia in the OR. *AORN Journal, 103*(2), 215–223.

Seller, R. H., & Symons, A. B. (2012). *Differential diagnosis of common complaints* (6th ed.). Philadelphia, PA: Elsevier.

Swift, J. (2013). Assessment and treatment of patients with acute unstable bradycardia. *Nursing Standard*, 27(22), 48–56.

Uphold, C. R., & Graham, M. V. (2013). *Clinical guidelines in family practice* (5th ed.). Gainesville, FL: Barmarrae Books.

Wung, S. F. (2016). Bradyarrhythmias: Clinical presentation, diagnosis, and management. *Critical Care Nursing Clinics of North America,* 28(3), 297–308.

CHAPTER 5

Chest Pain

Chest pain is a common and very distressing symptom for patients with a wide range of etiologies, including diseases of the respiratory, cardiac, musculoskeletal, GI, and psychological systems. The most common causes of chest pain are musculoskeletal or gastrointestinal in nature, but it is important that life-threatening causes of chest pain, including MI, unstable angina, aortic dissection, PE, tension pneumothorax, pericardial tamponade, and mediastinitis, are ruled out first. Typically, the patient's description of the chest pain can help the provider differentiate cardiac from noncardiac etiologies; however, women can present with atypical cardiac symptoms, such as fatigue, back pain, nausea, and abdominal pain, making differentiation more difficult.

Patients with the highest risk of cardiac issues include (but are not limited to) the following: males, 60 years or older, those with a known history of cardiac disease, pain that is worse with activity that is not reproducible by palpation, and pain that radiates to the arm, neck, or jaw. Comorbidities including diabetes, hyperlipidemia, hypertension, and tobacco use also put the patient at higher risk for a cardiac emergency. It is the nurse's priority to stabilize the patient's airway, breathing, and circulation, perform an ECG, assess the patient's risk factors, work quickly to help the provider figure out the underlying cause of the patient's chest pain, and call a rapid response or code team if the patient appears unstable. In this chapter, nursing intervention considerations and plan of care recommendations should reflect whatever the suspected cause is.

Differential Diagnosis Considerations

Common: anxiety, arrhythmia, asthma exacerbation, cocaine use, COPD exacerbation, costochondritis, esophageal spasm, esophagitis, GERD, heart failure, MI, PE, pneumonia, pneumothorax, PUD, rib pain, stable angina, unstable angina

Consider: acute chest syndrome, aortic dissection, biliary disease, cervical disc disease, cholecystitis, esophageal rupture, herpes zoster, hiatal hernia, mediastinitis, MVP, myocarditis, pancreatitis, pericardial tamponade, pericarditis, pleuritis, pulmonary HTN, sarcoidosis, sickle cell crisis

Questions to Ask the Patient/Family/Witness/Yourself

- When did the chest pain start? Did it start gradually or suddenly?
- What were you doing before/when the symptoms started?
- Where is the pain exactly? Can you point to it?
- Is the pain constant or does it come and go? If intermittent, how long does it last? How often is it happening per hour/day?
- Can you describe the pain (pressure, sharp, cramping, dull, achy, ripping, burning, heavy)?
- What makes the chest pain better (certain positions, eating, medication, rest)?
- What triggers the pain or makes it worse (activity, breathing, certain positions, changing positions, coughing, eating, touching, psychological stress)?
- Does the pain radiate to the abdomen, back, flank, arm, jaw, or neck?
- How severe is your pain? Can you rate it on a scale from 0 to 10? Is it waxing and waning in severity?
- Do you have a history of chest pain? If so, does it feel similar? What have you done or used to treat it?
- Have you had any recent: CV/GI/orthopedic/thoracic surgery? immobilization such as prolonged time spent in bed or sitting? respiratory illness? trauma to the abdomen, back, or chest?
- Do you take any medication for your chest pain issues? If so, have you been taking your medication as prescribed? (if applicable)
- Do you use any inhalers? If so, have you been taking them as prescribed? (if applicable)
- Have you taken any new prescribed or over-the-counter medications? Have there been any recent changes to your current medication?

- Do you have a family history of heart disease or heart attacks?
- Do you smoke? How much (ppd)? How long have you been smoking? (if applicable)
- Do you have a history of drug use? What types and how much? Do you use on a daily basis? When was your last use? (if applicable)

Associated Signs/Symptoms: PAIN: pain anywhere else; GENERAL: fatigue, fever, weakness; CARDIOVASCULAR: edema, palpitations, PND, orthopnea; RESPIRATORY: cough, hemoptysis, painful breathing/coughing, dyspnea, sputum production, wheezing; GASTROINTESTINAL: belching, heartburn, nausea, swallowing difficulties, vomiting; NEUROLOGICAL: dizziness, syncope; PSYCHOLOGICAL: anxiety, confusion, feelings of impending doom

Recommended Assessments

- Vital signs
- Temperature
- Weight and nutritional status
- I/O
- Pain scale
  - Tolerable pain level
- General
  - Level of consciousness and orientation
  - Inspect: signs of acute distress, acute illness, affect, restlessness
  - Difficulty speaking due to breathlessness
- Skin
  - Inspect: cyanosis, diaphoresis, mottling, pallor, vesicular rash
  - Palpate: temperature
- Head/face/neck
  - Inspect: JVD, tracheal deviation
  - Auscultate: carotid bruits
- Cardiovascular
  - Auscultate: heart sounds, rate, rhythm
  - Palpate: heaves, thrills

- Respiratory
  - Inspect: chest asymmetry, respiratory effort, depth, pattern, use of accessory muscles
  - Auscultate: lung sounds, stridor
- Gastrointestinal
  - Auscultate: bowel sounds
  - Palpate: tenderness
- Musculoskeletal
  - Palpate: chest wall tenderness
- Extremities
  - Inspect: IV site
  - Palpate: capillary refill, edema, pulses

Past Medical History Considerations
Puts the patient at risk for differential considerations

- Bleeding/clotting disorder
- CAD
- Cancer
- Cardiac valve disorders
- Cardiomyopathy
- Cholelithiasis
- Diabetes
- Drug abuse/use
- DVT
- HTN
- Hyperlipidemia
- Immobilization
- Nicotine use
- PVD
- Sickle cell anemia

Reoccurrence/exacerbation should be considered

- Arrhythmias (various)
- Asthma
- COPD

- Heart failure
- Herpes zoster
- MI
- PE

Chronic conditions that can cause chest pain
- Angina (stable)
- Anxiety
- Arrhythmias (various)
- Cervical DDD
- GERD
- Heart failure
- MVP
- Pancreatitis
- PUD
- Pulmonary HTN
- Sarcoidosis

Medication Evaluation
Has GI tract inflammation as a side effect
- Ascorbic acid
- Bisphosphonates
- Chemotherapy
- Iron supplements
- NSAIDs
- Potassium supplements

Puts the patient at risk for differential considerations
- Birth control/HRT → PE

Used to treat common differential considerations
- Antibiotics → various respiratory infections
- Benzodiazepines → acute anxiety
- Beta blockers → arrhythmias, cardioprotection

- CCBs → arrhythmias
- Corticosteroids → airway inflammation
- Diuretics → fluid overload
- ICS, LABA, LAMA, SABA, SAMA, and combination inhalers → chronic lung disease
- Nitrates → angina
- NSAIDs → chest wall inflammation
- Opioids → acute pain
- PPIs, H2 antagonists, antacids → upper GI tract inflammation
- SSRIs → chronic anxiety

Lab Evaluation and Trends

- BMP/CMP
- BNP
- Cardiac enzymes
- CBC

Nursing Intervention Considerations

- Call for help or rapid response/code team if vital signs are unstable or there are signs of urgent distress
- Maintain a patent airway
  - Apply oxygen if hypoxic
  - Encourage cough and deep breathing
  - Chest splinting with a pillow to promote more effective coughing
  - Encourage slow relaxed deep breathing if hyperventilating
  - Suction as needed
  - Call respiratory therapy for signs of respiratory distress
- Verify patent IV if IVF or IV medication treatment is anticipated
  - Flush according to facility protocol; watch for swelling, erythema, pain, and other signs of infiltration
- ECG STAT

- Medications (if ordered or protocol allows)
  - ASA 324mg chewed if MI is suspected
  - NTG 0.4mg SL every 5 minutes × 3 doses if MI is suspected
  - PRN IV push morphine for severe chest pain if MI is suspected (should be avoided if possible)
  - PRN bronchodilator treatment per respiratory therapy if the patient is coughing or short of breath
- Diet
  - NPO if procedure or surgery is anticipated
  - Restrict fluids until discussion with the provider, if there are signs of fluid overload
  - Offer bland, simple foods that the patient can tolerate
  - Encourage heart healthy, low-sodium food choices
  - Avoid foods that trigger symptoms
  - Avoid caffeine
- Activity
  - Keep the patient in bed until discussion with the provider
- Positioning
  - HOB raised to comfort for respiratory distress
  - HOB raised for 2–3 hours after meals or at night for GI symptomology
  - Reposition every 2–4 hours or establish an individualized turning schedule
- Monitor
  - Stay with the patient until stable
  - Pain levels
  - Vital signs and trends
  - Weight trends
  - Oxygen saturation/pulse oximetry
  - Temperature trends
  - Telemetry/cardiac monitor
  - I/O
  - Orientation status changes

- Agitation levels
- Peripheral pulses
- Skin assessment every 8–24 hours
- Signs of decreased cardiac output such as weak pulses, cool skin, altered mental status, hypotension, oliguria, and mottling
- Signs of respiratory distress such as cyanosis, tachypnea, hypoxia, use of accessory muscles, diaphoresis, and adventitious lung sounds
- Signs and symptoms of fluid overload such as cough, adventitious lung sounds, dyspnea, tachypnea, weight gain, edema, JVD, and ascites
- Safety
  - Perform a fall risk assessment and implement the appropriate strategies
- Environment
  - Provide a calm, quiet environment and reduce stimulation
  - Maintain a well-lit environment
  - Provide distractions
  - Maintain a comfortable room temperature
  - Offer aromatherapy and/or music therapy (if appropriate)
  - Utilize a fan (if appropriate)
- Supportive care
  - Maintain effective communication between yourself, patient, and family
  - Provide emotional support and reassurance to the patient and family
  - Maintain a calm manner during patient interactions
  - Discuss plan of care with the patient and decide reasonable goals together
  - Notify the patient and family of changes in the plan of care
  - Identify barriers to care and compliance

- Promote skin care and integrity
- Provide light clothing and bed linen
- **Educational topics (as applicable to the patient):**
  - General information regarding the patient's chest pain and differential diagnosis considerations
  - Procedure and intervention explanation and justification
  - Explanation regarding referrals and specialist who may see them for this issue
  - New medication education including reason, side effects, and administration needs
  - Medication changes
  - Medication compliance
  - NTG home use
  - Pain scale and pain goals
  - Cough and deep-breathing techniques
  - Oxygen therapy and maintenance
  - Relaxation techniques and breathing exercises
  - Trigger avoidance
  - Telemetry
  - Energy conservation techniques: placing items within reach, sitting to do tasks, taking breaks in between activities, sliding rather than lifting, pushing rather than pulling
  - Proper positioning and turning schedule
  - Skin care
  - Stress reduction and management
  - Safety needs and fall risk
  - Fluid restriction
  - Caffeine restriction
  - DASH diet, BRAT diet, NPO diet
  - Avoidance of food/fluid that trigger symptoms
  - Weight loss, physical activity, and exercise needs
  - Home blood pressure monitoring

- Smoking cessation
- Drug cessation and support
- When to notify the nurse or provider
- Signs and symptoms of cardiac emergencies
- Signs and symptoms of respiratory emergencies
- Signs and symptoms of fluid overload
- Pressure injury prevention

ISBARR Recommendation Considerations

- Ask the provider to come assess the patient STAT if they are symptomatic, unstable, or at high risk for cardiac emergencies
- Transfer to the ICU if hemodynamically unstable, advanced medication management is required, or closer monitoring is needed
- Medication
  - Discontinue/change suspected causative medication
  - Hold oral medications if the patient is unable to tolerate or NPO
  - Discuss changing medication routes with the provider (and pharmacy) if the patient is NPO
  - Add ASA if indicated for MI
  - Add PPI, H2 antagonist or antacid for dyspepsia, heartburn, or other signs/symptoms of GERD
  - Add/change diuretics for signs of fluid overload
  - Add corticosteroids for airway inflammation
  - Add PRN NTG if indicated for MI or angina
  - Add PRN antiemetic for nausea
  - Add PRN and/or scheduled medication for anxiety or irritability
  - Add PRN and/or scheduled bronchodilator nebulizer treatments per respiratory therapy for coughing, dyspnea, or other signs of respiratory distress
  - Add PRN and/or scheduled pain medication

- IV fluid needs if oral intake is poor, there are signs of dehydration, and the patient is NPO or hypotensive
- ECG if repeat testing is needed
- Imaging (depending on the suspected cause)
  - Chest CT scan, chest X-ray
- Labs (depending on the suspected cause)
  - ABG
  - BMP/CMP
  - BNP
  - Cardiac enzymes
  - CBC
  - D-dimer
- Safety
  - Activity level changes
  - Fall risk protocol
- Monitoring needs
  - Daily weights
  - Strict I/O
  - Continuous O_2 monitoring
  - Telemetry/continuous cardiac monitoring
  - Vital signs including frequency and parameters to call the provider
- Supportive cares
  - Compression stockings or SCDs
- Change diet to (depending on the suspected cause)
  - NPO
  - BRAT or bland
  - Caffeine restriction
  - DASH, low sodium
  - Fluid restriction
- Referrals
  - Cardiology
- Ask if the provider wants anything else done
- Read back orders; ask that they enter all orders into the electronic medical record

ISBARR Template

I **Introduction**	**Introduce Yourself and the Patient** • "Hello, Dr. Mirhoseini. This is Mina Nordness. I am the nurse for your patient Andrea Zimmerman in Room 603."
S **Situation**	**Sign/Symptom You Are Concerned About** • "I am calling because Ms. Zimmerman developed severe constant 10/10-chest pain five minutes ago. She is describing it as a pressure that is worse with deep breaths." **Associated Signs/Symptoms** • "She is also having constant shortness of breath and intermittent palpitations that are happening every two to three minutes."
B **Background**	**Vitals** • "She is tachypnic with a respiratory rate of 45, and tachycardic with a heart rate of 120. O_2 sat is 90% on room air and blood pressure is 160/92." **Exam** • "She is diaphoretic, pale, and her lungs are clear," **Past Medical History** • "and has no history of blood clots, CAD, or anxiety." **Labs and Medications** • "Her CBC and CMP had no abnormalities this morning, and she is not on any anticoagulants or estrogen replacements. She has been fairly immobile since being hospitalized and is rarely out of bed."
A **Assessment**	**Assessment** • "I am concerned about a pulmonary embolism."

ISBARR Template	
R **Recommendations** **R** **Read Back**	**Nurse's Recommendations, Interventions, and Read Back** • "I have placed her on four liters nasal cannula and her oxygen saturation is now at 95%. Twelve-lead ECG showed sinus rhythm, and there were no ST elevations. I have been taking vital signs every five minutes. Respiratory therapy is in the room monitoring the patient with me. Would you like cardiac enzymes, D-dimer, or other lab work? What about a chest CT or other imaging? Do you want anything else done at this time?" • "Dr. Mirhoseini, if I could read back your orders. You would like a STAT CT of the chest, CMP, CBC, D-dimer, and troponin. Call with results when they are available. Place patient on telemetry and keep her on continuous O_2 monitoring."

Disclaimer: This dialogue is factitious and any resemblance to actual persons, living or dead, or actual events is purely coincidental.

In order to avoid order discrepancies, it is recommended that all orders be entered by the provider in the electronic medical record.

Select Differential Diagnosis Presentations

Acute Chest Syndrome

Overview: vaso-occlusive crisis of the pulmonary vasculature in patients with sickle cell anemia

Patient may complain of: chills, fever, fatigue, chest pain, dyspnea, wheezing, coughing, sputum production

Objective findings: signs of acute distress/illness, fever, lethargy, warm skin, hypoxia, tachypnea, cough, sputum, use of accessory muscles, adventitious breath sounds

PMH considerations/risk factors: hx of sickle cell anemia, asthma, recent respiratory illness

Diagnostics: CBC, ECG, chest X-ray, chest CT

Angina (Stable)

Overview: chest pain caused by a decrease in myocardial oxygen supply that is improved with rest

Patient may complain of: fatigue, chest pain/tightness/heaviness that is worse with activity, better with rest or NTG, radiation of the pain to the left arm/neck/jaw, palpitations, dyspnea, activity intolerance, nausea, dyspepsia, dizziness, feelings of impending doom, anxiety; symptoms have a short duration

Objective findings: signs of acute distress, lethargy, diaphoresis, hypertension, tachycardia, murmur, weak pulses, sluggish capillary refill, tachypnea

PMH considerations/risk factors: hx of angina, CAD, HTN, heart failure, hyperlipidemia, diabetes, cardiac valve disorders, obesity, increased psychological stress, nicotine use, family hx of heart disease

Diagnostics: cardiac enzymes, ECG, stress test, coronary angiography

Angina (Unstable)

Overview: chest pain caused by a decrease in myocardial oxygen supply that is not improved with rest

Patient may complain of: fatigue, chest pain/tightness/heaviness that is worse with activity, not improved with rest or NTG, radiation of the pain to the left arm/neck/jaw, palpitations, dyspnea, activity intolerance, nausea, dyspepsia, dizziness, feelings of impending doom, anxiety; symptoms have a longer duration than stable angina

Objective findings: signs of acute distress, lethargy, diaphoresis, hypertension, tachycardia, murmur, weak pulses, sluggish capillary refill, tachypnea

PMH considerations/risk factors: hx of angina, CAD, HTN, heart failure, hyperlipidemia, diabetes, cardiac valve disorders, obesity, increased psychological stress, nicotine use, family hx of heart disease

Diagnostics: cardiac enzymes, ECG, stress test, coronary angiography

Anxiety

Overview: psychiatric disorder that can cause intense fear and worry

Patient may complain of: fatigue, chest pain, palpitations, dyspnea, nausea, vomiting, abdominal pain, constipation/diarrhea, paresthesias, tremors, headache, insomnia, dizziness, mind racing, feelings of impending doom

Objective findings: signs of acute distress, irritability, inability to focus, diaphoresis, tachycardia, hypertension, tachypnea, muscle tension

PMH considerations/risk factors: hx of anxiety, depression, PTSD, insomnia, substance abuse, physical abuse, recent physical or emotional trauma, family hx of psychiatric diseases

Diagnostics: clinical diagnosis; workup to rule out more emergent causes may be indicated

Aortic Dissection

Overview: a tear in the intima layer of the aorta

Patient may complain of: severe chest/back pain described as ripping or tearing, abdominal pain, flank pain, dyspnea, nausea, dizziness, (pre)syncope, paresthesias, feelings of impending doom

Objective findings: signs of acute distress, altered mental status, diaphoresis, cool clammy skin, syncope, JVD, murmur, hypotension/hypertension, weak pulses or pulse deficit, sluggish capillary refill, tachypnea

PMH considerations/risk factors: hx of HTN, heart failure, cardiac valve disorders, connective tissue disorders, diabetes, substance abuse, pregnancy, nicotine use, male gender, older age

Diagnostics: ECG, TEE, chest X-ray, chest CT, aortography

Arrhythmia

Overview: any irregular heart rhythm

Patient may complain of: fatigue, generalized weakness, (pre)syncope, palpitations, chest pain, dyspnea, dizziness, anxiety

Objective findings: signs of acute distress, lethargy, irritability, diaphoresis, irregular heart rhythm, bradycardia/tachycardia, murmur, hypotension, tachypnea, seizures

PMH considerations/risk factors: hx of arrhythmia, CAD, HTN, heart failure, MI, cardiac valve disorders, diabetes, previous CV surgery, substance abuse, increased psychological stress, nicotine use, family hx of heart disease

Diagnostics: BMP/CMP, CBC, TSH, ECG, ECHO, Holter monitor/loop recorder/event recorder

Asthma Exacerbation

Overview: acute inflammation and swelling of the airway, progressively worsening asthma symptomology

Patient may complain of: activity intolerance, chest pain/tightness, coughing, dyspnea, wheezing, sputum production, insomnia

Objective findings: signs of acute distress, irritability, diaphoresis, cyanosis, breathlessness, hypoxia, tachypnea, cough, sputum, use of accessory muscles, adventitious breath sounds

PMH considerations/risk factors: hx of asthma, allergies, obesity, eczema, recent respiratory illness, nicotine use

Diagnostics: clinical diagnosis; chest X-ray, spirometry, and PEF may be considered

Cholecystitis

Overview: inflammation of the gallbladder

Patient may complain of: fever, chills, fatigue, RUQ/epigastric pain, right shoulder pain, nausea, vomiting, anorexia, dyspepsia

Objective findings: signs of acute distress/illness, lethargy, fever, diaphoresis, jaundice, tachycardia, RUQ/epigastric tenderness with guarding, positive Murphy's sign, palpable gallbladder

PMH considerations/risk factors: hx of cholelithiasis, obesity, female gender

Diagnostics: CBC, CMP, abdominal CT/US, HIDA scan

COPD Exacerbation

Overview: acute inflammation and swelling of the airway, progressively worsening COPD symptomology

Patient may complain of: worsening fatigue, activity intolerance and sputum production from baseline, chest pain/tightness, coughing, dyspnea, wheezing, hemoptysis, insomnia

Objective findings: signs of acute distress, lethargy, cyanosis, diaphoresis, hypoxia, breathlessness, cough, adventitious breath sounds, sputum, prolonged expirations, use of accessory muscles, barrel chest, digital clubbing

PMH considerations/risk factors: hx of COPD, asthma, allergies, GERD, recent respiratory illness, nicotine use

Diagnostics: clinical diagnosis; chest X-ray and spirometry may be considered

Costochondritis

Overview: inflammation of the cartilage that connects the ribs to the sternum

Patient may complain of: chest pain that is worse with deep breaths, movement, or touching; symptoms have a longer duration

Objective findings: tenderness over chest wall along sternum; exam is otherwise unremarkable

PMH considerations/risk factors: hx of chronic pain, trauma to the chest, recent CV/thoracic surgery, or respiratory illness

Diagnostics: clinical diagnosis; workup to rule out more emergent causes may be indicated

Esophagitis (Various Types)

Overview: inflammation of the esophagus

Patient may complain of: painful swallowing, dysphagia, chest pain, heartburn, upper abdominal/epigastric pain, dyspepsia, nausea, vomiting, signs of GI bleeding, dry coughing

Objective findings: oral herpes or thrush (depending on etiology), poor dentition, cough; exam is typically unremarkable

PMH considerations/risk factors: hx of esophagitis; GERD; hiatal hernia; cancer; immunosuppression; allergic diseases (food allergies, asthma, eczema); obesity; radiation therapy of the head, neck, and chest; alcohol abuse/use; nicotine use; NSAID use

Diagnostics: endoscopy with biopsy

Gastroesophageal Reflux Disease (GERD)

Overview: abnormal reflux of acid from the stomach back into the esophagus

Patient may complain of: sore throat, sour taste in mouth, dysphagia, chest pain or heartburn that may be worse lying flat or after meals, nausea, dyspepsia, epigastric pain, chronic coughing, insomnia

Objective findings: epigastric tenderness; exam is typically unremarkable

PMH considerations/risk factors: hx of GERD, hiatal hernia, obesity, diabetes, pregnancy, nicotine use, alcohol abuse/use

Diagnostics: clinical diagnosis

Heart Failure

Overview: broad term to describe pumping malfunction of the heart

Patient may complain of: fatigue, activity intolerance, chest pain, palpitations, dyspnea, orthopnea, PND, coughing, sputum production, weight gain/loss, anorexia, nausea, nocturia, insomnia

Objective findings: signs of acute distress, lethargy, diaphoresis, cyanosis, JVD, bradycardia/tachycardia, hypertension/

hypotension, displaced PMI, murmur, gallop, weak pulses, sluggish capillary refill, digital clubbing, edema, breathlessness, tachypnea, cough, adventitious lung sounds, sputum, hepatomegaly, ascites

PMH considerations/risk factors: hx of heart failure, HTN, CAD, cardiac valve disorders, MI, diabetes, arrhythmias, hyper/hypothyroidism, obesity, nicotine use, substance abuse, family hx of heart disease

Diagnostics: BNP, BMP/CMP, TSH, ECG, I/O, chest X-ray, ECHO, cardiac catheterization

Myocardial Infarction

Overview: decreased or no blood flow through the coronary arteries causing cardiac muscle death

Patient may complain of: fatigue, chest pain not improved with rest, radiation of the pain to the left arm/neck/jaw, palpitations, dyspnea, activity intolerance, abdominal pain, nausea, dizziness, anxiety, feelings of impending doom; symptoms have longer duration than stable angina

Objective findings: signs of acute distress, lethargy, irritability, altered mental status, diaphoresis, cool clammy skin, hypertension/hypotension, tachycardia/bradycardia, arrhythmia, murmur, ST elevations, pathologic Q waves, weak pulses, sluggish capillary refill, tachypnea

PMH considerations/risk factors: hx of MI, CAD, HTN, heart failure, hyperlipidemia, diabetes, cardiac valve disorders, sedentary lifestyle, NSAID use, nicotine use, substance abuse, family hx of heart disease, older age

Diagnostics: cardiac enzymes, ECG, stress test, coronary angiography

Pancreatitis

Overview: inflammation of the pancreas

Patient may complain of: fatigue, chills, fever, epigastric/upper abdominal pain, radiation of the pain to the back, worse with movement, nausea, vomiting, dyspepsia, diarrhea

Objective findings: signs of acute distress/illness, lethargy, fever, diaphoresis, pallor, jaundice, tachycardia, hypotension, upper abdominal/epigastric tenderness, abdominal distention, positive Cullen's sign or Grey Turner sign (abdominal ecchymosis)

PMH considerations/risk factors: hx of chronic pancreatitis, hypertriglyceridemia, cholelithiasis, GI cancer, recent GI surgery or trauma to the abdomen, nicotine use, alcohol abuse/use

Diagnostics: amylase, lipase, abdominal CT/US

Peptic Ulcer Disease

Overview: ulcers that develop in the lining of a stomach and/or duodenum

Patient may complain of: chest pain, dyspepsia, epigastric pain, heartburn, pain relief with food or antacids, nausea, signs of GI bleeding

Objective findings: nonspecific epigastric tenderness; exam is typically unremarkable

PMH considerations/risk factors: hx of PUD, *Helicobacter pylori* infection, NSAID use, recent travel outside of the United States, nicotine use, alcohol abuse/use

Diagnostics: CBC, *H. pylori* serum/breath/stool testing, occult stool, endoscopy with biopsy

Pneumonia

Overview: infection of the air sacs in one or both lungs causing inflammation and fluid accumulation

Patient may complain of: chills, fever, fatigue, chest pain/tightness, dyspnea, wheezing, coughing, sputum production, hemoptysis, activity intolerance, anorexia, nausea, vomiting, headache

Objective findings: signs of acute distress/illness, lethargy, altered mental status (elderly), fever, tachycardia, tachypnea, use of accessory muscles, cough, sputum, hypoxia, adventitious breath sounds, dullness to percussion over consolidation, pleural friction rub

PMH considerations/risk factors: hx of COPD, asthma, immunosuppression, dysphagia, immunization status, recent/current hospitalization, intubation, nicotine use, alcohol abuse, older/younger age

Diagnostics: CBC, sputum culture, chest X-ray

Pneumothorax

Overview: abnormal air or fluid in the pleural cavity causing lung collapse

Patient may complain of: sudden onset of chest pain, palpitations, dyspnea, coughing, anxiety, feelings of impending doom

Objective findings: signs of acute distress, tachycardia, hypotension, tachypnea, diminished/absent/unilateral breath sounds, uneven chest excursion, tracheal deviation, hypoxia, cough

PMH considerations/risk factors: hx of Marfan syndrome, COPD, cystic fibrosis, asthma, TB, trauma to the chest/back, thin body habitus, recent thoracentesis or pulmonary biopsy, family hx of pneumothorax, nicotine use, male gender

Diagnostics: chest X-ray

Pulmonary Embolism

Overview: a blood clot in the pulmonary vasculature

Patient may complain of: chills, fever, chest pain, pain with deep breaths, palpitations, activity intolerance, dyspnea, coughing, hemoptysis, abdominal pain, dizziness

Objective findings: signs of acute distress, fever, pallor, cyanosis, diaphoresis, tachycardia, hypotension, S3/S4 heart sounds, tachypnea, hypoxia, cough, signs of DVT

PMH considerations/risk factors: hx of DVT, PE or CVA, bleeding/clotting disorder, cancer, pregnancy, HRT/birth control use, IV drug use, recent surgery, immobility, nicotine use

Diagnostics: D-dimer, chest CT, V/Q scan, chest X-ray

References

American Medical Directors Association. (2010). *Know-it-all before you call: Data collection system.* Columbia, MD: Author.

Amsterdam, E. A., Wenger, N. K., Brindis, R. G., Casey, D. E., Ganiats, T. G., Holmes, D. R., . . . Zieman, S. J. (2014). 2014 AHA/ACC guideline for the management of patients with non-ST elevation acute coronary syndromes. *Circulation, 130*(25), 344–426.

Anderson, J. L., Adams, C. D., Antman, E. M., Bridges, C. R., Califf, R. M., Casey, D. E.,. . .Wright, S. (2013). 2012 ACCF/AHA focused update incorporated into the ACCF/AHA 2007 guidelines for the management of patient with unstable angina/non-ST elevation myocardial infarction. *Circulation, 127*, 1–168.

Beygui, F., Castren, M., Brunetto, N. D., Rosell-Ortiz, F., Christ, M., Zeymer, U., . . . Goldstein, P. (2015). Pre-hospital management of patients with chest pain and/or dyspnea of cardiac origin: A position paper of the acute cardiovascular care association (ACCA) of the ESC. *European Heart Journal: Acute Cardiovascular Care,* 1–23. doi: 10.1177/2048872615604119

Bulechek, G. M., Butcher, H. K., Dochterman, J. M., & Wagner, C. (2013). *Nursing Intervention Classification (NIC).* St. Louis, MO: Elsevier Mosby.

Desai, S. P. (2009). *Clinician's guide to laboratory medicine* (3rd ed.). Houston, TX: MD2B.

Gulanick, M., & Myers, J. L. (2017). *Nursing care plans: Diagnosis, interventions, & outcomes* (9th ed.). St. Louis, MO: Elsevier.

Hale, A., & Hovey, M. J. (2014). *Fluid, electrolyte and acid-base imbalances.* Philadelphia, PA: F.A. Davis Company.

Hollander, J. E., & Chase, M. (2016). Evaluation of the adult with chest pain in the emergency department. In J. Grayzel (Ed.), *UpToDate.* Retrieved from https://www.uptodate.com/contents/evaluation-of-the-adult-with-chest-pain-in-the-emergency-department

Hollander, J. E., Than, M., & Mueller, C. (2016). State-of-the-art evaluation of emergency department patients presenting with potential acute coronary syndromes. *Circulation, 134,* 547–564.

Jarvis, C. (2015). *Physical examination & health assessment.* St. Louis, MO: Elsevier.

LeBlond, R. F., Brown, D. D., Suneja, M., & Szot, J. F. (2015). *DeGowin's diagnostic examination* (10th ed.). New York, NY: McGraw-Hill.

McCance, K. L., Huether, S. E., Brashers, V. L., & Rote, N. S. (2014). *Pathophysiology: The biologic basis for disease in adults and children* (7th ed.). St. Louis, MO: Elsevier

McConaghy, J. R., & Oza, R. S. (2013). Outpatient diagnosis of acute chest pain in adults. *American Family Physician, 87*(3), 177–182.

Miller, C., & Granger, C. B. (2016). Evaluation of patients with chest pain at low or intermediate risk for acute coronary syndrome. In G. M. Saperia (Ed.), *UpToDate.* Retrieved from https://www.uptodate.com/contents/evaluation -of-patients-with-chest-pain-at-low-or-intermediate-risk-for-acute-coronary -syndrome

Mokhtari, A., Lindahl, B., Smith, J. G., Holzmann, M. J., Khoshnood, A., & Ekelund, U. (2016). Diagnostic accuracy of high-sensitivity cardiac troponin T at presentation combined with history and ECG for ruling out major adverse cardiac events. *Annals of Emergency Medicine, 68*(6), 649–658. doi:10.1016/j.annemergmed.2016.06.008

National Institute for Health and Care Excellence (NICE). (2014). *Myo-cardial infarction (acute): Early rule out using high-sensitivity troponin tests.* Retrieved from https://www.nice.org.uk/guidance/dg15

O'Castell, D. (2016). Evaluation of the adult with chest pain of esophageal origin. In S. Grover (Ed.), *UpToDate.* Retrieved from https://www.uptodate .com/contents/evaluation-of-the-adult-with-chest-pain-of-esophageal -origin

O'Gara, P., Kushner, F., Ascheim, D., Casey, D. E., Chung, M. K., de Lemos, J. A., &... Yancy, C. W. (2013). 2013 ACCF/AHA guideline for the management of ST-elevation myocardial infarction: A report of the American college of cardiology foundation/American heart association task force on practice guidelines. *Circulation, 127*(4), 362–425. doi:10.1161/CIR.0b013e3182742cf6

Papadakis, M. A., & McPhee, S. J. (2017). *Current medical diagnosis and treatment* (56th ed.). New York, NY: McGraw-Hill.

Raftery, A. T., Lim, E., & Ostor, A. J. (2014). *Differential diagnosis* (4th ed.). London, UK: Elsevier.

Rybicki, F. J., Udelson, J. E., Peacock, W. F., Goldhaber, S. Z., Issel-bacher, E. M., Kazerooni, E.,... Woodard, P. K. (2016). 2015 ACR/ACC/AHA/AATS/ACEP/ASNC/NASCI/SAEM/SCCT/SCMR/SCPC/SNMMI/STR/STS appropriate utilization of cardiovascular imaging in emergency department patients with chest pain: A joint document of the American college of radiology appropriateness criteria committee and the American college of cardiology appropriate use criteria task force. *Journal of The American College of Cardiology, 67*(7), 853–879. doi:10.1016/j.jacc.2015.09.011

Seller, R. H., & Symons, A. B. (2012). *Differential diagnosis of common complaints* (6th ed.). Philadelphia, PA: Elsevier.

Uphold, C. R., & Graham, M. V. (2013). *Clinical guidelines in family practice* (5th ed.). Gainesville, FL: Barmarrae Books.

Wertli, M. M., Ruchti, K. B., Steurer, J., & Held, U. (2013). Diagnostic indicators of non-cardiovascular chest pain: A systematic review and meta-analysis. *BMC Medicine, 11*(239), 1–35.

Wilbeck, J. & Evans, D. (2015). Acute chest pain and pulmonary embolism. *The Nurse Practitioner, 40*(1), 43–45.

Yelland, M. J. (2018). Outpatient evaluation of the adult with chest pain. In H. Libman (Ed.), *UpToDate.* Retrieved from https://www.uptodate.com/contents/outpatient-evaluation-of-the-adult-with-chest-pain

CHAPTER 6

Constipation

Constipation is a common and usually benign issue. According to the American Gastroenterological Association, constipation is defined as "infrequent stools" that occur less than three times per week. That definition can be expanded to include symptoms of hard stools, bloating, distension, incomplete, and/or painful defecation. A patient may describe themselves as constipated because of the hardness of their stools and bloating, but have a bowel movement every day. It can be an acute self-limiting issue or a chronic problem that causes frequent distress. The diagnosis is usually made clinically and does not require an extensive workup. Gastroenterology consults are not typically needed unless the patient is due for an age-appropriate colonoscopy or is presenting with red flag signs and symptoms, such as signs of GI bleeding, weight changes, dramatic changes in bowel habits, severe abdominal pain, and anemia.

Constipation can be well-managed with dietary changes and medications. Any secondary causes of constipation, such as medication, psychological issues, or certain chronic diseases, should also be evaluated. Priorities of the nurse include monitoring for red flag signs and symptoms, managing pain and discomfort, and providing constipation prevention and dietary education. Goals for constipation treatment should be discussed with the patient before a plan of care is established.

Differential Diagnosis Considerations

Common: anxiety, behavioral stool retention, dehydration, IBS, idiopathic constipation, (post-surgical) ileus, inactivity, intestinal obstruction, low-fiber diet, medication induced, pregnancy, travel

Consider: anorexia nervosa, Chagas disease, CVA, diabetes, diverticulosis, GI malignancy, Hirschsprung's

disease, hypercalcemia, hyperparathyroidism, hypokalemia, hypothyroidism, IBD, MS, Ogilvie syndrome, Parkinson's disease, pelvic floor dysfunction, perianal abscess, spinal cord injury, starvation

Questions to Ask the Patient/Family/Witness/Yourself

- When did the constipation start?
- When was your last bowel movement? What did it look like (consistency, amount, color)? How often do you (typically) have a bowel movement per day/week?
- Is there blood within the stool? Streaked on the side of the stool? On toilet paper with wiping?
- How easy is it to have a bowel movement? Do you have any straining or pain?
- Do you feel like you are having complete bowel movements?
- Does anything trigger your bowel movements (food, caffeine, medication, psychological stress)?
- Are you able to pass gas?
- Do you have abdominal/epigastric bloating or fullness with or after eating?
- How is your appetite? Are you able to keep down food and/or fluids?
- How much fluid are you drinking on a daily basis?
- Do you have a history of constipation? If so, what have you done or used to treat it?
- Have you had any recent: dietary changes or eaten anything out of the ordinary? immobilization such as prolonged time spent in bed or sitting? surgery or anesthesia?
- Do you use pain medication on a daily basis?
- Have you taken any new prescribed or over-the-counter medications? Have there been any recent changes to your current medication?

Associated Signs/Symptoms: PAIN: pain anywhere; GENERAL: fever, weight changes; GASTROINTESTINAL: bloating, diarrhea, heartburn, nausea, signs of GI bleeding, swallowing difficulties, rectal pain, vomiting

Recommended Assessments

- Vital signs
- Weight and nutritional status
- I/O
- Pain scale (if applicable)
  - Tolerable pain level
- General
  - Inspect: signs of acute distress, affect, restlessness
- Skin
  - Inspect: dryness
  - Palpate: turgor
- Mouth
  - Inspect: mucous membrane moisture level
- Gastrointestinal
  - Inspect: distention, scarring
  - Auscultate: bowel sounds
  - Palpate: guarding, masses, organomegaly, hernias, (rebound) tenderness
- Rectal
  - Inspect: bleeding, erythema, fissures, hemorrhoids, swelling
  - Palpate: stool impaction, masses, tenderness
- Extremities
  - Inspect: IV site (if applicable)

Past Medical History Considerations
Puts the patient at risk for differential considerations

- Abdominal surgery
- Chronic pain
- Hernia
- Immobilization
- Laxative abuse
- Radiation therapy to the abdomen/pelvis

Reoccurrence/exacerbation should be considered

- Intestinal obstruction

Chronic conditions that can cause constipation

- Anorexia nervosa
- Anxiety
- Constipation (primary)
- CVA
- Diabetes
- Diverticulosis
- GI malignancy
- Hyperparathyroidism
- IBD
- IBS
- Lumbar disk herniation
- MS
- Parkinson's disease
- Pregnancy
- Spinal cord injury
- Thyroid disease

Medication Evaluation

Most common causative/exacerbating medication

- Aluminum salts
- Anticholinergics
- Antidepressants
- Antidiarrheals
- Antihistamines
- Antispasmodics
- Atropine
- Beta blockers
- Calcium supplements
- CCBs
- Diuretics

- Iron supplements
- Opioids

Used to treat constipation

- Enemas
- Fiber supplements
- Laxatives
- Linaclotide
- Lubiprostone
- Naloxegol
- Stool softeners
- Suppositories

Lab Evaluation and Trends

- BMP/CMP

Nursing Intervention Considerations

- Medications (if ordered or protocol allows)
  - Hold suspected causative medication until discussion with the provider
  - PRN stool softener, laxative, enema, suppository
  - PRN anti-emetic for nausea, IV/IM if vomiting
- Diet
  - NPO if intestinal obstruction is suspected
  - Push fluids if there are no contraindications (>2,000mL/day)
  - Offer warm fluids before elimination attempts
  - Encourage high-fiber food choices
- Activity
  - Encourage activity and ambulation if safety permits
- Positioning
  - Supine or side lying position with knees flexed to chest to take tension off the abdominal wall if the patient has active abdominal pain

- - Reposition every 2–4 hours or establish an individualized turning schedule
- Collect
  - Stool sample for signs of GI bleeding (if applicable)
- Monitor
  - Pain levels
  - I/O
  - Agitation levels
  - Weight trends
  - Bowel sounds
  - Skin assessment every 8–24 hours
  - Signs of dehydration such as lethargy, decreased skin turgor, dry mucous membranes, tachycardia, and (orthostatic) hypotension
  - Signs and symptoms of GI bleeding such as fatigue, dizziness, dyspnea, melena, hematochezia, hematemesis, pallor, ecchymosis, altered mental status, hypotension, tachycardia, and tachypnea
  - Stool output color, consistency, frequency, and volume
- Environment
  - Provide a calm, quiet environment and reduce stimulation
  - Remove distractions during elimination attempts
  - Provide privacy and "Do Not Disturb" notice on the patient's door during elimination if safety permits
  - Maintain a comfortable room temperature
  - Utilize a fan (if appropriate)
- Supportive care
  - Maintain effective communication between yourself, patient, and family
  - Provide emotional support and reassurance to the patient and family
  - Maintain a calm manner during patient interactions
  - Discuss plan of care with the patient and decide reasonable goals together
  - Notify the patient and family of changes in the plan of care

- Identify barriers to elimination patterns
- Promote skin care and integrity
- Encourage frequent attempts to void
- **Educational topics (as applicable to the patient):**
  - General information regarding the patient's constipation and differential diagnosis considerations
  - New medication education including reason, side effects, and administration needs
  - Medication changes
  - Pain scale and pain goals
  - Relaxation techniques and breathing exercises
  - Bristol stool scale
  - Age-appropriate colonoscopy recommendations
  - Bowel schedule
  - Peri-care and proper hygiene
  - Proper positioning and turning schedule
  - Skin care
  - High-fiber diet, NPO diet
  - Increased fluid intake
  - Increased physical activity
  - When to notify the nurse or provider
  - Signs and symptoms of GI bleeding
  - Constipation prevention
  - Dehydration prevention
  - Pressure injury prevention

ISBARR Recommendation Considerations

- Medication
  - Hold oral medications if the patient is unable to tolerate or NPO
  - Discuss changing medication routes with the provider (and pharmacy) if the patient is NPO
  - Discontinue/change suspected causative medication
  - Add PRN anti-emetic for nausea

- Add PRN and/or scheduled enema, fiber supplement, stool softener, laxative, or suppository
- IV fluid needs if oral intake is poor, there are signs of dehydration, and the patient is NPO or hypotensive
- Imaging (depending on the suspected cause)
  - KUB
- Labs
  - Occult stool
- Safety
  - Activity level changes
- Change diet to (depending on the suspected cause)
  - NPO
  - High fiber
  - Push oral fluids
- Ask if the provider wants anything else done
- Read back orders; ask that they enter all orders into the electronic medical record

ISBARR Template	
I **Introduction**	**Introduce Yourself and the Patient** • "Hello Dr. Piacentine, this is Craig Schutta. I am your nurse for Amanda Kutil at Still Young Assisted Living."
S **Situation**	**Sign/Symptom You Are Concerned About** • "I am calling because Ms. Kutil has been complaining of constipation. She has not had a bowel movement in four days, her last bowel movement was hard, small, she had to strain a lot, and didn't feel like it was a complete bowel movement." **Associated Signs/Symptoms** • "She's also been feeling bloated but denies any severe abdominal pain, nausea, or vomiting."

Constipation

ISBARR Template	
B **Background**	**Vitals** • "Vitals are stable. Blood pressure is 126/90, heart rate is 70, respirations are 14, and temperature is 97.4." **Exam** • "Her abdomen looks distended but she has no tenderness, and bowel sounds are normoactive throughout." **Past Medical History** • "She has no history of constipation but her fluid intake has been poor and she only drinks a small glass of water with her meals." **Labs and Medications** • "I noticed she was started on Tylenol #3 for post-op back pain a week ago. She also has oral docusate ordered and has been taking it on a daily basis with no results."
A **Assessment**	**Assessment** • "I think the Tylenol #3 and her poor fluid intake is causing her constipation."
R **Recommendations** **R** **Read Back**	**Nurse's Recommendations, Interventions, and Read Back** • "I have been pushing her to drink more fluids. Can you order a high-fiber diet and another laxative? Would you like anything else done at this time?" • "Thanks Dr. Piacentine, let me read those orders back to you. You want 17g PO Miralax dose now and then PRN once daily. Continue current docusate dose. Start a high-fiber diet and continue to push fluids."

Disclaimer: This dialogue is factitious and any resemblance to actual persons, living or dead, or actual events is purely coincidental.

In order to avoid order discrepancies, it is recommended that all orders be entered by the provider in the electronic medical record.

Select Differential Diagnosis Presentations

Dehydration

Overview: abnormal loss of extracellular fluid volume

Patient may complain of: fatigue, thirst, dry mouth, constipation, palpitations, oliguria, muscle cramps, dizziness, headache

Objective findings: fever, altered mental status, lethargy, irritability, decreased skin turgor, generalized skin dryness, dry mucous membranes, (orthostatic) hypotension, tachycardia, oliguria

PMH considerations/risk factors: hx of liver or renal disease/failure, recent vomiting and/or diarrhea, GI bleeding, polyuria, diuretic use, burn injury, or intense physical activity

Diagnostics: BMP/CMP, CBC, urine Na, I/O

Diverticulosis

Overview: abnormal outpouchings or sacs that develop in the GI tract wall

Patient may complain of: constipation, abdominal pain, and rectal bleeding if diverticular bleeding is present; patient is typically asymptomatic

Objective findings: vague abdominal tenderness, hematochezia if diverticular bleeding is present; exam is typically unremarkable

PMH considerations/risk factors: hx of diverticulosis, obesity, low-fiber diet, nicotine use

Diagnostics: occult stool, colonoscopy

Hypercalcemia

Overview: elevated serum calcium

Patient may complain of: fatigue, generalized weakness, anorexia, constipation, nausea, dyspepsia, vomiting, muscle aches; patient is typically asymptomatic unless severe

Objective findings: altered mental status, lethargy, hypertension, bradycardia, shortened QT interval, hypoactive bowel
sounds, decreased reflexes; exam is typically unremarkable
unless severe

PMH considerations/risk factors: hx of cancer, AIDS/HIV, Addison's disease, hyperparathyroidism

Diagnostics: serum Ca, ECG

Hypokalemia

Overview: low serum potassium

Patient may complain of: fatigue, palpitations, nausea, vomiting, constipation, muscle weakness and cramping, seizures,
anxiety; patient is typically asymptomatic unless severe

Objective findings: lethargy, irritability, altered mental status, wide QRS, arrhythmia, bradypnea, hypoactive bowel
sounds, decreased reflexes; exam is typically unremarkable
unless severe

PMH considerations/risk factors: hx of CKD, diabetes, diarrhea,
alcohol abuse/use, eating disorders, NPO status, diuretic use

Diagnostics: serum K, ECG

Hypothyroidism

Overview: underactive thyroid gland

Patient may complain of: fatigue, cold intolerance, constipation, weight gain, irregular menstrual cycles, headaches,
paresthesias

Objective findings: lethargy, skin dryness, facial swelling,
goiter, bradycardia, hypotension, hypoactive bowel sounds,
decreased reflexes

PMH considerations/risk factors: hx of thyroid dysfunction,
autoimmune diseases, radiation therapy of the head and
neck, previous thyroidectomy, female gender

Diagnostics: TSH, T3, free T4, TPO; thyroid US may be
considered

Inflammatory Bowel Disease

> *Overview:* chronic inflammation of all or different parts of the GI tract
>
> *Patient may complain of:* chills, fever, fatigue, weight loss, anorexia, abdominal pain/cramping, nausea, vomiting, dyspepsia, constipation/diarrhea, change in bowel habits, signs of GI bleeding
>
> *Objective findings:* signs of acute distress/illness, lethargy, fever, signs of malnourishment, diaphoresis, pallor, tachycardia, abdominal tenderness, hematochezia
>
> *PMH considerations/risk factors:* hx of Crohn's disease or ulcerative colitis, food intolerance/allergies, bleeding/clotting disorders, NSAID use, recent travel outside of the United States, nicotine use, family hx of IBS, younger age
>
> *Diagnostics:* occult stool, CRP, CBC, endoscopy with biopsy

Intestinal Obstruction

> *Overview:* inability of digestive material to move through the GI tract normally
>
> *Patient may complain of:* abdominal pain, anorexia, nausea, vomiting, inability to pass gas, constipation/diarrhea
>
> *Objective findings:* signs of acute distress/illness, decreased skin turgor, dry mucous membranes, tachycardia, abdominal distention and tenderness, hypoactive or absent bowel sounds, fecal impaction (rectal exam)
>
> *PMH considerations/risk factors:* hernia, GI cancer, IBD, previous GI surgery, radiation therapy to the abdomen, opioid use
>
> *Diagnostics:* KUB, abdominal CT

Irritable Bowel Syndrome

> *Overview:* recurrent benign intestinal pain syndrome with associated bowel habit changes
>
> *Patient may complain of:* abdominal pain and cramping, diarrhea and/or constipation, bloating, dyspepsia, heartburn, nausea, sensation of incomplete bowel movements

Objective findings: irritable, mild abdominal bloating and generalized tenderness; exam is typically unremarkable

PMH considerations/risk factors: hx of IBS, IBD, depression, anxiety, family hx of IBS, female gender, younger age

Diagnostics: may not require any diagnostic testing; colonoscopy with biopsy, stool cultures, and CRP may be considered

References

Anastasi, J. K., Capili, B., & Chang, M. (2013). Managing irritable bowel syndrome. *American Journal of Nursing, 113*(7), 42–53. doi:10.1097/01.NAJ.0000431921.70418.ff\

Bardsley, A. (2015). Approaches to managing chronic constipation in older people within the community setting. *British Journal of Community Nursing, 20*(9), 444–450. doi:10.12968/bjcn.2015.20.9.444

Bharucha, A. E., Dorn, S. D., Lembo, A., & Pressman, A. (2013). American Gastroenterological Association medical position statement on constipation. *Gastroenterology, 144*(1), 211–217.

Bulechek, G. M., Butcher, H. K., Dochterman, J. M., & Wagner, C. (2013). *Nursing intervention classification (NIC).* St. Louis, MO: Elsevier Mosby.

Day, M. R., Wills, T., & Coffey, A. (2014). Constipation and the pros and cons of laxatives for older adults. *Nursing & Residential Care, 16*(4), 196–200.

Desai, S. P. (2009). *Clinician's guide to laboratory medicine* (3rd ed.). Houston, TX: MD2B.

Gulanick, M., & Myers, J. L. (2017). *Nursing care plans: Diagnosis, interventions, & outcomes* (9th ed.). St. Louis, MO: Elsevier.

Hale, A., & Hovey, M. J. (2014). *Fluid, electrolyte and acid-base imbalances.* Philadelphia, PA: F.A. Davis Company.

Holl, R. M. (2014). Bowel movement: The sixth vital sign. *Holistic Nursing Practice, 28*(3), 195–197. doi:10.1097/HNP.0000000000000024

Jarvis, C. (2015). *Physical examination & health assessment.* St. Louis, MO: Elsevier.

LeBlond, R. F., Brown, D. D., Suneja, M., & Szot, J. F. (2015). *DeGowin's diagnostic examination* (10th ed.). New York, NY: McGraw-Hill.

McCance, K. L., Huether, S. E., Brashers, V. L., & Rote, N. S. (2014). *Pathophysiology: The biologic basis for disease in adults and children* (7th ed.). St. Louis, MO: Elsevier.

Mitchell, G. (2014). Managing constipation in primary care. *Primary Health Care, 24*(5), 18–22.

Mounsey, A., Raleigh, M., & Wilson, A. (2015). Management of constipation in older adults. *American Family Physician, 92*(6), 500–504.

Papadakis, M. A., & McPhee, S. J. (2017). *Current medical diagnosis and treatment* (56th ed.). New York, NY: McGraw-Hill.

Portenoy, R. K., Mehta, Z., & Admed, E. (2017). Cancer pain management with opioids: Prevention and management of side effects. In D. M. Savarese (Ed.), *UpToDate*. Retrieved from https://www.uptodate .com/contents/prevention-and-management-of-side-effects-in-patients -receiving-opioids-for-chronic-pain

Prichard, D., & Bharucha, A. (2015). Management of opioid-induced constipation for people in palliative care. *International Journal of Palliative Nursing, 21*(6), 272–280.

Raftery, A. T., Lim, E., & Ostor, A. J. (2014). *Differential diagnosis* (4th ed.). London, UK: Elsevier.

Rao, S. (2017). Constipation in the older adult. In S. Grover (Ed.), *UpToDate*. Retrieved from https://www.uptodate.com/contents/ constipation-in-the-older-adult

Schuster, B. G., Kosar, L., & Kamrul, R. (2015). Constipation in older adults: Stepwise approach to keep things moving. *Canadian Family Physician, 61*(2), 152–158.

Seller, R. H., & Symons, A. B. (2012). *Differential diagnosis of common complaints* (6th ed.). Philadelphia, PA: Elsevier.

Uphold, C. R., & Graham, M. V. (2013). *Clinical guidelines in family practice* (5th ed.). Gainesville, FL: Barmarrae Books.

Wald, A. (2016). Etiology and evaluation of chronic constipation in adults. In S. Grover (Ed.), *UpToDate*. Retrieved from https://www.uptodate .com/contents/etiology-and-evaluation-of-chronic-constipation-in-adults

Wald, A. (2018). Management of chronic constipation in adults. In S. Grover (Ed.), *UpToDate*. Retrieved from https://www.uptodate.com/contents /management-of-chronic-constipation-in-adults

Weinberg, D. S., Smalley, W., Heidelbaugh, J. J., & Sultan, S. (2014). American gastroenterological association institute guideline on the pharmacological management of irritable bowel syndrome. *Gastroenterology, 147*(5), 1146–1148.

CHAPTER 7

Cough

Coughing is a normal defensive reflex that clears secretions and protects the airway from aspiration of food and other foreign matter. Acute coughing, lasting less than 3 weeks, is usually self-limiting and is because of an upper respiratory tract infection or exacerbation of a chronic lung disease. It rarely requires an extensive workup unless red flag signs and symptoms are present, which include hemoptysis, dyspnea, weight loss/gain, fever, hypoxia, and chest pain.

It is the nurse's priority to protect the patient's airway, monitor for red flag signs and symptoms, and administer medication to provide symptomatic relief. It will also be important to educate the patient on infection prevention and chronic lung disease management (if applicable). If coughing is not managed well with common treatment modalities, further testing by pulmonology may be required. In this chapter, nursing intervention considerations and plan of care recommendations should reflect whatever the suspected cause is.

Differential Diagnosis Considerations

Common acute (<3 weeks) causes: allergies, asthma exacerbation, bronchitis, COPD exacerbation, heart failure exacerbation, influenza, post-nasal drip (UACS), pneumonia, sinusitis (acute), URI

Common subacute (3–8 weeks) causes: pertussis, post-infectious cough, post-nasal drip (UACS)

Common chronic (>8 weeks) causes: asthma, COPD, GERD, post-nasal drip (UACS), smoking

Consider: aspiration, bronchiectasis, cystic fibrosis, heart failure, interstitial lung disease, medication induced, PE, pneumothorax, psychogenic, pulmonary malignancy, sarcoidosis, SARS, sinusitis (chronic), TB

Questions to Ask the Patient/ Family/Witness/Yourself

- When did the coughing start? Did it start gradually or suddenly?
- Is the coughing constant or does it come and go?
- What makes the coughing better (certain positions, medication, rest)?
- Does anything trigger the coughing or make it worse (activity, certain positions, certain times of the day, eating)?
- Do you have any pain with coughing?
- Are you coughing up sputum/phlegm? If so, is the phlegm/sputum clear, white, purulent, pink? Is there any blood?
- Do you have a history of coughing issues? If so, what have you done or used to treat it?
- Have you had any recent: respiratory illness? exposure to respiratory infection or been around anyone that is sick? exposure to chemicals, smoke, or toxins? hospitalization? immobilization such as prolonged time spent in bed or sitting? surgery? trauma to the back, chest, or neck? travel outside of the United States?
- Have you had any recent invasive interventions such as intubation?
- Do you use any inhalers? If so, have you been taking them as prescribed?
- Have you taken any new prescribed or over-the-counter medications? Have there been any recent changes to your current medication?
- What are you allergic to? Have you been exposed to a known allergen?
- Do you smoke? How much (ppd)? How long have you been smoking? (if applicable)

Associated Signs/Symptoms: PAIN: pain anywhere; GENERAL: chills, fatigue, fever, weakness, weight changes; EENT: ear pain, eye drainage, eye itching, nasal congestion, nasal drainage, sneezing, sore throat; NECK: stiffness, swollen glands; CARDIOVASCULAR: chest pain/tightness, edema, PND, orthopnea; RESPIRATORY:

hemoptysis, painful breathing/coughing, dyspnea, wheezing;
GASTROINTESTINAL: heartburn, nausea, swallowing difficulties, vomiting; NEUROLOGICAL: headache

Recommended Assessments

- Vital signs
- Temperature
- Weight and nutritional status
- I/O
- Pain scale (if applicable)
  - Tolerable pain level
- General
  - Level of consciousness and orientation
  - Inspect: signs of acute distress, acute illness, affect, restlessness
  - Difficulty speaking due to breathlessness
- Skin
  - Inspect: cyanosis, diaphoresis, dryness, pallor
  - Palpate: temperature
- Eyes
  - Inspect: conjunctival erythema, lid swelling, drainage
- Mouth
  - Inspect: halitosis, posterior pharynx erythema or swelling, tonsillar exudates, mucous membrane moisture level
- Nose
  - Inspect: drainage, turbinate swelling
- Head/face/neck
  - Inspect: JVD, tracheal deviation, signs of trauma
  - Palpate: lymphadenopathy, swelling, tenderness
- Cardiovascular
  - Auscultate: heart sounds, rate, rhythm
- Respiratory
  - Inspect: chest asymmetry, respiratory effort, depth, pattern, use of accessory muscles
  - Auscultate: lung sounds, stridor

- Extremities
  - Inspect: IV site (if applicable)
  - Palpate: capillary refill, edema, pulses

Past Medical History Considerations

- Allergies
- Immunization status: influenza, pertussis, pneumonia

Puts the patient at risk for differential considerations

- AIDS/HIV
- Cancer
- DVT
- Dysphagia
- Eczema
- HTN
- Immobilization
- Nicotine use

Reoccurrence/exacerbation should be considered

- Asthma
- COPD
- Heart failure
- PE
- Sinusitis

Chronic conditions that can cause cough

- Allergies
- Asthma
- COPD
- Cystic fibrosis
- GERD
- Heart failure
- Interstitial lung disease
- Post-nasal drip (UACS)
- Pulmonary malignancy

- Sarcoidosis
- Sinusitis

Medication Evaluation
Most common causative/exacerbating medication
- ACE inhibitors

Used to treat common differential considerations
- Antibiotics → various respiratory infections
- Antihistamines → allergies, UACS
- Antitussives → acute cough
- Corticosteroids → airway inflammation
- Decongestants → upper respiratory congestion
- Diuretics → fluid overload
- Expectorants → acute cough
- ICS, LABA, LAMA, SABA, SAMA, and combination inhalers → chronic lung disease
- PPIs, H2 antagonists, antacids → upper GI tract inflammation

Lab Evaluation and Trends
- BNP
- CBC

Nursing Intervention Considerations
- Call for help or rapid response/code team if vital signs are unstable or there are signs of urgent distress
- Maintain a patent airway
  - Apply oxygen if hypoxic
  - Encourage cough and deep breathing
  - Encourage slow relaxed breathing if hyperventilating
  - Chest splinting with a pillow to promote more effective coughing
  - Suction as needed

- Provide oral care throughout the day (q2–4hrs)
- Call respiratory therapy for signs of respiratory distress
- Verify patent IV if IVF or IV medication treatment is anticipated
  - Flush according to facility protocol; watch for swelling, erythema, pain, and other signs of infiltration
- Medications (if ordered or protocol allows)
  - PRN cough suppressant
  - PRN bronchodilator treatment per respiratory therapy
- Diet
  - NPO until discussion with the provider, if aspiration is suspected
  - Restrict fluids until discussion with the provider, if there are signs of fluid overload
  - Push fluids if there are no contraindications (>2000mL/day)
- Activity
  - Encourage activity and ambulation if safety permits
- Positioning
  - HOB raised to comfort for respiratory distress
  - Reposition every 2–4 hours or establish an individualized turning schedule
- Collect
  - Sputum sample
- Monitor
  - Vital signs and trends
  - Pain levels
  - Oxygen saturation/pulse oximetry
  - Telemetry/cardiac monitor
  - Temperature trends
  - I/O
  - Weight trends
  - Agitation levels
  - Skin assessment every 8–24 hours
  - Signs of decreased cardiac output such as weak pulses, cool skin, altered mental status, hypotension, oliguria, and mottling

- Signs of respiratory distress such as cyanosis, tachypnea, hypoxia, use of accessory muscles, diaphoresis, and adventitious lung sounds
- Signs and symptoms of aspiration such as coughing, throat clearing, dyspnea, drooling, and voice changes
- Signs and symptoms of sepsis such as fever, chills, hypotension, altered mental status, hypoxia, cool clammy skin, dyspnea, oliguria, tachycardia, and tachypnea
- Signs and symptoms of fluid overload such as cough, adventitious lung sounds, dyspnea, tachypnea, weight gain, edema, JVD, and ascites
- Sputum output color, consistency, frequency, and volume
- Environment
  - Provide a calm, quiet environment and reduce stimulation
  - Maintain a comfortable room temperature
  - Initiate isolation precautions: droplet, airborne
- Supportive care
  - Maintain effective communication between yourself, patient, and family
  - Provide emotional support and reassurance to the patient and family
  - Maintain a calm manner during patient interactions
  - Discuss plan of care with the patient and decide reasonable goals together
  - Notify the patient and family of changes in the plan of care
  - Identify barriers to care and compliance
  - Promote skin care and integrity
  - **Educational topics (as applicable to the patient):**
    - General information regarding the patient's cough and differential diagnosis considerations
    - Explanation regarding referrals and specialist who may see them for this issue
    - New medication education including reason, side effects, and administration needs
    - Medication changes

- Medication compliance
- MDI administration techniques
- Pain scale and pain goals
- Oxygen therapy and maintenance
- Trigger avoidance
- Relaxation techniques and breathing exercises
- Cough and deep-breathing techniques
- Telemetry
- Proper positioning and turning schedule
- Skin care
- Handwashing and infection control measures
- Isolation precaution needs
- Increased physical activity
- NPO diet, dysphagia diet
- Swallow precautions
- Increased fluid intake
- Fluid restriction
- Immunization needs
- Smoking cessation
- When to notify the nurse or provider
- Signs and symptoms of aspiration
- Signs and symptoms of respiratory emergencies
- Signs and symptoms of cardiac emergencies
- Signs and symptoms of fluid overload
- Pressure injury prevention

ISBARR Recommendation Considerations

- Ask the provider to come assess the patient STAT if they are unstable or red flag symptoms are present
- Medication
  - Discontinue/change suspected causative medication
  - Hold oral medications if the patient is unable to tolerate or NPO
  - Discuss changing medication routes with the provider (and pharmacy) if the patient is NPO

Cough

- Add corticosteroids for airway inflammation
- Add/change diuretics for signs of fluid overload
- Add PPI, H2 antagonist, or antacid for dyspepsia, heartburn, or other signs/symptoms of GERD
- Add PRN and/or scheduled bronchodilator nebulizer treatments per respiratory therapy for coughing, dyspnea, or other signs of respiratory distress
- Add PRN cough suppressant
- IV fluid needs if oral intake is poor, there are signs of dehydration, and the patient is NPO or hypotensive
- Imaging (depending on the suspected cause)
  - Chest X-ray, chest CT scan
- Labs (depending on the suspected cause)
  - ABG
  - BNP
  - CBC
  - D-dimer
  - Sputum culture
- Safety
  - Activity level changes
  - Aspiration precautions
  - Isolation precautions: airborne, droplet
- Monitoring needs
  - Continuous O_2 monitoring
  - Daily weights
  - Strict I/O
  - Telemetry/continuous cardiac monitoring
  - Vital signs including frequency and parameters to call the provider
- Supportive cares
  - Compression stockings or SCDs
- Change diet to (depending on the suspected cause)
  - NPO
  - Dysphagia diet per speech pathology's recommendations
  - Fluid restriction
  - Push oral fluids

- Referrals
  - Pulmonology
  - Respiratory therapy
  - Speech pathology
- Ask if the provider wants anything else done
- Read back orders; ask that they enter all orders into the electronic medical record

ISBARR Template	
I **Introduction**	**Introduce Yourself and the Patient** • "Hi, Dr. Henschel, this is Joel Robers. I am the nurse for Abby Ventzke in Room 302. She is a patient of Dr. Hirsch's. She is a 66-year-old, admitted a week ago after she broke her right femur and had an internal fixation. I understand you are covering for Dr. Hirsch this evening?"
S **Situation**	**Sign/Symptom You Are Concerned About** • "Mrs. Ventzke has been complaining of a new productive cough that started a few hours ago." **Associated Signs/Symptoms** • "She also feels fatigued and is having the chills, but denies shortness of breath or chest pain."
B **Background**	**Vitals** • "I just took her temperature and it was 101.2. Other vitals are stable. Blood pressure is 110/89, heart rate is 70, respiratory rate is 16, and oxygen saturation is 95% on room air." **Exam** • "She has crackles in her right posterior lower lobe and her sputum looks yellow and thick." **Past Medical History** • "She has no history of smoking, COPD, or asthma, and is up to date on her flu and pneumonia vaccines. She has been getting up out of bed three times a day with physical therapy."

ISBARR Template	
	Labs and Medications • "Her CBC is being drawn this morning at 0800. Yesterday, the WBC count was 9,000. She does not have any PRNs ordered for cough."
A **Assessment**	**Assessment** • "I am concerned about pneumonia."
R **Recommendations** **R** **Read Back**	**Nurse's Recommendations, Interventions, and Read Back** • "I have her doing cough and deep-breathing exercises. I also collected a sputum sample. Did you want a chest X-ray or a sputum culture? Can you order something for her coughing symptoms?" • "Thank you, Dr. Henschel, I would like to read those orders back to you. You would like a chest X-ray; call with the results when available. Dextromethorphan 10mg/5mL, 20mg every six hours PRN for cough. PRN TID Duoneb nebulizer treatments per respiratory therapy and you do not want a sputum culture at this time?"

Disclaimer: This dialogue is factitious and any resemblance to actual persons, living or dead, or actual events is purely coincidental.

In order to avoid order discrepancies, it is recommended that all orders be entered by the provider in the electronic medical record.

Select Differential Diagnosis Presentations

Allergies (Allergic Rhinitis/Conjunctivitis)

Overview: hypersensitive immune response after exposure to an allergen

Patient may complain of: facial pain/congestion, sneezing, nasal congestion, nasal drainage, itchy and watery eyes, sore throat, post-nasal drip, dry coughing

Objective findings: conjunctival erythema, eye lid erythema and swelling, clear stringy watery eye drainage, inflamed nasal turbinates, rhinorrhea, posterior pharyngeal cobblestoning and post-nasal drip, cough

PMH considerations/risk factors: hx of seasonal allergies, asthma, eczema, food allergies, family hx of allergies

Diagnostics: clinical diagnosis; skin testing by an allergist may be considered

Aspiration

Overview: inhalation of foreign object, food, or liquid into the airway

Patient may complain of: fever, fatigue, inability/difficulty swallowing, chest pain, coughing, dyspnea, wheezing, sputum production, heartburn, nausea, vomiting

Objective findings: signs of acute distress, fever, irritability, diaphoresis, cyanosis, drooling, hoarseness, choking, hypoxia, cough, tachypnea, adventitious lung sounds, sputum

PMH considerations/risk factors: hx of dysphagia, myasthenia gravis, Parkinson's disease, CVA, esophageal stricture, GERD, asthma, ENT/GI cancer, dementia, trauma to the neck, dentition issues, radiation therapy to the head and neck, intubation, NG tube, immobility, nicotine use, alcohol abuse/use

Diagnostics: CBC, swallow study, chest X-ray

Asthma Exacerbation

Overview: acute inflammation and swelling of the airway, progressively worsening asthma symptomology

Patient may complain of: activity intolerance, chest pain/tightness, coughing, dyspnea, wheezing, sputum production, insomnia

Objective findings: signs of acute distress, irritability, diaphoresis, cyanosis, breathlessness, hypoxia, tachypnea, cough, sputum, use of accessory muscles, adventitious breath sounds

PMH considerations/risk factors: hx of asthma, allergies, obesity, eczema, recent respiratory illness, nicotine use

Diagnostics: clinical diagnosis; chest X-ray, spirometry, PEF may be considered

Bronchitis

Overview: inflammation of the bronchioles typically due to an infection

Patient may complain of: fever, chills, fatigue, sore throat, nasal congestion, chest pain/tightness, coughing, dyspnea, wheezing, sputum production, hemoptysis

Objective findings: signs of acute illness, lethargy, low-grade fever, rhinorrhea, pharyngeal erythema, cough, sputum, adventitious breath sounds, tachypnea

PMH considerations/risk factors: hx of asthma, COPD, allergies, GERD, exposure to lung irritants, nicotine use, older age

Diagnostics: clinical diagnosis; ABG, chest X-ray, spirometry may be considered

COPD Exacerbation

Overview: acute inflammation and swelling of the airway, progressively worsening COPD symptomology

Patient may complain of: worsening fatigue, activity intolerance and sputum production from baseline, chest pain/tightness, coughing, dyspnea, wheezing, hemoptysis, insomnia

Objective findings: signs of acute distress, lethargy, cyanosis, diaphoresis, hypoxia, breathlessness, cough, adventitious breath sounds, sputum, prolonged expirations, use of accessory muscles, barrel chest, digital clubbing

PMH considerations/risk factors: hx of COPD, asthma, allergies, GERD, recent respiratory illness, nicotine use

Diagnostics: clinical diagnosis; chest X-ray, spirometry may be considered

Gastroesophageal Reflux Disease

Overview: abnormal reflux of acid from the stomach back into the esophagus

Patient may complain of: sore throat, sour taste in mouth, dysphagia, chest pain, or heartburn that may be worse lying flat or after meals, nausea, dyspepsia, epigastric pain, chronic coughing, insomnia

Objective findings: epigastric tenderness; exam is typically unremarkable

PMH considerations/risk factors: hx of GERD, hiatal hernia, obesity, diabetes, pregnancy, nicotine use, alcohol abuse/use

Diagnostics: clinical diagnosis

Heart Failure

Overview: broad term to describe pumping malfunction of the heart

Patient may complain of: fatigue, activity intolerance, chest pain, palpitations, dyspnea, orthopnea, PND, coughing, sputum production, weight gain/loss, anorexia, nausea, nocturia, insomnia

Objective findings: signs of acute distress, lethargy, diaphoresis, cyanosis, JVD, bradycardia/tachycardia, hypertension/hypotension, displaced PMI, murmur, gallop, weak pulses, sluggish capillary refill, digital clubbing, edema, breathlessness, tachypnea, cough, adventitious lung sounds, sputum, hepatomegaly, ascites

PMH considerations/risk factors: hx of heart failure, HTN, CAD, cardiac valve disorders, MI, diabetes, arrhythmias, hyper/hypothyroidism, obesity, nicotine use, substance abuse, family hx of heart disease

Diagnostics: BNP, BMP/CMP, TSH, ECG, I/O, chest X-ray, ECHO, cardiac catheterization

Influenza

Overview: viral respiratory illness

Patient may complain of: chills, fever, fatigue, body aches, sore throat, nasal congestion, nasal drainage, dry coughing, headache

Objective findings: signs of acute distress/illness, lethargy, altered mental status (elderly), fever, tachycardia, pharyngeal erythema, conjunctival erythema, nasal turbinate swelling, rhinorrhea, lymphadenopathy, cough

PMH considerations/risk factors: recent exposure to influenza, pregnancy, hx of immunosuppression, older/younger age, influenza season, immunization status

Diagnostics: clinical diagnosis; rapid flu test and CBC may be considered

Pneumonia

Overview: infection of the air sacs in one or both lungs causing inflammation and fluid accumulation

Patient may complain of: chills, fever, fatigue, chest pain/tightness, dyspnea, wheezing, coughing, sputum production, hemoptysis, activity intolerance, anorexia, nausea, vomiting, headache

Objective findings: signs of acute distress/illness, lethargy, altered mental status (elderly), fever, tachycardia, tachypnea, use of accessory muscles, cough, sputum, hypoxia, adventitious breath sounds, dullness to percussion over consolidation, pleural friction rub

PMH considerations/risk factors: hx of COPD, asthma, immunosuppression, dysphagia, immunization status, recent/current hospitalization, intubation, nicotine use, alcohol abuse, older/younger age

Diagnostics: CBC, sputum culture, chest X-ray

Pneumothorax

Overview: abnormal air or fluid in the pleural cavity causing lung collapse

Patient may complain of: sudden onset of chest pain, palpitations, dyspnea, coughing, anxiety, feelings of impending doom

Objective findings: signs of acute distress, tachycardia, hypotension, tachypnea, diminished/absent unilateral breath sounds, uneven chest excursion, tracheal deviation, hypoxia, cough

PMH considerations/risk factors: hx of Marfan syndrome, COPD, cystic fibrosis, asthma, TB, trauma to the chest/back, thin body habitus, recent thoracentesis or pulmonary biopsy, family hx of pneumothorax, nicotine use, male gender

Diagnostics: chest X-ray

Post-Nasal Drip

Overview: excessive mucous produced by the nasal mucosa that accumulates in the back of the nose or throat

Patient may complain of: sneezing, nasal congestion, nasal drainage, sore throat, coughing, headache

Objective findings: nasal turbinate swelling, rhinorrhea, halitosis, posterior pharyngeal erythema, cobblestoning and drainage, cough

PMH considerations/risk factors: hx of allergies, asthma, GERD, recent respiratory illness

Diagnostics: clinical diagnosis

Pulmonary Embolism

Overview: a blood clot in the pulmonary vasculature

Patient may complain of: chills, fever, chest pain, pain with deep breaths, palpitations, activity intolerance, dyspnea, coughing, hemoptysis, abdominal pain, dizziness

Objective findings: signs of acute distress, fever, pallor, cyanosis, diaphoresis, tachycardia, hypotension, S3/S4 heart sounds, tachypnea, hypoxia, cough, signs of DVT

PMH considerations/risk factors: hx of DVT, PE or CVA, bleeding/clotting disorder, cancer, pregnancy, HRT/birth control use, IV drug use, recent surgery, immobility, nicotine use

Diagnostics: D-dimer, chest CT, V/Q scan, chest X-ray

Sinusitis

Overview: inflammation of the sinuses typically due to an infection

Patient may complain of: chills, fever, fatigue, facial pain, nasal congestion, nasal drainage, ear pain, dental pain, sore throat, coughing, sputum production, nausea, headache; acute symptoms last <4 weeks

Objective findings: signs of acute illness, low-grade fever, lethargy, frontal/maxillary tenderness, nasal turbinate swelling, rhinorrhea (purulent can indicate bacterial infection), halitosis, pharyngeal erythema, cough, sputum; signs and symptoms are more severe with a bacterial infection

PMH considerations/risk factors: hx of chronic sinusitis, allergies, asthma, immunosuppression, nicotine use

Diagnostics: clinical diagnosis; workup to rule out more emergent causes may be indicated

Upper Respiratory Infection

Overview: broad term for infection of the upper respiratory tract including the nose, throat, and upper airway

Patient may complain of: chills, fever, fatigue, nasal congestion, nasal drainage, sore throat, coughing, sputum production, nausea, vomiting, headache; symptoms have a short duration (<10 days)

Objective findings: signs of acute illness, low-grade fever, lethargy, conjunctival erythema, nasal turbinate swelling, rhinorrhea, halitosis, pharyngeal erythema, cough, sputum; signs and symptoms are typically mild in nature

PMH considerations/risk factors: hx of asthma, COPD, immunosuppression, allergies, nicotine use

Diagnostics: clinical diagnosis; workup to rule out more emergent causes may be indicated

References

American Medical Directors Association. (2010). *Know-it-all before you call: Data collection system.* Columbia, MD: Author.

Bulechek, G. M., Butcher, H. K., Dochterman, J. M., & Wagner, C. (2013). *Nursing intervention classification (NIC).* St. Louis, MO: Elsevier Mosby.

Desai, S. P. (2009). *Clinician's guide to laboratory medicine* (3rd ed.). Houston, TX: MD2B.

File, T. M. (2018). Acute bronchitis in adults. In S. Bond (Ed.), *UpToDate.* Retrieved from https://www.uptodate.com/contents/acute-bronchitis -in-adults

Gibson, P., Wang, G., McGarvey, L., Vertigan, A. E., Altman, K. W., Birring, S. S., & . . . Diekemper, R. L. (2016). Treatment of unexplained chronic cough: CHEST guideline and expert panel report. *Chest, 149*(1), 27–44. doi:10.1378 /chest.15-1496

Guirguis-Blake, J. M., Senger, C. A., Webber, E. M., Mularski, R. A., & Whitlock, E. P. (2016). Screening for chronic obstructive pulmonary disease: Evidence report and systematic review for the US preventive services task force. *Journal of The American Medical Association, 315*(13), 1378–1393. doi:10.1001/jama.2016.2654

Hale, A., & Hovey, M. J. (2014). *Fluid, electrolyte and acid-base imbalances.* Philadelphia, PA: F.A. Davis Company.

Holzinger, F., Beck, S., Dini, L., Stoter, C., & Heintze, C. (2014). The diagnosis and treatment of acute cough in adults. *Deutsches Arzteblatt International, 111,* 356–363.

Irwin, R. S., French, C., Zelman, S., Diekemper, R. L, & Gold, P. M. (2014). Overview of the management of cough. *Chest, 146*(4), 885–889.

Jarvis, C. (2015). *Physical examination & health assessment.* St. Louis, MO: Elsevier.

Jiang, M., Guan, W. J., Fang, Z. F., Xie, Y. Q., Xie, J. X., Chen, H., . . . Zhong, N. S. (2016). A critical review of the quality of cough clinical practice guideline. *Chest, 150*(4), 777–788.

Kahrilas, P. J., Altman, K. W., Chang, A. B., Field, S. K., Harding, S. M., Lane, A. P., . . . Irwin, R. S. (2016). Chronic cough due to gastroesophageal reflux in adults: CHEST guideline and expert panel report. *Chest, 150*(6), 1341–1360. doi:10.1016/j.chest.2016.08.1458

LeBlond, R. F., Brown, D. D., Suneja, M., & Szot, J. F. (2015). *DeGowin's diagnostic examination* (10th ed.). New York, NY: McGraw-Hill.

McCance, K. L., Huether, S. E., Brashers, V. L., & Rote, N. S. (2014). *Pathophysiology: The biologic basis for disease in adults and children* (7th ed.). St. Louis, MO: Elsevier.

McIntosh, K. (2016). Severe acute respiratory syndrome (SARS). In A. R. Thorner (Ed.), *UpToDate.* Retrieved from https://www.uptodate .com/contents/severe-acute-respiratory-syndrome-sars

Molassiotis, A., Bailey, C., Caress, A., Brunton, L., & Smith, J. (2015). Interventions for cough in cancer. *Cochrane Database of Systematic Reviews*, (5), 1–53. doi:10.1002/14651858.CD007881.pub3

Molassiotis, A., Smith, J. A., Mazzone, P., Blackhall, F., & Irwin, R. S. (2017). Symptomatic treatment of cough among adult patients with lung cancer. *Chest, 151*(4), 861–874.

Papadakis, M. A., & McPhee, S. J. (2017). *Current medical diagnosis and treatment* (56th ed.). New York, NY: McGraw-Hill.

Raftery, A. T., Lim, E., & Ostor, A. J. (2014). *Differential diagnosis* (4th ed.). London, UK: Elsevier.

Seller, R. H., & Symons, A. B. (2012). *Differential diagnosis of common complaints* (6th ed.). Philadelphia, PA: Elsevier.

Sexton, D. J., & McClain, M. T. (2018). The common cold in adults: Treatment and prevention. In H. Libman (Ed.), *UpToDate*. Retrieved from https://www.uptodate.com/contents/the-common-cold-in-adults-treatment-and-prevention

Short, S., Bashir, H., Marshall, P., Miller, N., Olmschenk, D., Prigge, K., & Solyntjes, L. (2017). Diagnosis and treatment of respiratory illness in children and adults. *Institute for Clinical Systems Improvement*. Retrieved from https://www.icsi.org/_asset/pwyrky/RespIllness.pdf

Silvestri, R. C., & Weinberger, S. E. (2017). Evaluation of subacute and chronic cough in adults. In H. Hollingsworth (Ed.), *UpToDate*. Retrieved from https://www.uptodate.com/contents/evaluation-of-subacute-and-chronic-cough-in-adults

Strickland, S. L., Rubin, B. K., Haas, C. F., Volsko, T. A., Drescher, G. S., & O'Malley, C. A. (2015). AARC clinical practice guideline: Effectiveness of pharmacologic airway clearance therapies in hospitalized patients. *Respiratory Care, 60*(7), 1071–1077. doi:10.4187/respcare.04165

Uphold, C. R., & Graham, M. V. (2013). *Clinical guidelines in family practice* (5th ed.). Gainesville, FL: Barmarrae Books.

Von Gunten, C., & Buckholz, G. (2018). Palliative care: Overview of cough, stridor, and hemoptysis. In D. M. Savarese (Ed.), *UpToDate*. Retrieved from https://www.uptodate.com/contents/palliative-care-overview-of-cough-stridor-and-hemoptysis

Weinberger, S. E., & Silvestri, R. C. (2017). Treatment of subacute and chronic cough in adults. In H. Hollingsworth (Ed.), *UpToDate*. Retrieved from https://www.uptodate.com/contents/treatment-of-subacute-and-chronic-cough-in-adults

CHAPTER 8

Delirium

Acute delirium is a common issue among hospitalized patients and poses increased risk of mortality if not treated quickly. Risk factors for delirium include older age, polypharmacy, infections, traumatic brain injury, underlying cognitive disorders, organ failure, dehydration, immobility, and malnutrition. Reasons for delirium include substance intoxication, side effects of medication, and various medical conditions; however, an obvious cause may not always be found. The American Psychiatric Association defines delirium as follows:

- A change in consciousness with a reduced ability to focus, sustain, or shift attention
- A change in cognition or the development of a perceptual disturbance that is not accounted for by a preexisting dementia
- A cognitive disturbance that develops over a short period of time
- The presence of other cognitive disturbances such as memory changes, disorientation, and/or speech changes

It is important to determine whether the patient's delirium is related to a chronic dementia or a new underlying process. If the nurse is unfamiliar with the patient, it is essential they gather a baseline cognitive description from a family member or caregiver. It is the nurse's priority to collect thorough history and assessment information, help the provider find the underlying cause, monitor for infection, and maintain the patient's safety. In this chapter, nursing intervention considerations and plan of care recommendations should reflect whatever the suspected cause is.

Differential Diagnosis Considerations

Common: CVA/TIA, benzodiazepine withdrawal, dehydration, electrolyte disturbances, fever, hypercapnia, hyperglycemia, hypoglycemia, hypoxia, ICU delirium, increased ICP, infectious process (influenza, meningitis, pneumonia, pyelonephritis, soft tissue infection, UTI), liver failure, medication induced, pain, post-operative state, renal failure, seizures, sepsis, shock (various types), sundowning, TBI, withdrawal from alcohol/drugs

Consider: anemia, anxiety, brain malignancy, burn injury, cerebral edema, CO poisoning, depression, digoxin toxicity, DKA, encephalitis, encephalopathy, fat embolism, folate deficiency, heart failure, hypothermia, MI, Parkinson's disease, sleep deprivation, thiamine deficiency, thyroid dysfunction, vitamin B12 deficiency

Questions to Ask the Patient/Family/Witness/Yourself

- When did the delirium start? Did it start gradually or suddenly?
- Is the delirium constant, or does it come and go?
- Is it worse at certain times of the day?
- How is their appetite? Are they able to keep down food and/or fluids?
- How much fluid are they drinking on a daily basis?
- Do they have a history of delirium? If so, what was the cause? What was done or used to treat it?
- Have they had any recent: illness/infection? exposure to CO, chemicals, smoke, or toxins? hospitalization/ICU stay? immobilization such as prolonged time spent in bed or sitting? surgery? trauma to the head?
- Have they taken any new prescribed or over-the-counter medications? Have there been any recent changes to their current medication?
- Do they drink alcohol? How many drinks per day/week? What kind and amount of alcohol do they drink? When was their last drink? (if applicable)
- Do they have a history of drug use? What types and how much? Do they use on a daily basis? When was their last use? (if applicable)

Associated Signs/Symptoms: PAIN: pain anywhere; GENERAL: chills, fatigue, fever, insomnia, weakness; EENT: vision changes; NECK: stiffness, swollen glands; CARDIOVASCULAR: chest pain/

tightness, palpitations; RESPIRATORY: cough, dyspnea, sputum production; GASTROINTESTINAL: diarrhea, nausea, signs of GI bleeding, vomiting; GENITOURINARY: dysuria, hematuria, incontinence, urinary frequency, urinary retention; MUSCULOSKELETAL: muscle cramps; NEUROLOGICAL: dizziness, headache, numbness/tingling, seizures, syncope, tremors; SKIN: erythema, rash, swelling; ENDOCRINE: hot/cold intolerance, polydipsia, polyphagia, polyuria; PSYCHOLOGICAL: anxiety, depression, hallucinations, restlessness

Recommended Assessments

There are several scales available to screen and diagnose delirium, including the Confusion Assessment Method (CAM), NEECHAM Confusion Scale, Delirium Rating Scale-revised version, Nursing Delirium Screening Scale, Delirium Observation Screening Scale, and Memorial Delirium Assessment Scale. The CAM is strongly

Confusion Assessment Method	
1. Acute onset	Have they had an acute change in mental status from baseline? Does it fluctuate during the day? (change in severity, or come and go?)
2. Inattention	Does the patient have difficulty focusing? Are they easily distracted or having difficulty keeping track of what is being said?
3. Disorganized thinking	Is the patient's thought process disorganized? Are they rambling or switching from subject to subject? Is the flow of the conversation logical?
4. Altered level of consciousness	How do you rate the patient's level of consciousness? It is considered abnormal if the patient scores anything but alert. 1. Alert 2. Hyper alert (overly sensitive to environment) 3. Lethargic (easy to arouse) 4. Stupor (difficult to arouse) 5. Coma

Data from Inouye, S., van Dyck, C., Alessi, C., Balkin, S., Siegal, A. & Horwitz, R. (1990). Clarifying confusion: The confusion assessment method. *Annals of Internal Medicine, 113*(12), 941-948.

supported in the literature and is the most commonly used tool to aid in the diagnosis of delirium. A diagnosis requires the presence of 1 AND 2, plus 3 OR 4.

- Vital signs
- Temperature
- I/O
- Pain scale (if applicable)
  - Tolerable pain level
- General
  - Level of consciousness and orientation
  - Inspect: signs of acute distress, acute illness, affect, restlessness
  - Speech changes
  - GCS
- Skin
  - Inspect: cyanosis, diaphoresis, dryness, jaundice, pallor, rash, wounds, surgical site (if applicable)
  - Palpate: temperature, turgor
- Eyes
  - Inspect: nystagmus, ptosis, pupillary response
- Mouth
  - Inspect: abnormal mouth movements, acetone breath, dentition, exudates, mucous membrane moisture level
  - Gag reflex
- Head/face/neck
  - Inspect: ROM of neck, signs of trauma
  - Palpate: lymphadenopathy, swelling, tenderness
- Cardiovascular
  - Auscultate: heart sounds, rate, rhythm
- Respiratory
  - Inspect: respiratory effort, depth, pattern, use of accessory muscles
  - Auscultate: lung sounds
- Gastrointestinal
  - Inspect: distention

- Auscultate: bowel sounds
- Palpate: ascites, guarding, masses, organomegaly, (rebound) tenderness
- Genitourinary
  - Palpate: bladder distention, CVAT
- Neurological
  - Inspect: facial droop, gait, tremors
  - Palpate: extremity strength, sensation
  - Cranial nerve exam
- Extremities
  - Inspect: IV site
  - Palpate: capillary refill, edema, pulses

Past Medical History Considerations

Puts the patient at risk for differential considerations

- Alcohol abuse/use
- Chronic pain
- CKD
- COPD
- Diabetes
- Drug abuse/use
- HTN
- Immobilization
- Liver disease

Reoccurrence/exacerbation should be considered

- UTI

Chronic conditions that can cause or mimic delirium

- Alzheimer's disease/dementia
- Anemia
- Anxiety
- Brain malignancy
- Chronic pain

- CVA/TIA
- Depression
- Epilepsy
- Heart failure
- Insomnia
- Malnutrition
- Parkinson's disease
- TBI
- Thyroid disease

Medication Evaluation

Most common causative/exacerbating medication

- Antiarrhythmics
- Antibiotics
- Anticholinergics
- Anticonvulsants
- Antidepressants
- Antiemetics
- Antihistamines
- Antipsychotics
- Benzodiazepines (withdrawal)
- Beta blockers
- Clonidine
- Corticosteroids
- Digoxin
- Diuretics
- Insulin
- Lithium
- Muscle relaxants
- Opioids

Lab Evaluation and Trends

- Bedside capillary glucose trends
- BMP/CMP
- CBC

Nursing Intervention Considerations

- Call for help or rapid response/code team if vital signs are unstable or there are signs of urgent distress
- Maintain a patent airway
  - Apply oxygen if hypoxic
  - Encourage slow relaxed deep breathing if hyperventilating
- Verify patent IV if IVF or IV medication treatment is anticipated
  - Flush according to facility protocol; watch for swelling, erythema, pain, and other signs of infiltration
- Check blood sugar if hypo- or hyperglycemia is suspected
- Medications (if ordered or protocol allows)
  - Hold suspected causative medication until discussion with the provider
  - If opioid overdose is suspected, give Naloxone 0.5mg IV push, may repeat if necessary
  - If hypoglycemic and has altered mental status or unable to swallow, give 1mg IV/IM/SQ glucagon, and/or 25–50mL IV 50% dextrose, or follow your facility's hypoglycemia protocol (goal is >100)
- Diet
  - Push fluids if there are no contraindications (>2000mL/day)
  - If hypoglycemic, alert, and can swallow, give a fast-acting carbohydrate like a glucose tablet, 4oz of fruit juice, 8oz of milk, 4oz of non-diet soda, hard candy, or teaspoon of honey/sugar. Repeat until sugar is normalized (goal is >100).
- Activity
  - Encourage activity and ambulation if safety permits
- Positioning
  - HOB raised to comfort
  - Lay supine with feet elevated if the patient is hypotensive
  - Reposition every 2–4 hours or establish an individualized turning schedule

- Collect
  - Urine sample if there are signs/symptoms of UTI
- Monitor
  - Stay with the patient until stable
  - Pain levels
  - Vital signs and trends
  - Oxygen saturation/pulse oximetry
  - Temperature trends
  - I/O
  - Blood sugar trends (if applicable)
  - Orientation status changes, GCS, CAM
  - Agitation levels
  - Neurological exam
  - Skin assessment every 8–24 hours
  - Signs of decreased cardiac output such as weak pulses, cool skin, altered mental status, hypotension, oliguria, and mottling
  - Signs of respiratory distress such as cyanosis, tachypnea, hypoxia, use of accessory muscles, diaphoresis, and adventitious lung sounds
  - Signs of dehydration such as lethargy, decreased skin turgor, dry mucous membranes, tachycardia, and (orthostatic) hypotension
  - Signs and symptoms of increased ICP such as worsening headache, nausea, vomiting, hypertension, bradypnea, altered mental status, vision changes, fixed or sluggish pupillary response, and GCS changes
  - Signs and symptoms of blood loss such as fatigue, dizziness, dyspnea, melena, hematochezia, hematemesis, hematuria, epistaxis, pallor, ecchymosis, altered mental status, hypotension, tachycardia, tachypnea, and hemoptysis
  - Signs and symptoms of sepsis such as fever, chills, hypotension, altered mental status, hypoxia, cool clammy skin, dyspnea, oliguria, tachycardia, and tachypnea

- Urine output color, frequency, and volume
- Safety
  - Perform a fall risk assessment and implement the appropriate strategies
  - Initiate frequent checks or 1:1 care if needed
- Environment
  - Provide a calm, quiet environment and reduce stimulation
  - Maintain a well-lit environment
  - Provide distractions
  - Utilize ways to reorient the patient with clocks, calendars, frequent family/friend interaction, and personal items from home
  - Maintain a comfortable room temperature
  - Offer aromatherapy and/or music therapy (if appropriate)
  - Utilize a fan (if appropriate)
- Supportive care
  - Maintain effective communication between yourself, patient, and family
  - Provide emotional support and reassurance to the patient and family
  - Maintain a calm manner during patient interactions
  - Notify the patient and family of changes in the plan of care
  - Refrain from correcting or arguing with the patient during periods of confusion and reorient the patient as needed
  - Identify barriers to care and compliance
  - Promote skin care and integrity
  - Offer back rubs, warmed blankets, warm drinks, and new bed linens
  - Allow the patient to wear their own nighttime clothes
  - Encourage the use of hearing aids and glasses (if applicable)

- **Educational topics (as applicable to the patient):**
  - General information regarding the patient's delirium and differential diagnosis considerations
  - Procedure and intervention explanation and justification
  - Medication changes
  - Oxygen therapy and maintenance
  - Relaxation techniques and breathing exercises
  - Stimulus control
  - Peri-care and proper hygiene
  - Skin care
  - Proper positioning and turning schedule
  - Safety needs and fall risk
  - 1:1 care
  - Home safety modifications and injury prevention
  - Handwashing and infection control measures
  - Trigger avoidance
  - Sleep hygiene
  - Blood glucose measurement techniques and frequency
  - Increased fluid intake
  - Increased physical activity (if applicable)
  - Alcohol and/or drug cessation and support
  - Signs and symptoms of hypoglycemia
  - Signs and symptoms of various infections
  - Pressure injury prevention
  - Dehydration prevention

ISBARR Recommendation Considerations

- Ask the provider to come assess the patient STAT if delirium is a new issue and the patient is unstable
- Transfer to the ICU if hemodynamically unstable, advanced medication management is required or closer monitoring is needed
- Medication
  - Discontinue/change suspected causative medication

- IV fluid needs if oral intake is poor, there are signs of dehydration, and the patient is NPO or hypotensive
- ECG if cardiac etiology is suspected
- Imaging (depending on what is suspected)
  - Head CT scan, chest X-ray
- Labs (depending on the suspected cause)
  - ABG
  - Blood culture
  - BMP/CMP
  - CBC
  - Digoxin
  - Magnesium
  - TSH
  - Toxicology screening
  - Urinalysis
  - Urine culture
- Safety
  - 1:1 monitoring
  - Activity level changes
  - Fall risk protocol
  - Restraints (avoid if possible)
- Monitoring needs
  - Blood sugars including frequency and parameters to call the provider (if applicable)
  - Continuous O_2 monitoring
  - Telemetry/continuous cardiac monitoring
  - Vital signs including frequency and parameters to call the provider
- Change diet to
  - Push oral fluids
- Protocols
  - CIWA-Ar if alcohol withdrawal is suspected
- Ask if the provider wants anything else done
- Read back orders; ask that they enter all orders into the electronic medical record

	ISBARR Template
I **Introduction**	**Introduce Yourself and the Patient** • "Hello, Dr. Bertrandt, this is Ben Uher. I am your nurse for Theo James in Room 402. He was transferred to me from the ICU this morning after being admitted for pneumonia three days ago."
S **Situation**	**Sign/Symptom You Are Concerned About** • "Upon admission to the floor, after a few hours I noticed he seemed confused. According to the nurse that had him in the ICU, he was alert and had no baseline confusion. I performed a CAM assessment that was positive for delirium. He is alert but is having disorganized thought processes, is jumping from subject to subject, and is unable to focus. His wife agrees that his cognition has changed today." **Associated Signs/Symptoms** • "He is denying any headaches, dizziness, chest pain, shortness of breath, pain, urinary frequency, or dysuria."
B **Background**	**Vitals** • "Vitals are stable, his temperature is 99.1 and O_2 sat is 98% on room air." **Exam** • "He is oriented to self and occasionally place. He does appear to be drowsy and falling asleep easily. He is following directions and has no signs of facial droop, speech changes, or one-sided weakness." **Past Medical History** • "He doesn't have a history of any psychiatric issues or dementia. He does have a history of diabetes," **Labs and Medications** • "so I checked blood sugar, which was 94. His CBC and CMP had no abnormalities this morning. He has been taking scheduled oral Percocet every four hours since last night, and his last dose was at 0800."

ISBARR Template

A Assessment	**Assessment** • "I am concerned about delirium, but I'm un-sure of the cause. I am wondering if it is related to the use of Percocet in the past 24 hours."
R Recommendations R Read Back	**Nurse's Recommendations, Interventions, and Read Back** • "I implemented the fall risk protocol. Can you come assess him? Did you want any other labs or imaging done at this time? Should I hold his Percocet dose?" • "Thank you, Dr. Bertrandt. At this time, you want me to collect a urine for UA and cul-ture, yes?"

Disclaimer: This dialogue is factitious and any resemblance to actual persons, living or dead, or actual events is purely coincidental.

In order to avoid order discrepancies, it is recommended that all orders be entered by the provider in the electronic medical record.

Select Differential Diagnosis Presentations

Anxiety

Overview: psychiatric disorder that can cause intense fear and worry

Patient may complain of: fatigue, chest pain, palpitations, dys-pnea, nausea, vomiting, abdominal pain, constipation, diar-rhea, paresthesias, tremors, headache, insomnia, dizziness, mind racing, feelings of impending doom

Objective findings: signs of acute distress, irritability, inability to focus, diaphoresis, tachycardia, hypertension, tachypnea, muscle tension

PMH considerations/risk factors: hx of anxiety, depression, PTSD, insomnia, substance abuse, physical abuse, recent physi-cal or emotional trauma, family hx of psychiatric diseases

Diagnostics: clinical diagnosis; workup to rule out more emer-gent causes may be indicated

Cerebral Vascular Accident

Overview: partial or complete obstruction of blood flow to the brain due to ischemia or hemorrhage causing brain tissue death

Patient may complain of: vision changes, nausea, vomiting, dysphagia, headache, dizziness, seizures, insomnia, difficulty with memory, speaking, focusing, and understanding; unilateral paralysis of the face, arms, and legs

Objective findings: signs of acute distress, altered mental status, ptosis, dysarthria, hypertension, carotid bruit(s), facial droop, seizures, unilateral weakness and sensation disturbances, immobility, gait disturbances

PMH considerations/risk factors: hx of HTN, CAD, heart failure, hyperlipidemia, arrhythmia, cardiac valve disease, diabetes, obesity, nicotine use, substance abuse, family hx of heart disease

Diagnostics: Head CT/MRI

Dehydration

Overview: abnormal loss of extracellular fluid volume

Patient may complain of: fatigue, thirst, dry mouth, palpitations, constipation, oliguria, muscle cramps, dizziness, headache

Objective findings: fever, altered mental status, lethargy, irritability, decreased skin turgor, generalized skin dryness, dry mucous membranes, (orthostatic) hypotension, tachycardia, oliguria

PMH considerations/risk factors: hx of liver or renal disease/failure, recent vomiting and/or diarrhea, GI bleeding, polyuria, diuretic use, burn injury, or intense physical activity

Diagnostics: BMP/CMP, CBC, urine Na, I/O

Diabetic Ketoacidosis

Overview: lack of insulin leads to extreme hyperglycemia and the production of ketones, causing the blood to be more acidic

Patient may complain of: fatigue, generalized abdominal pain, dyspnea, nausea, vomiting, polyuria, polyphagia, polydipsia

Objective findings: altered mental status, lethargy, acetone breath, decreased skin turgor, dry mucous membranes, tachycardia, hypotension, tachypnea

PMH considerations/risk factors: hx of type 1 diabetes, medication noncompliance, substance abuse, recent major illness or stress

Diagnostics: anion gap, BMP/CMP, ABG, hemoglobin A1C, urine ketones

Hypercalcemia

Overview: elevated serum calcium

Patient may complain of: fatigue, generalized weakness, anorexia, constipation, nausea, dyspepsia, vomiting, muscle aches; patient is typically asymptomatic unless severe

Objective findings: altered mental status, lethargy, hypertension, bradycardia, shortened QT interval, hypoactive bowel sounds, decreased reflexes; exam is typically unremarkable unless severe

PMH considerations/risk factors: hx of cancer, AIDS/HIV, Addison's disease, hyperparathyroidism

Diagnostics: serum Ca, ECG

Hypermagnesemia

Overview: elevated serum magnesium

Patient may complain of: fatigue, palpitations, nausea, vomiting, muscle spasms, headache; patient is typically asymptomatic unless severe

Objective findings: lethargy, altered mental status, diaphoresis, flushing, hypotension, bradycardia, arrhythmia, prolonged PR interval, wide QRS complex, bradypnea, decreased reflexes; exam is typically unremarkable unless severe

PMH considerations/risk factors: hx of gastroparesis, ileus, intestinal obstruction, CKD, AKI, hypothyroidism, magnesium supplementation

Diagnostics: serum Mg, ECG

Hypernatremia

Overview: elevated serum sodium

Patient may complain of: thirst, muscle spasms and cramps, tremors, seizures, anxiety; patient is typically asymptomatic unless severe

Objective findings: irritability, altered mental status, decreased skin turgor, dry mucous membranes, tachycardia, hypotension, bradypnea, decreased reflexes; exam is typically unremarkable unless severe

PMH considerations: hx of AKI, Cushing's syndrome, GI loss, burn injury, diabetes, diuretic use

Diagnostics: serum Na

Hypocalcemia

Overview: low serum calcium

Patient may complain of: fatigue, diarrhea, muscle cramps, paresthesias, seizures, anxiety; patient is typically asymptomatic unless severe

Objective findings: lethargy, altered mental status, irritability, positive Trousseau's and Chvostek's sign, prolonged QT interval, hypotension, bradycardia, tachypnea, hyperactive bowel sounds, hyperactive reflexes; exam is typically unremarkable unless severe

PMH considerations/risk factors: hx of cancer, immobility, malnutrition, hypoparathyroidism, alcohol abuse/use, vitamin D deficiency

Diagnostics: serum Ca, ECG

Hypokalemia

Overview: low serum potassium

Patient may complain of: fatigue, palpitations, nausea, vomiting, constipation, muscle weakness and cramping, seizures, anxiety; patient is typically asymptomatic unless severe

Objective findings: lethargy, irritability, altered mental status, wide QRS, arrhythmia, bradypnea, hypoactive bowel sounds, decreased reflexes; exam is typically unremarkable unless severe

PMH considerations/risk factors: hx of CKD, diabetes, diarrhea, alcohol abuse/use, eating disorders, NPO status, diuretic use

Diagnostics: serum K, ECG

Hypomagnesemia

Overview: low serum magnesium

Patient may complain of: fatigue, generalized weakness, nausea, vomiting, constipation, confusion, paresthesias, tremors, seizures; patient is typically asymptomatic unless severe

Objective findings: altered mental status, lethargy, bradycardia, hypotension, wide QRS, peaked T waves, prolonged PR interval, arrhythmia, bradypnea, hypoactive bowel sounds, hyperactive reflexes, tremors; exam is typically unremarkable unless severe

PMH considerations/risk factors: hx of diarrhea, burn injury, alcohol abuse/use, malnutrition, DKA, pancreatitis

Diagnostics: serum Mg, ECG

Hyponatremia

Overview: low serum sodium

Patient may complain of: fatigue, thirst, nausea, vomiting, anorexia, muscle cramps and weakness, headache; patient is typically asymptomatic unless severe

Objective findings: altered mental status, lethargy, irritability, tachycardia, weak pulses, bradypnea, decreased reflexes; exam is typically unremarkable unless severe

PMH considerations/risk factors: hx of GI loss, CKD, heart failure, diuretic use, SIADH, dehydration

Diagnostics: serum Na

Increased Intracranial Pressure

Overview: rise in pressure within the cranial cavity

Patient may complain of: vision changes, nausea, vomiting, headache, confusion, seizures, dizziness

Objective findings: signs of acute distress, altered mental status, GCS changes, sluggish/fixed pupillary response, hypertension, bradycardia, bradypnea

PMH considerations/risk factors: hx of TBI, CVA, CNS infections, hydrocephalus, cancer, seizures, HTN

Diagnostics: ICP monitoring, head CT/MRI

Liver Disease/Failure

Overview: broad term to describe damage and malfunction of the liver

Patient may complain of: fatigue, itching, anorexia, nausea, vomiting, RUQ abdominal pain, bloating, signs of GI bleeding

Objective findings: altered mental status, lethargy, jaundice, edema, hypotension, ascites, abdominal distention, hepatomegaly, spider angiomas; exam may be unremarkable

PMH considerations/risk factors: hx of liver disease, hepatitis, diabetes, sepsis, obesity, cancer, Wilson's disease, IV drug use, alcohol abuse

Diagnostics: CMP, hepatitis panel, ammonia, PT/INR, abdominal US/CT, biopsy

Meningitis

Overview: inflammation and infection of the meninges surrounding the brain and spinal cord

Patient may complain of: chills, fever, fatigue, photophobia, neck pain, anorexia, nausea, vomiting, headache, confusion, dizziness

Objective findings: signs of acute distress/illness, lethargy, fever, irritability, altered mental status, petechial rash, nuchal rigidity (positive Brudzinski, Kernig sign), seizures, signs of increased ICP

PMH considerations/risk factors: hx of TBI, immunosuppression, pregnancy, close quarter living situations, recent travel outside of the United States, alcohol abuse, older/younger age

Diagnostics: CBC, lumbar puncture, head CT

Myocardial Infarction

Overview: decreased or no blood flow through the coronary arteries causing cardiac muscle death

Patient may complain of: fatigue, chest pain not improved with rest, radiation of the pain to the left arm/neck/jaw, palpitations, dyspnea, activity intolerance, abdominal pain, nausea, dizziness, anxiety, feelings of impending doom; symptoms have longer duration than stable angina

Objective findings: signs of acute distress, lethargy, irritability, altered mental status, diaphoresis, cool clammy skin, hypertension/hypotension, tachycardia/bradycardia, arrhythmia, murmur, ST elevations, pathologic Q waves, weak pulses, sluggish capillary refill, tachypnea

PMH considerations/risk factors: hx of MI, CAD, HTN, heart failure, hyperlipidemia, diabetes, cardiac valve disorders, sedentary lifestyle, NSAID use, nicotine use, substance abuse, family hx of heart disease, older age

Diagnostics: cardiac enzymes, ECG, stress test, coronary angiography

Parkinson's Disease

Overview: progressive movement disorder of the central nervous system

Patient may complain of: fatigue, generalized weakness, vision changes, dysphagia, constipation, urinary retention, gait instability, joint rigidity, tremors, confusion, hallucinations, insomnia; symptoms are progressive in nature

Objective findings: altered mental status, lethargy, flat affect, dysarthria, (orthostatic) hypotension, bradykinesia, generalized muscle and joint rigidity, postural instability, resting tremor, psychosis

PMH considerations/risk factors: hx of Parkinson's disease, trauma to the head, family hx of Parkinson's, male gender, older age

Diagnostics: clinical diagnosis; head MRI may be ordered initially

Pneumonia

Overview: infection of the air sacs in one or both lungs causing inflammation and fluid accumulation

Patient may complain of: chills, fever, fatigue, chest pain/tightness, dyspnea, wheezing, coughing, sputum production, hemoptysis, activity intolerance, anorexia, nausea, vomiting, headache

Objective findings: signs of acute distress/illness, lethargy, altered mental status (elderly), fever, tachycardia, tachypnea, use of accessory muscles, cough, sputum, hypoxia, adventitious breath sounds, dullness to percussion over consolidation, pleural friction rub

PMH considerations/risk factors: COPD, asthma, immunosuppression, dysphagia, immunization status, recent/current hospitalization, intubation, nicotine use, alcohol abuse, older/younger age

Diagnostics: CBC, sputum culture, chest X-ray

Pyelonephritis

Overview: bacterial infection of the kidney

Patient may complain of: fever; chills; nausea; vomiting; abdominal/back/flank pain; increased urinary frequency, retention, and urgency; dysuria; hematuria; urine odor; confusion (elderly)

Objective findings: signs of acute distress/illness, altered mental status (elderly), fever, tachycardia, CVAT, abdominal tenderness, bladder distention

PMH considerations: hx of frequent UTIs, diabetes, urolithiasis, urinary retention, immunosuppression, pregnancy, poor fluid intake, immobility, recent catheter use or GU surgery, female gender

Diagnostics: CBC, urinalysis, urine culture, renal US

Renal Disease/Failure

Overview: broad term to describe damage and malfunction of the kidneys

Patient may complain of: fatigue, itching, dyspnea, anorexia, nausea, vomiting, oliguria, confusion

Objective findings: lethargy, altered mental status, arrhythmia, edema, pericardial rub, adventitious lung sounds, oliguria or anuria; exam is typically unremarkable unless severe

PMH considerations/risk factors: hx of CKD, diabetes, HTN, CAD, sepsis, BPH, burn injury, heart failure, dehydration, GI/blood loss, NSAID use, ACE inhibitor use, diuretic use, older age

Diagnostics: BMP/CMP, anion gap, urinalysis, renal US

Sepsis

Overview: severe inflammatory response due to an infection causing organ dysfunction

Patient may complain of: chills, fever, fatigue, generalized weakness, palpitations, (pre)syncope, dyspnea, oliguria; symptoms of whatever infection is suspected (i.e., appendicitis, diverticulitis, cholecystitis, pneumonia, cellulitis, meningitis, UTI)

Objective findings: signs of acute distress/illness, lethargy, fever, altered mental status, cyanosis, cool clammy skin or warm to the touch, tachycardia, hypotension, tachypnea, hypoxia, oliguria; signs of whatever infection is suspected

PMH considerations/risk factors: hx of immunosuppression, diabetes, cancer, recent infection or hospitalization, older/younger age

Diagnostics: blood culture, lactate, CBC, BMP/CMP, PT/INR; workup may also relate to whatever infection is suspected

Transient Ischemic Attack

Overview: transient obstruction of blood flow to the brain mimicking a CVA

Patient may complain of: vision changes, nausea, vomiting, dysphagia, headache, dizziness, seizures, insomnia, difficulty with memory, speaking, focusing, and understanding; unilateral paralysis of face, arms, and legs; signs and symptoms are transient in nature

Objective findings: signs of acute distress, altered mental status, ptosis, dysarthria, hypertension, carotid bruit(s), facial droop, seizures, unilateral weakness and sensation disturbances, immobility, gait disturbances; may not have abnormal exam findings due to transient nature of the issue

PMH considerations/risk factors: hx of HTN, CAD, heart failure, hyperlipidemia, arrhythmia, cardiac valve disease, diabetes, obesity, nicotine use, substance abuse, family hx of heart disease

Diagnostics: Head CT/MRI

Urinary Tract Infection

Overview: broad term for infection of the urinary tract including the urethra, bladder, ureters, and kidneys

Patient may complain of: fever; chills; abdominal/back/flank/pelvic pain; nausea; vomiting; dysuria; increased urinary frequency, retention, and urgency; hematuria; incontinence; urine odor; confusion (elderly)

Objective findings: fever, altered mental status (elderly), pelvic tenderness, bladder distention; exam is typically unremarkable

PMH considerations/risk factors: hx of frequent UTIs, diabetes, interstitial cystitis, urinary retention, immunosuppression, dehydration, pregnancy, incontinence, recent catheter use, GU surgery or sexual activity, immobility, female gender

Diagnostics: urinalysis/urine dipstick, urine culture

Withdrawal (Alcohol)

Overview: rapid or abrupt decrease in alcohol intake causing physical and psychological disturbances

Patient may complain of: fever, chills, palpitations, anorexia, nausea, vomiting, seizures, headache, alcohol craving, insomnia, anxiety

Objective findings: signs of acute distress, fever, irritability, altered mental status, diaphoresis, tachycardia, hypertension, hepatomegaly, ascites, seizures, tremors, hallucinations/delirium

PMH considerations: hx of alcohol abuse, longer cessation (>48 hrs) since last drink, other substance abuse

Diagnostics: toxicology screen; workup to rule out more emergent causes may be indicated

Withdrawal (Opioids)

Overview: rapid or abrupt decrease in opioid intake causing physical and psychological disturbances

Patient may complain of: fever, body aches, nasal congestion, nasal drainage, anorexia, abdominal cramping, diarrhea, nausea, vomiting, tremors, opioid craving, anxiety, insomnia

Objective findings: signs of acute distress, fever, irritability, altered mental status, diaphoresis, piloerection, frequent yawning, pupil dilatation, rhinorrhea, hypertension, tachycardia, hyperactive bowel sounds

PMH considerations/risk factors: hx of daily opioid use, chronic pain, other substance abuse

Diagnostics: toxicology screen; workup to rule out more emergent causes may be indicated

References

American Geriatrics Society. (2015a). Abstracted clinical practice guideline for postoperative delirium in older adults. *Journal of the American Geriatrics Society*, 63(1), 142–150. doi:10.1111/jgs.13281

American Geriatrics Society. (2015b). American geriatrics society 2015 updated beers criteria for potentially inappropriate medication use in older adults. *Journal of the American Geriatrics Society*, *63*(11), 2227–2246. doi:10.1111/j.1532-5415.2012.03923.x

American Medical Directors Association. (2010). *Know-it-all before you call: Data collection system.* Columbia, MD: Author.

American Psychiatric Association. (2013). *Diagnostic and statistical manual of mental disorders* (5th *ed.*). Washington DC: PA Press.

Barbateskovic, M., Larsen, L. K., Oxenboll-Collet, M., Jakobsen, J. C., Perner, A., & Wetterslev, J. (2016). Pharmacological interventions for delirium in intensive care patients: A protocol for an overview of reviews. *Systematic Reviews, 5*(211), 1–12. doi 10.1186/s13643-016- 0391-5

Barr, J., Fraser, G. L., Puntillo, K., Ely, E. W., Gelinas, C., Dasta, J. F., . . . Skrobik, Y. (2013). Clinical practice guidelines for the management of pain, agitation, and delirium in adult patients in the intensive care unit: Executive summary. *American Journal of Health-System Pharmacy*, *70*(1), 53–58.

Chalela, J. A., & Kasner, S. E. (2016). Acute toxic-metabolic encephalopathy in adults. In J. L. Wilterdink (Ed.), *UpToDate.* Retrieved from https://www .uptodate.com/contents/acute-toxic-metabolic-encephalopathy-in-adults

Chang, V. T. (2018). Approach to symptom assessment in palliative care. In D. M. Savarese (Ed.), *UpToDate.* Retrieved from https://www.uptodate .com/contents/approach-to-symptom-assessment-in-palliative-care

Davidson, J. E., Winkelman, C., Gélinas, C., & Dermenchyan, A. (2015). Pain, agitation, and delirium guidelines: Nurses' involvement in development and implementation. *Critical Care Nurse*, *35*(3), 17–32. doi:10.4037/ccn2015824

Desai, S. P. (2009). *Clinician's guide to laboratory medicine* (3rd ed.). Houston, TX: MD2B.

DiSabatino-Smith, C. (2017). Feasibility and effectiveness of a delirium prevention bundle in critically ill patients. *American Journal of Critical Care*, *26*(1), 19–27. doi:10.4037/ajcc2017374

El Hussein, M., Hirst, S., & Salyers, V. (2015). Factors that contribute to underrecognition of delirium by registered nurses in acute care settings: A scoping review of the literature to explain this phenomenon. *Journal of Clinical Nursing*, *24*(7/8), 906–915. doi:10.1111/jocn.12693

Francis, J. (2014). Delirium and acute confusional states: Prevention, treatment, and prognosis. In J. L. Wilterdink (Ed.), *UpToDate.* Retrieved from https://www.uptodate.com/contents/delirium-and-acute-confusional -states-prevention-treatment-and-prognosis

Francis, J., & Young, G. B. (2014). Diagnosis of delirium and confusional states. In J. L. Wilterdink (Ed.), *UpToDate.* Retrieved from https://www .uptodate.com/contents/diagnosis-of-delirium-and-confusional-states

Gion, T., & Leclaire-Thoma, A. (2014). Delirium in the brain-injured patient. *Rehabilitation Nursing, 39*(5), 232–239. doi:10.1002/rnj.128

Grover, S., & Kate, N. (2012). Assessment scales for delirium: A review. *World Journal of Psychiatry, 2*(4), 58–70.

Hale, A., & Hovey, M. J. (2014). *Fluid, electrolyte and acid-base imbalances.* Philadelphia: F.A. Davis Company.

Inouye, S. K., van Dyck, C.H., Alessi, C. A., Blakin, S., Siegal, A.P., & Horwitz, R. I. (1990). Clarifying confusion: The confusion assessment method. A new method for detection of delirium. *Annals of Internal Medicine, 133,* 941–948.

Jarvis, C. (2015). *Physical examination & health assessment.* St. Louis, MO: Elsevier.

Kalish, V. B., Gillham, J. E., & Unwin, B. K. (2014). Delirium in older persons: Evaluation and management. *American Family Physician, 90*(3), 150–158.

LeBlond, R. F., Brown, D. D., Suneja, M., & Szot, J. F. (2015). *DeGowin's diagnostic examination* (10th ed.). New York, NY: McGraw-Hill.

Lippmann, S., & Perugula, M. L. (2016). Delirium or dementia? *Innovation in Clinical Neuroscience, 13*(9-10), 56–57.

McCance, K. L., Huether, S. E., Brashers, V. L., & Rote, N. S. (2014). *Pathophysiology: The biologic basis for disease in adults and children* (7th ed.). St. Louis, MO: Elsevier.

Pai, S. L. (2018). Delayed emergence and emergence delirium in adults. In N. A. Nussmeier (Ed.), *UpToDate.* Retrieved from https://www.uptodate.com/contents/delayed-emergence-and-emergence-delirium-in-adults

Papadakis, M. A., & McPhee, S. J. (2017). *Current medical diagnosis and treatment* (56th ed.). New York, NY: McGraw-Hill.

Raftery, A. T., Lim, E., & Ostor, A. J. (2014). *Differential diagnosis* (4th ed.). London, UK: Elsevier.

Schuckit, M. A. (2014). Recognition and management of withdrawal delirium (delirium tremens). *New England Journal of Medicine, 371*(22), 2109–2113. doi:10.1056/NEJMra1407298

Seller, R. H., & Symons, A. B. (2012). *Differential diagnosis of common complaints* (6th ed.). Philadelphia, PA: Elsevier.

Stolbach, A., & Hoffman, R. S. (2017). Acute opioid intoxication in adults. In J. Grayzel (Ed.), *UpToDate.* Retrieved from https://www.uptodate.com/contents/acute-opioid-intoxication-in-adults

Uphold, C. R., & Graham, M. V. (2013). *Clinical guidelines in family practice* (5th ed.). Gainesville, FL: Barmarrae Books.

CHAPTER 9

Diarrhea (Acute)

According to the World Gastroenterology Organization, acute diarrhea is defined as three loose or watery bowel movements within a 24-hour period, and symptoms lasting less than 2 weeks. Most acute diarrhea episodes are related to an infectious process. Viral pathogens are the most common cause, while bacterial and parasitic pathogens occur more often in those with risk factors and typically cause more severe symptoms. Risk factors for these infections include an age older than 70 years, antibiotic use, cancer treatment, cirrhosis, corticosteroid use, heart disease, hemochromatosis, recent or current hospitalization, IBD, immunosuppression, MSM, pancreatitis, pregnancy, and workplace exposure (food handlers, daycare workers, health care workers). It is important for the nurse to determine if the patient has a history of chronic diarrhea, as well as to assess the patient for the presence of risk factors for contracting these pathogens. The nurse's highest priority is to maintain the patient's hydration status and monitor them for GI bleeding. It will also be important to give the patient education on infection prevention. A GI referral is rarely required unless the cause for diarrhea remains unclear or symptoms are prolonged.

Differential Diagnosis Considerations

Common:

- **Most common:** bacterial etiology (*Bacteroides fragilis, Campylobacter, Clostridium difficile, Clostridium perfringens, Escherichia coli, Salmonella, Shigella, Staphylococcus aureus, Yersinia*), viral etiology (adenovirus, astrovirus, CMV, norovirus, rotavirus)
- **Less common:** parasitic etiology (*Cryptosporidium, Cyclospora, Entamoeba histolytica, Giardia lamblia*)
- **Consider:** food allergies, intestinal obstruction, lactose intolerance, medication induced, tube feeding

Chronic/secondary diarrhea considerations: Addison's disease, anxiety, carcinoid syndrome, celiac disease, diverticulitis, factitious diarrhea, food/lactose intolerance, functional diarrhea, gastroenteritis, GI malignancy, hepatitis A, hyperthyroidism, IBD, IBS, ischemic bowel disease, laxative abuse, medication induced, microscopic colitis, pancreatitis, short bowel syndrome, SIBO, withdrawal from alcohol/drugs

Questions to Ask the Patient/Family/Witness/Yourself

- When did the diarrhea start? Did it start gradually or suddenly?
- How often do you (typically) have a bowel movement per day/week?
- When was your last bowel movement? What did it look like (consistency, amount, color)?
- Was there blood within the stool? Streaked on the side of the stool? On toilet paper with wiping?
- How easy is it to have a bowel movement? Do you have any straining or pain?
- Does anything trigger your bowel movements (food, caffeine, medication, movement, psychological stress)?
- Does the diarrhea awake you from your sleep?
- Do you feel like you are having complete bowel movements?
- How is your appetite? Are you able to keep down food and/or fluids?
- Do you have abdominal/epigastric bloating or fullness with or after eating?
- How much fluid are you drinking on a daily basis?
- In the past 2 days, have you ingested fried rice, raw milk, uncooked shellfish, undercooked beef, pork, or poultry?
- Do you have a history of lactose intolerance? If so, have you recently ingested any milk, cheese, yogurt, ice cream, or other dairy products?
- Do you have a history of chronic diarrhea issues? If so, what have you done or used to treat it?
- Have you had any recent: exposure to GI infection, contaminated drinking water, or have been around anyone who is sick?

GI surgery? hospitalization? radiation therapy? travel outside of the United States?

- Have you had any recent invasive interventions such as tube feeding?
- Have you taken any new prescribed or over-the-counter medications? Have there been any recent changes to your current medication?
- Do you work in a daycare, the medical field, or food service?
- What are you allergic to? Have you been exposed to a known allergen?
- Do you drink alcohol? How many drinks per day/week? What kind and amount of alcohol do you drink? When was your last drink? (if applicable)
- Do you have a history of drug use? What types and how much? Do you use on a daily basis? When was your last use? (if applicable)

Associated Signs/Symptoms: PAIN: pain anywhere; GENERAL: chills, fatigue, fever, weight changes; GASTROINTESTINAL: heartburn, fecal incontinence, nausea, vomiting; NEUROLOGICAL: dizziness

Recommended Assessments

- Vital signs
- Temperature
- Weight and nutritional status
- I/O
- Pain scale (if applicable)
  - Tolerable pain level
- General
  - Inspect: signs of acute distress, acute illness, affect, restlessness
- Skin
  - Inspect: diaphoresis, dryness, jaundice, pallor
  - Palpate: temperature, turgor
- Mouth
  - Inspect: mucous membrane moisture level

- Cardiovascular
  - Auscultate: heart sounds, rate, rhythm
- Gastrointestinal
  - Inspect: distention, scarring
  - Auscultate: bowel sounds
  - Palpate: guarding, masses, organomegaly, (rebound) tenderness
- Rectal (if applicable)
  - Inspect: bleeding, erythema, lesions, swelling
  - Palpate: tenderness
- Extremities
  - Inspect: IV site (if applicable)

Past Medical History Considerations

- Allergies

Puts the patient at risk for differential considerations

- Abdominal surgery (gastric bypass, colectomy)
- AIDS/HIV
- Alcohol abuse/use
- Diabetes
- Drug use/abuse
- IBD
- Laxative abuse
- Liver disease
- Radiation therapy to the abdomen/pelvis

Reoccurrence/exacerbation should be considered

- Diverticulitis
- GI bleed
- Intestinal obstruction

Chronic conditions that can cause diarrhea

- Addison's disease
- Anxiety

- Celiac disease
- GI malignancy
- Hepatitis
- IBD
- IBS
- Lactose intolerance
- Pancreatitis
- Short bowel syndrome
- Thyroid disease

Medication Evaluation

Most common causative/exacerbating medication

- Antacids
- Antibiotics
- Chemotherapy
- Digoxin
- Diuretics
- H2 antagonists
- Laxatives
- Metformin
- NSAIDs
- PPIs
- Stool softeners

Puts the patient at higher risk for contracting a diarrhea-causing pathogen

- Antibiotics
- Chemotherapy
- Corticosteroids
- PPIs

Lab Evaluation and Trends

- BMP/CMP
- CBC

Nursing Intervention Considerations

- Verify patent IV if IVF or IV medication treatment is anticipated
  - Flush according to facility protocol; watch for swelling, erythema, pain, and other signs of infiltration
- Medications (if ordered or protocol allows)
  - Hold suspected causative medication until discussion with the provider
  - PRN antiemetic for nausea, IV/IM if vomiting
- Diet
  - NPO if intestinal obstruction is suspected
  - NPO if procedure or surgery is anticipated
  - Push fluids if there are no contraindications (>2,000mL/day)
  - Offer bland, simple foods that the patient can tolerate
  - Avoid foods that trigger symptoms
  - Avoid caffeine
  - Avoid foods/fluids that can darken stool such as blueberries, red wine, beets, and black licorice
- Positioning
  - Supine or side lying position with knees flexed to chest to take tension off the abdominal wall if the patient has active abdominal pain
  - Reposition every 2–4 hours or establish an individualized turning schedule
- Collect
  - Stool sample
- Monitor
  - Pain levels
  - Vital signs and trends
  - Temperature trends
  - I/O
  - Bowel sounds
  - Weight trends
  - Orientation status changes
  - Agitation levels

- Skin assessment every 8–24 hours, or more frequently if the patient is incontinent
- Signs of dehydration such as lethargy, decreased skin turgor, dry mucous membranes, tachycardia, and (orthostatic) hypotension
- Signs and symptoms of GI bleeding such as fatigue, dizziness, dyspnea, melena, hematochezia, hematemesis, pallor, ecchymosis, altered mental status, hypotension, tachycardia, and tachypnea
- Stool output color, consistency, frequency, and volume
- Safety
  - Perform a fall risk assessment and implement the appropriate strategies
- Environment
  - Provide a calm, quiet environment and reduce stimulation
  - Provide privacy and "Do Not Disturb" notice on the patient's door during elimination if safety permits
  - Maintain a comfortable room temperature
  - Utilize a fan (if appropriate)
  - Initiate isolation precautions: contact
- Supportive care
  - Maintain effective communication between yourself, patient, and family
  - Provide emotional support and reassurance to the patient and family
  - Maintain a calm manner during patient interactions
  - Discuss plan of care with the patient and decide reasonable goals together
  - Notify the patient and family of changes in the plan of care
  - Promote skin care and integrity
  - **Educational topics (as applicable to the patient):**
    - General information regarding the patient's diarrhea and differential diagnosis considerations

- Explanation regarding referrals and specialist who may see them for this issue
- New medication education including reason, side effects, and administration needs
- Medication changes
- Pain scale and pain goals
- Relaxation techniques and breathing exercises
- Bristol stool scale
- Age-appropriate colonoscopy recommendations
- Proper positioning and turning schedule
- Skin care
- Peri-care and proper hygiene
- Safety needs and fall risk
- Handwashing and infection control measures
- Isolation precaution needs
- NPO diet, BRAT diet
- Avoidance of food/fluid that trigger symptoms
- Avoidance of food/fluid that can discolor the stool
- Increased fluid intake
- Caffeine restriction
- Alcohol and/or drug cessation and support
- Signs and symptoms of GI infection
- Signs and symptoms of GI bleeding
- Pressure injury prevention
- Dehydration prevention

ISBARR Recommendation Considerations

- Medication
  - Discontinue/change suspected causative medication
  - Hold oral medications if the patient is unable to tolerate or NPO
  - Discuss changing medication routes with the provider (and pharmacy) if the patient is NPO

- Add PRN antiemetic for nausea
- Add PRN loperamide for afebrile patients with non-bloody stool and no abdominal pain
- IV fluid needs if oral intake is poor, there are signs of dehydration, and the patient is NPO or hypotensive
- Imaging (depending on the suspected cause)
  - KUB
- Labs (depending on the suspected cause)
  - Amylase, lipase
  - BMP/CMP
  - CBC
  - Occult stool
  - Stool culture with *C. difficile* testing
  - Toxicology screening
  - TSH
- Safety
  - Fall risk protocol
  - Isolation precautions: contact
- Monitoring needs
  - Daily weights
  - Strict I/O
  - Vital signs including frequency and parameters to call the provider
- Change diet to (depending on the suspected cause)
  - NPO
  - Caffeine restriction
  - BRAT or bland
  - Push oral fluids
- Protocols
  - CIWA-Ar if alcohol withdrawal is suspected
- Referrals
  - Gastroenterology
- Ask if the provider wants anything else done
- Read back orders; ask that they enter all orders into the electronic medical record

Diarrhea (Acute)

ISBARR Template	
I **Introduction**	**Introduce Yourself and the Patient** • "Hello, Dr. Grey, this is Jena Cruciani. I am the nurse for your patient Kim Vukovic in Room 202. As you know, she is 72 years old who was admitted four days ago for cellulitis."
S **Situation**	**Sign/Symptom You Are Concerned About** • "During my shift, Ms. Vukovic has had three small watery stools. She told me she had eight similar stools in the past 24 hours. There have been no signs of blood." **Associated Signs/Symptoms** • "She is also having some generalized mild abdominal cramping with defecation."
B **Background**	**Vitals** • "Her vital signs are stable. Blood pressure is 105/82, heart rate is 90, respiratory rate is 14, she is 96% on room air, and her temperature is 98.0." **Exam** • "Her oral mucosa is dry. She has normoactive bowel sounds and her abdomen was non-tender and non-distended when I examined her." **Past Medical History** • "She has no history of chronic diarrhea and denied any recent travel or ingesting any undercooked meats." **Labs and Medications** • "I know she has been on antibiotics for her cellulitis. Her CBC showed a normal WBC count this morning."
A **Assessment**	**Assessment** • "With her age, and the fact she has been in the hospital on antibiotics for the past four days, I am concerned about *C. difficile* infection."

ISBARR Template	
R Recommendations R Read Back	**Nurse's Recommendations, Interventions, and Read Back** • "I collected a stool sample and I have been trying to push oral fluids. Did you want to send the stool for any testing for *C. difficile*? I also recommend we put her on contact precautions. Did you want to start any IV fluids or other medication?" • "Thank you Dr. Grey, please let me read those orders back to you. You would like me to send the stool for cultures, GDH antigen, and *C. difficile* toxin A and B. Start normal saline IVF at 100cc per hour and contact precautions. Is all that correct?"

Disclaimer: This dialogue is factitious and any resemblance to actual persons, living or dead, or actual events is purely coincidental.

In order to avoid order discrepancies, it is recommended that all orders be entered by the provider in the electronic medical record.

Select Differential Diagnosis Presentations

Diverticulitis

Overview: inflammation of diverticulum

Patient may complain of: fever, chills, LLQ abdominal pain (typically), constipation/diarrhea, nausea, vomiting

Objective findings: signs of acute distress/illness, fever, palpable abdominal mass, LLQ tenderness with guarding

PMH considerations/risk factors: hx of IBD, IBS, diverticulosis, GI cancer, obesity, nicotine use, older age

Diagnostics: CBC, occult stool, abdomen CT/US

Gastroenteritis

Overview: broad term for infection (typically viral) of the stomach and intestines

Patient may complain of: chills, fever, fatigue, anorexia, nausea, vomiting, diarrhea, generalized abdominal pain, dyspepsia

Objective findings: fever, lethargy, decreased skin turgor, dry mucous membranes, generalized abdominal tenderness without guarding

PMH considerations/risk factors: hx of ingestion of undercooked food/contaminated water, immunosuppression, recent antibiotic use, older age

Diagnostics: clinical diagnosis; stool cultures may be considered if symptoms are severe or prolonged

Hyperthyroidism

Overview: overactive thyroid gland

Patient may complain of: anxiety, heat intolerance, fatigue, generalized weakness, palpitations, diarrhea, nausea, vomiting, weight loss, muscle cramps, tremors, seizures, insomnia

Objective findings: lethargy, irritability, diaphoresis, hair thinning, exophthalmos, goiter, tachycardia, hypertension, tremors, seizures

PMH considerations/risk factors: hx of Grave's disease, thyroiditis, pregnancy, thyroid cancer, family hx of thyroid dysfunction, female gender, older age

Diagnostics: TSH, T3, T4, thyroid US, radioactive iodine uptake scan

Inflammatory Bowel Disease

Overview: chronic inflammation of all or different parts of the GI tract

Patient may complain of: chills, fever, fatigue, weight loss, anorexia, abdominal pain/cramping, nausea, vomiting, dyspepsia, constipation/diarrhea, change in bowel habits, signs of GI bleeding

Objective findings: signs of acute distress/illness, lethargy, fever, signs of malnourishment, diaphoresis, pallor, tachycardia, abdominal tenderness, hematochezia

PMH considerations/risk factors: hx of Crohn's disease or ulcerative colitis, food intolerance/allergies, bleeding/clotting disorders, NSAID use, recent travel outside of the United States, nicotine use, family hx of IBS, younger age

Diagnostics: occult stool, CRP, CBC, endoscopy with biopsy

Intestinal Obstruction

Overview: inability of digestive material to move through the GI tract normally

Patient may complain of: abdominal pain, anorexia, nausea, vomiting, inability to pass gas, constipation/diarrhea

Objective findings: signs of acute distress/illness, decreased skin turgor, dry mucous membranes, tachycardia, abdominal distention and tenderness, hypoactive or absent bowel sounds, fecal impaction (rectal exam)

PMH considerations/risk factors: hx of hernia, GI cancer, IBD, previous GI surgery, radiation therapy to the abdomen, opioid use

Diagnostics: KUB, abdominal CT

Irritable Bowel Syndrome

Overview: recurrent benign intestinal pain syndrome with associated bowel habit changes

Patient may complain of: abdominal pain and cramping, diarrhea/constipation, bloating, dyspepsia, heartburn, nausea, sensation of incomplete bowel movements

Objective findings: irritable, mild abdominal bloating and generalized tenderness; exam is typically unremarkable

PMH considerations/risk factors: hx of IBS, IBD, depression, anxiety, family hx of IBS, female gender, younger age

Diagnostics: may not require any diagnostic testing; colonoscopy with biopsy, stool cultures, and CRP may be considered

Pancreatitis

Overview: inflammation of the pancreas

Patient may complain of: fatigue, chills, fever, epigastric/upper abdominal pain, radiation of the pain to the back, worse with movement, nausea, vomiting, dyspepsia, diarrhea

Objective findings: signs of acute distress/illness, lethargy, fever, diaphoresis, pallor, jaundice, tachycardia, hypotension, upper abdominal/epigastric tenderness, abdominal distention, positive Cullen's sign or Grey Turner sign (abdominal ecchymosis)

PMH considerations/risk factors: hx of chronic pancreatitis, hypertriglyceridemia, cholelithiasis, GI cancer, recent GI surgery or trauma to the abdomen, nicotine use, alcohol abuse/use

Diagnostics: amylase, lipase, abdominal CT/US

Withdrawal (Alcohol)

Overview: rapid or abrupt decrease in alcohol intake causing physical and psychological disturbances

Patient may complain of: fever, chills, palpitations, anorexia, nausea, vomiting, diarrhea, seizures, headache, alcohol craving, insomnia, anxiety

Objective findings: signs of acute distress, fever, irritability, altered mental status, diaphoresis, tachycardia, hypertension, hepatomegaly, ascites, seizures, tremors, hallucinations/delirium

PMH considerations: hx of alcohol abuse, longer cessation (>48 hrs) since last drink, other substance abuse

Diagnostics: toxicology screen; workup to rule out more emergent causes may be indicated

Withdrawal (Opioids)

Overview: rapid or abrupt decrease in opioid intake causing physical and psychological disturbances

Patient may complain of: fever, body aches, nasal congestion, nasal drainage, anorexia, abdominal cramping, diarrhea, nausea, vomiting, tremors, opioid craving, anxiety, insomnia

Objective findings: signs of acute distress, fever, irritability, altered mental status, diaphoresis, piloerection, frequent yawning, pupil dilatation, rhinorrhea, hypertension, tachycardia, hyperactive bowel sounds

PMH considerations/risk factors: hx of daily opioid use, chronic pain, other substance abuse

Diagnostics: toxicology screen; workup to rule out more emergent causes may be indicated

References

American Medical Directors Association. (2010). *Know-it-all before you call: Data collection system.* Columbia, MD: Author.

Barr, W., & Smith, A. (2014). Acute diarrhea in adults. *American Family Physician, 89*(3), 180–189. Retrieved from http://www.aafp.org/afp/2014/0201/p180.pdf

Bulechek, G. M., Butcher, H. K., Dochterman, J. M., & Wagner, C. (2013). *Nursing intervention classification (NIC).* St. Louis, MO: Elsevier Mosby.

Desai, S. P. (2009). *Clinician's guide to laboratory medicine* (3rd ed.). Houston, TX: MD2B.

Gulanick, M., & Myers, J. L. (2017). *Nursing care plans: Diagnosis, interventions, & outcomes* (9th ed.). St. Louis, MO: Elsevier.

Hale, A., & Hovey, M. J. (2014). *Fluid, electrolyte and acid-base imbalances.* Philadelphia, PA: F.A. Davis Company.

Jarvis, C. (2015). *Physical examination & health assessment.* St. Louis, MO: Elsevier.

Lamont, J. T., Kelly, C. P., & Bakken, J. S. (2018). *Clostridium difficile* infection in adults: Clinical manifestations and diagnosis. In E. L. Baron (Ed.), *UpToDate.* Retrieved from https://www.uptodate.com/contents/clostridium-difficile-infection-in-adults-clinical-manifestations-and-diagnosis

LaRocque, R., & Harris, J. B. (2017). Approach to the adult with acute diarrhea in resource-rich settings. In A. Bloom (Ed.), *UpToDate.* Retrieved from https://www.uptodate.com/contents/approach-to-the-adult-with-acute-diarrhea-in-resource-rich-settings

LaRocque, R., & Pietroni, M. (2017). Approach to the adult with acute diarrhea in resource- limited countries. In A. Bloom (Ed.), *UpToDate.* Retrieved from https://www.uptodate.com/contents/approach-to-the-adult-with-acute-diarrhea-in-resource-limited-countries

LeBlond, R. F., Brown, D. D., Suneja, M., & Szot, J. F. (2015). *DeGowin's diagnostic examination* (10th ed.). New York, NY: McGraw-Hill.

McCance, K. L., Huether, S. E., Brashers, V. L., & Rote, N. S. (2014). *Pathophysiology: The biologic basis for disease in adults and children* (7th ed.). St. Louis, MO: Elsevier.

Mitchell, B. G., Russo, P. L., & Race, P. (2014). *Clostridium difficile* infection: Nursing considerations. *Nursing Standard, 28*(47), 43–48. doi:10.7748/ns.28.47.43.e8857

Papadakis, M.A., & McPhee, S. J. (2017). *Current medical diagnosis and treatment* (56th ed.). New York, NY: McGraw-Hill.

Pimentel, M. (2016). Small intestinal bacterial overgrowth. In S. Grover (Ed.), *UpToDate.* Retrieved from https://www.uptodate.com/contents/small-intestinal-bacterial-overgrowth-management

Raftery, A. T., Lim, E., & Ostor, A. J. (2014). *Differential diagnosis* (4th ed.). London, UK: Elsevier.

Riddle, M. S., DuPont, H. L., & Conner, B. A. (2016). ACG clinical guideline: Diagnosis, treatment, and prevention of acute diarrheal infections in adults. *The American Journal of Gastroenterology, 111,* 602–622.

Seller, R. H., & Symons, A. B. (2012). *Differential diagnosis of common complaints* (6th ed.). Philadelphia, PA: Elsevier.

Shane, A. L., Mody, R. K., Crump, J. A., Tarr, P. I., Steiner, T. S., Kotloff, K., . . .Pickering, L. K. (2017). 2017 Infectious Diseases Society of American clinical practice guidelines for the diagnosis and management of infectious diarrhea. *Clinical Infectious Diseases,* 1–31.

Surawicz, C. M., Brandt, L. J., Binion, D. G., Ananthakrishnan, A. N., Curry, S. R., Gilligan, P. H., . . . Zuckerbraun, B. S. (2013). Guidelines for diagnosis, treatment, and prevention of *Clostridium difficile* infections. *The American Journal of Gastroenterology, 108*(4), 478–498.

Uphold, C. R., & Graham, M. V. (2013). *Clinical guidelines in family practice* (5th ed.). Gainesville, FL: Barmarrae Books.

Wald, A. (2017). Factitious diarrhea: Clinical manifestations, diagnosis, and management. In S. Grover (Ed.), *UpToDate.* Retrieved from https://www.uptodate.com/contents/factitious-diarrhea-clinical-manifestations-diagnosis-and-management

Walters, P. R., & Zuckerman, B. S. (2014). *Clostridium difficile* infection: Clinical challenges and management strategies. *Critical Care Nurse, 34*(4), 24–35. doi:10.4037/ccn2014822

Wanke, C. A. (2016a). Approach to the adult with acute diarrhea in resource-rich settings. In A. Bloom (Ed.), *UpToDate.* Retrieved from

https://0-www.uptodate.com.libus.csd.mu.edu/contents/approach-to
-the-adult-with-acute-diarrhea-in-resource-rich-settings?source=search
_result&search=diarrhea&selectedTitle=1~150

Wanke, C. A. (2016b). Epidemiology and causes of acute diarrhea in
resource-rich countries. In A. Bloom (Ed.), *UpToDate*. Retrieved from
https://0-www.uptodate.com.libus.csd.mu.edu/contents/epidemiology-and
-causes-of-acute- diarrhea-in-resource-rich-countries?source=search
_result&search=diarrhea&selectedTitle=9~150

Weinberg, D. S., Smalley, W., Heidelbaugh, J. J., & Sultan, S. (2014).
American gastroenterological association institute guidelines on the
pharmacological management of irritable bowel syndrome. *Gastroenterology, 147,* 1146–1148.

World Gastroenterology Organization. (2012). *Acute diarrhea in adults
and children: A global perspective*. Retrieved from http://www.world
gastroenterology.org/guidelines/global-guidelines/acute-diarrhea/acute
-diarrhea-english

CHAPTER 10

Dizziness

Dizziness is a subjective sensation of the room spinning, lightheadedness, (pre)syncope, or disequilibrium. The differential diagnosis considerations for dizziness are complex and encompass a large spectrum of etiologies. Referrals to neurology, cardiology, physical therapy, and ENT may be necessary, depending on the cause. A new sudden onset of dizziness or imbalance can be a sign of CVA and requires rapid attention. The provider will also need to come and assess the patient urgently if any red flag symptoms are present, such as weakness, chest pain, palpitations, dyspnea, numbness/tingling, and seizures. The nurse is responsible for assessing for a more readily reversible cause of dizziness, including dehydration, hyperventilation, hypoglycemia, hypoxia, orthostatic hypotension, and medication-induced dizziness. The nurse's main priorities include collecting a thorough history, obtaining a detailed description of the symptom for the provider, performing a full neurological exam, and maintaining the patient's safety. In this chapter, nursing intervention considerations and plan of care recommendations should reflect whatever the suspected cause is.

Differential Diagnosis Considerations

Common: anxiety, arrhythmia, BPPV, dehydration, disequilibrium, hyperventilation, hypoglycemia, hypoxia, increased ICP, medication induced, Ménière's disease, migraine headache, orthostatic hypotension, otitis media, Parkinson's disease, peripheral neuropathy, (pre)syncope, TBI, vasovagal reflex, vestibular migraine, vestibular neuritis

Consider: AAA rupture, acoustic neuroma, alcohol abuse/use, anaphylaxis, anemia, aortic dissection, brainstem ischemia, CANVAS, carcinoid syndrome, cardiac valve disorder, cerebellar infarction, cerebral hemorrhage, Chiari malformation, Cogan's syndrome, CO poisoning, CVA/TIA, ectopic pregnancy, MI, meningitis, MS, PE, perilymphatic fistula, pregnancy, psychogenic, Ramsay Hunt syndrome, seizures, semicircular canal dehiscence syndrome

Questions to Ask the Patient/Family/Witness/Yourself

- When did the dizziness start? Did it start gradually or suddenly?
- What were you doing before/when the symptoms started?
- Is the dizziness constant, or does it come and go? If intermittent, how long does it last? How often is it happening per hour/day?
- What does your dizziness feel like (room spinning, lightheaded, feeling like you are going to faint)?
- What makes the dizziness better (certain positions, medication, rest)?
- What triggers or makes the dizziness worse (activity, bearing down, certain positions, changing positions, coughing, head movements)?
- Do you have a history of dizziness? If so, what have you done or used to treat it?
- How much fluid are you drinking on a daily basis?
- When was the last time you ate? What did you eat?
- When was your last menstrual period? (If applicable)
- Have you had any recent: ENT/respiratory illness? exposure to CO? trauma to the head?
- Have you taken any new prescribed or over-the-counter medications? Have there been any recent changes to your current medication?
- What are you allergic to? Have you been exposed to a known allergen?
- Do you drink alcohol? How many drinks per day/week? What kind and amount of alcohol do you drink? When was your last drink? (if applicable)

Associated Signs/Symptoms: PAIN: pain anywhere; GENERAL: fever, weakness; EENT: ear pain, hearing changes, tinnitus, vision changes; NECK: stiffness; CARDIOVASCULAR: chest pain/tightness, palpitations; RESPIRATORY: dyspnea; GASTROINTESTINAL:

nausea, signs of GI bleeding, vomiting; MUSCULOSKELETAL: gait imbalance/instability; NEUROLOGICAL: headaches, numbness/tingling, photophobia, phonophobia, seizures, tremors; PSYCHOLOGICAL: anxiety, confusion

Recommended Assessments

- Vital signs
  - Orthostatic blood pressure
- Temperature
- Weight and nutritional status
- I/O
- Pain scale (if applicable)
  - Tolerable pain level
- General
  - Level of consciousness and orientation
  - Inspect: signs of acute distress, acute illness, affect, restlessness
  - Speech changes
  - GCS
- Skin
  - Inspect: cyanosis, diaphoresis, dryness, pallor
  - Palpate: turgor
- Eyes
  - Inspect: nystagmus, ptosis, pupillary response
- Mouth
  - Inspect: mucous membrane moisture level
- Ears
  - Inspect: erythema, external drainage
  - Palpate: external tenderness
- Head/face/neck
  - Inspect: ROM of neck, signs of trauma
  - Auscultate: carotid bruits
  - Palpate: swelling, tenderness
- Cardiovascular
  - Auscultate: heart sounds, rate, rhythm
  - Palpate: heaves, thrills

- Respiratory
  - Inspect: respiratory effort, depth, pattern, use of accessory muscles
  - Auscultate: lung sounds
- Neurological
  - Inspect: facial droop, gait, tremors
  - Palpate: extremity strength, sensation
  - Cranial nerve exam
  - Romberg test (if safety permits)
- Extremities
  - Inspect: IV site
  - Palpate: capillary refill, pulses

Past Medical History Considerations

- Allergies

Puts the patient at risk for differential considerations

- Alcohol abuse/use
- COPD
- Diabetes
- Heart failure
- HTN
- Nicotine use

Reoccurrence/exacerbation should be considered

- Anaphylaxis
- Arrhythmias (various)
- MI
- Otitis media
- PE

Chronic conditions that can cause dizziness

- Anemia
- Anxiety
- Arrhythmias (various)

- BPPV
- Cardiac valve disorders
- CVA/TIA
- Epilepsy
- Ménière's disease
- Migraines
- MS
- Parkinson's disease
- Peripheral neuropathy
- TBI

Medication Evaluation

Most common causative/exacerbating medication

- ACE inhibitors
- Alpha adrenergic blockers
- Aminoglycosides
- Anticholinergics
- Antiparkinson agents
- Antipsychotics
- Beta blockers
- Benzodiazepines
- CCBs
- Digoxin
- Diuretics
- Insulin
- Muscle relaxers
- Nitrates
- Opioids
- SSRIs
- Tricyclic antidepressants

Used to treat BPPV

- Antiemetics
- Antihistamines
- Benzodiazepines

Lab Evaluation and Trends (If Available)

- Bedside capillary glucose trends
- BMP/CMP
- CBC

Nursing Intervention Considerations

- Call for help or rapid response/code team if vital signs are unstable or there are signs of urgent distress
- Maintain a patent airway
  - Apply oxygen if hypoxic
  - Encourage slow relaxed deep breathing if hyperventilating
- Verify patent IV if IVF or IV medication treatment is anticipated
  - Flush according to facility protocol; watch for swelling, erythema, pain, and other signs of infiltration
- ECG if cardiac etiology is suspected
- Blood sugar if hypoglycemia is suspected
- Medications (if ordered or protocol allows)
  - Hold suspected causative medication until discussion with the provider
  - PRN antiemetic for nausea, IV/IM if vomiting
  - If hypoglycemic and has altered mental status or unable to swallow, give 1mg IV/IM/SQ glucagon, and/or 25–50mL IV 50% dextrose, or follow your facility's hypoglycemia protocol (goal is >100)
- Diet
  - Push fluids if there are no contraindications (>2,000mL/day)
  - If hypoglycemic, alert, and can swallow, give a fast-acting carbohydrate like a glucose tablet, 4oz of fruit juice, 8oz of milk, 4oz of non-diet soda, hard candy, or teaspoon of honey/sugar. Repeat until sugar is normalized (goal is >100)

- Activity
  - Keep the patient in bed until discussion with the provider
- Positioning
  - HOB raised to comfort
  - Side lying position if there is a decrease in LOC or the patient is vomiting
  - Reposition every 2–4 hours or establish an individualized turning schedule
- Monitor
  - Stay with the patient until stable
  - Pain levels
  - Vital signs and trends
  - Temperature trends
  - Oxygen saturation/pulse oximetry
  - I/O
  - Telemetry/cardiac monitor
  - Blood sugar trends (if applicable)
  - Orientation status changes, GCS
  - Agitation levels
  - Neurological exam
  - Skin assessment every 8–24 hours
  - Signs of decreased cardiac output such as weak pulses, cool skin, altered mental status, hypotension, oliguria, and mottling
  - Signs of respiratory distress such as cyanosis, tachypnea, hypoxia, use of accessory muscles, diaphoresis, and adventitious lung sounds
  - Signs of dehydration such as lethargy, decreased skin turgor, dry mucous membranes, tachycardia, and (orthostatic) hypotension
  - Signs and symptoms of increased ICP such as worsening headache, nausea, vomiting, hypertension, bradypnea, altered mental status, vision changes, fixed or sluggish pupillary response, and GCS changes

- Signs and symptoms of blood loss such as fatigue, dizziness, dyspnea, melena, hematochezia, hematemesis, hematuria, epistaxis, pallor, ecchymosis, altered mental status, hypotension, tachycardia, tachypnea, and hemoptysis
- Safety
  - Perform a fall risk assessment and implement the appropriate strategies
- Environment
  - Provide a calm, quiet environment and reduce stimulation
  - Maintain a well-lit environment
  - Avoid bothersome odors in the room
  - Maintain a comfortable room temperature
  - Offer aromatherapy and/or music therapy (if appropriate)
  - Utilize a fan (if appropriate)
- Supportive care
  - Maintain effective communication between yourself, patient, and family
  - Provide emotional support and reassurance to the patient and family
  - Maintain a calm manner during patient interactions
  - Discuss plan of care with the patient and decide reasonable goals together
  - Notify the patient and family of changes in the plan of care
  - Promote skin care and integrity
  - Provide light clothing and bed linen
  - Avoid vagal maneuvers
  - Encourage the use of glasses (if applicable)
  - **Educational topics (as applicable to the patient):**
    - General information regarding the patient's dizziness and differential diagnosis considerations
    - Procedure and intervention explanation and justification

- Explanation regarding referrals and specialist who may see them for this issue
- New medication education, including reason, side effects, and administration needs
- Medication changes
- Oxygen therapy and maintenance
- Relaxation techniques and breathing exercises
- Trigger avoidance
- Telemetry
- Skin care
- Proper positioning and turning schedule
- Safety needs and fall risk
- Increased fluid intake
- Blood glucose measurement techniques and frequency
- Sleep hygiene
- Stress reduction and management
- Alcohol and/or drug cessation and support
- Home safety modifications and injury prevention
- When to notify the nurse or provider
- Signs and symptoms of hypoglycemia
- Signs and symptoms of respiratory emergencies
- Signs and symptoms of cardiac emergencies
- Signs and symptoms of abnormal bleeding
- Pressure injury prevention
- Dehydration prevention

ISBARR Recommendation Considerations

- Ask the provider to come assess the patient STAT if they are unstable or red flag symptoms are present
- Transfer to the ICU if hemodynamically unstable, advanced medication management is required or closer monitoring is needed

- Medication
  - Discontinue/change suspected causative medication
  - Add PRN antiemetic for nausea
  - If BPPV is an established diagnosis and other differentials have been ruled out, PRN antihistamine, benzodiazepine, and/or antiemetic can be used for symptom management
- IV fluid needs if oral intake is poor, there are signs of dehydration, and the patient is NPO or hypotensive
- ECG if not already done or repeat testing is needed
- Imaging (depending on the suspected cause)
  - Head CT scan/MRI, chest X-ray
- Labs (depending on the suspected cause)
  - ABG
  - BMP/CMP
  - CBC
- Safety
  - Activity level changes
  - Fall risk protocol
- Monitoring needs
  - Blood sugars including frequency and parameters to call the provider (if applicable)
  - Continuous O_2 monitoring
  - Telemetry/continuous cardiac monitoring
  - Vital signs including frequency and parameters to call the provider
- Supportive cares
  - Compression stockings or SCDs
- Change diet to
  - Push oral fluids
- Referrals
  - Cardiology
  - ENT
  - Neurology
- Ask if the provider wants anything else done
- Read back orders; ask that they enter all orders into the electronic medical record

ISBARR Template

I **Introduction**	**Introduce Yourself and the Patient** • "Hello, Dr. Schroeder, this is Janet Krejci. I am the nurse for Mrs. Madeline Schmidt at Golden Living Long Term Care."
S **Situation**	**Sign/Symptom You Are Concerned About** • "She started complaining of dizziness with positional changes today. It is worse when she goes from sitting to standing position but she denies it with head movements." **Associated Signs/Symptoms** • "The dizziness is making her nauseated but she has not vomited. She doesn't have a headache, hearing changes, numbness, tingling, or weakness."
B **Background**	**Vitals** • "Orthostatic blood pressures are 132/98 sitting and standing 102/80. Heart rate is 86 in both positions." **Exam** • "On exam, she has dry mucous membranes. Her gait is stable with a walker and she is alert and orientated." **Past Medical History** • "She said she has had similar dizziness episodes like this in the past week or so. In her chart, I do not see a previous diagnosis of vertigo or orthostatic hypotension." **Labs and Medications** • "She takes 40mg daily lisinopril, 50mg BID metoprolol, and 40mg BID Lasix for hypertension and CHF, which she took scheduled doses this morning. She has not had any recent lab work in the last month."
A **Assessment**	**Assessment** • "I am concerned the orthostatic hypotension is causing her dizziness. She also seems to be mildly dehydrated."

ISBARR Template	
R **Recommendations** R **Read Back**	**Nurse's Recommendations, Interventions, and Read Back** • "For safety, I have her up with one assist and changing positions slowly. I am also encouraging her to drink fluids but staying within her 2,000cc fluid restriction. Her next dose of metoprolol and Lasix is due at 1800. Do you want me to give those doses? Do you want to change any of her blood pressure medications? Can we initiate the fall risk protocol? Do you want any labs or anything else done at this time?" • "Thank you, Dr. Schroeder, I just wanted to verify your orders. You would like me to decrease the Lasix dose to 20mg BID, check her orthostatic blood pressure and weight daily, maintain 2,000cc fluid restriction, start fall risk protocol, and draw a CBC, BNP, and CMP. I will also make sure to call you if her symptoms worsen or persist."

Disclaimer: This dialogue is factitious and any resemblance to actual persons, living or dead, or actual events is purely coincidental.

In order to avoid order discrepancies, it is recommended that all orders be entered by the provider in the electronic medical record.

Select Differential Diagnosis Presentations

Abdominal Aortic Aneurysm Rupture

Overview: abnormal dilation of the abdominal aorta leads to vessel rupture

Patient may complain of: severe abdominal/back pain, palpitations, nausea, vomiting, dizziness

Objective findings: signs of acute distress, altered mental status, diaphoresis, tachycardia, hypotension, pulsating abdominal mass, abdominal bruit

PMH considerations/risk factors: CAD, HTN, heart failure, diabetes, connective tissue disorders, trauma to the abdomen, nicotine use, family hx of AAA, male gender, older age

Diagnostics: abdominal US/CT/MRI

Anxiety

Overview: psychiatric disorder that can cause intense fear and worry

Patient may complain of: fatigue, chest pain, palpitations, dyspnea, nausea, vomiting, abdominal pain, constipation/diarrhea, paresthesias, tremors, headache, insomnia, dizziness, mind racing, feelings of impending doom

Objective findings: signs of acute distress, irritability, inability to focus, diaphoresis, tachycardia, hypertension, tachypnea, muscle tension

PMH considerations/risk factors: hx of anxiety, depression, PTSD, insomnia, substance abuse, physical abuse, recent physical or emotional trauma, family hx of psychiatric diseases

Diagnostics: clinical diagnosis; workup to rule out more emergent causes may be indicated

Aortic Dissection

Overview: a tear in the intima layer of the aorta

Patient may complain of: severe chest/back pain described as ripping or tearing, abdominal pain, flank pain, dyspnea, nausea, dizziness, (pre)syncope, paresthesias, feelings of impending doom

Objective findings: signs of acute distress, altered mental status, diaphoresis, cool clammy skin, syncope, JVD, murmur, hypotension/hypertension, weak pulses or pulse deficit, sluggish capillary refill, tachypnea

PMH considerations/risk factors: hx of HTN, heart failure, cardiac valve disorders, connective tissue disorders, diabetes, substance abuse, pregnancy, nicotine use, male gender, older age

Diagnostics: ECG, TEE, chest X-ray, chest CT, aortography

Arrhythmia

Overview: any irregular heart rhythm

Patient may complain of: fatigue, generalized weakness, (pre)syncope, palpitations, chest pain, dyspnea, dizziness, seizures, anxiety

Objective findings: signs of acute distress, lethargy, irritability, diaphoresis, irregular heart rhythm, bradycardia/tachycardia, murmur, hypotension, tachypnea, seizures

PMH considerations/risk factors: hx of arrhythmia, CAD, HTN, heart failure, MI, cardiac valve disorders, diabetes, previous CV surgery, substance abuse, increased psychological stress, nicotine use, family hx of heart disease

Diagnostics: BMP/CMP, CBC, TSH, ECG, ECHO, Holter monitor/loop recorder/event recorder

Benign Paroxysmal Positional Vertigo

Overview: abnormal calcium debris within the inner ear causing obstruction of fluid movement, leading to acute dizziness

Patient may complain of: nausea, vomiting, dizziness with head position changes, balance disturbances; symptoms have a short duration

Objective findings: nystagmus, positive Dix-Hallpike maneuver, gait instability

PMH considerations/risk factors: hx of BPPV, orthostatic hypotension, recent head injury or ear infection, female gender

Diagnostics: clinical diagnosis; workup to rule out more emergent causes may be indicated

Cerebral Vascular Accident

Overview: partial or complete obstruction of blood flow to the brain due to ischemia or hemorrhage causing brain tissue death

Patient may complain of: vision changes, nausea, vomiting, dysphagia, headache, dizziness, seizures, insomnia, difficulty with memory, speaking, focusing, and understanding; unilateral paralysis of the face, arms, and legs

Objective findings: signs of acute distress, altered mental status, ptosis, dysarthria, hypertension, carotid bruit(s), facial droop, seizures, unilateral weakness and sensation disturbances, immobility, gait disturbances

PMH considerations/risk factors: hx of HTN, CAD, heart failure, hyperlipidemia, arrhythmia, cardiac valve disease, diabetes, obesity, nicotine use, substance abuse, family hx of heart disease

Diagnostics: Head CT/MRI

Dehydration

Overview: abnormal loss of extracellular fluid volume

Patient may complain of: fatigue, thirst, dry mouth, palpitations, oliguria, constipation, muscle cramps, dizziness, headache

Objective findings: fever, altered mental status, lethargy, irritability, decreased skin turgor, generalized skin dryness, dry mucous membranes, (orthostatic) hypotension, tachycardia, oliguria

PMH considerations/risk factors: hx of liver or renal disease/failure, recent vomiting and/or diarrhea, GI bleeding, polyuria, diuretic use, burn injury, or intense physical activity

Diagnostics: BMP/CMP, CBC, urine Na, I/O

Ectopic Pregnancy

Overview: fertilized egg implants outside of the uterus, typically in the fallopian tubes

Patient may complain of: chills, fever, breast tenderness, severe lower abdominal pain, nausea, vomiting, irregular vaginal bleeding, dizziness

Objective findings: signs of acute distress/illness, fever, hypotension, tachycardia, lower abdominal tenderness, vaginal bleeding

PMH considerations/risk factors: hx of infertility, IUD, previous GYN surgeries

Diagnostics: urine or serum Hcg, pelvic US, pelvic exam

Increased Intracranial Pressure

Overview: rise in pressure within the cranial cavity

Patient may complain of: vision changes, nausea, vomiting, headache, confusion, dizziness, seizures

Objective findings: signs of acute distress, altered mental status, GCS changes, sluggish/fixed pupillary response, hypertension, bradycardia, bradypnea

PMH considerations/risk factors: hx of TBI, CVA, CNS infections, hydrocephalus, cancer, seizures, HTN

Diagnostics: ICP monitoring, head CT/MRI

Ménière's Disease

Overview: inner ear disease thought to be caused by a buildup of fluid in the labyrinth

Patient may complain of: hearing changes, tinnitus, ear fullness, nausea, vomiting, dizziness

Objective findings if symptomatic: signs of acute distress/illness, nystagmus, hearing difficulty, Romberg positive

PMH considerations/risk factors: hx of Ménière's disease, allergies, TBI, migraines, CVA/TIA, MS, BPPV, younger age

Diagnostics: audiometry, MRI

Meningitis

Overview: inflammation and infection of the meninges surrounding the brain and spinal cord

Patient may complain of: chills, fever, fatigue, photophobia, neck pain, anorexia, nausea, vomiting, headache, confusion, dizziness

Objective findings: signs of acute distress/illness, lethargy, fever, irritability, altered mental status, petechial rash, nuchal rigidity (positive Brudzinski, Kernig sign), seizures, signs of increased ICP

PMH considerations/risk factors: hx of TBI, immunosuppression, pregnancy, close quarter living situations, recent travel outside of the United States, alcohol abuse, older/younger age

Diagnostics: CBC, lumbar puncture, head CT

Migraine Headache

Overview: recurrent head pain with or without aura

Patient may complain of: generalized weakness, photophobia, phonophobia, blurred vision, nausea, vomiting, throbbing lateralized headache, paresthesias, dizziness, presence of an aura

Objective findings: irritability, intolerance to light and sound; exam is typically unremarkable

PMH considerations/risk factors: hx of migraines, increased psychological stress, lack of sleep, nicotine use, alcohol abuse/use, family hx of migraines, female gender, younger age (<40 years)

Diagnostics: clinical diagnosis; head CT/MRI may be considered initially

Myocardial Infarction

Overview: decreased or no blood flow through the coronary arteries causing cardiac muscle death

Patient may complain of: fatigue, chest pain not improved with rest, radiation of the pain to the left arm/neck/jaw, palpitations, dyspnea, activity intolerance, abdominal pain, nausea, dizziness, anxiety, feelings of impending doom; symptoms have longer duration than stable angina

Objective findings: signs of acute distress, lethargy, irritability, altered mental status, diaphoresis, cool clammy skin, hypertension/ hypotension, tachycardia/bradycardia, arrhythmia, murmur, ST elevations, pathologic Q waves, weak pulses, sluggish capillary refill, tachypnea

PMH considerations/risk factors: hx of MI, CAD, HTN, heart failure, hyperlipidemia, diabetes, cardiac valve disorders, sedentary lifestyle, NSAID use, nicotine use, substance abuse, family hx of heart disease, older age

Diagnostics: cardiac enzymes, ECG, stress test, coronary angiography

Otitis Media

Overview: infection or inflammation of the middle ear

Patient may complain of: chills, fever, fatigue, otalgia, hearing changes, tinnitus, nasal congestion, nasal drainage, coughing, anorexia, nausea, headache, dizziness

Objective findings: signs of acute distress/illness, lethargy, fever, irritability, erythematous bulging tympanic membrane with or without effusion, otorrhea (perforation)

PMH considerations/risk factors: hx of otitis media, eustachian tube dysfunction, younger age

Diagnostics: clinical diagnosis

Pulmonary Embolism

Overview: a blood clot in the pulmonary vasculature

Patient may complain of: chills, fever, chest pain, pain with deep breaths, palpitations, activity intolerance, dyspnea, coughing, hemoptysis, abdominal pain, dizziness

Objective findings: signs of acute distress, fever, pallor, cyanosis, diaphoresis, tachycardia, hypotension, S3/S4 heart sounds, tachypnea, hypoxia, cough, signs of DVT

PMH considerations/risk factors: hx of DVT, PE or CVA, bleeding/clotting disorder, cancer, pregnancy, HRT/birth control use, IV drug use, recent surgery, immobility, nicotine use

Diagnostics: D-dimer, chest CT, V/Q scan, chest X-ray

Transient Ischemic Attack

Overview: transient obstruction of blood flow to the brain mimicking a CVA

Patient may complain of: vision changes, nausea, vomiting, dysphagia, headache, dizziness, seizures, insomnia, difficulty with memory, speaking, focusing, and understanding; unilateral paralysis of face, arms, and legs; signs and symptoms are transient in nature

Objective findings: signs of acute distress, altered mental status, ptosis, dysarthria, hypertension, carotid bruit(s), facial droop, seizures, unilateral weakness and sensation disturbances, immobility, gait disturbances; may not have abnormal exam findings due to transient nature of the issue

PMH considerations/risk factors: hx of HTN, CAD, heart failure, hyperlipidemia, arrhythmia, cardiac valve disease, diabetes, obesity, nicotine use, substance abuse, family hx of heart disease

Diagnostics: head CT/MRI

References

American Medical Directors Association. (2010). *Know-it-all before you call: Data collection system.* Columbia, MD: Author.

Bhattacharyya, N., Gubbels, S. P., Schwartz, S. R., Edlow, J. A., El-Kashlan, H., Fife, T.,. . .Corrigan, M. D. (2017). Clinical practice guideline: Benign paroxysmal positional vertigo. *Otolaryngology-Head and Neck Surgery, 156*(3), 1–47.

Bovo, R., Faccioli, C., & Martini, A. (2014). Dizziness in the elderly. *Hearing, Balance and Communication, 13*(2), 54–65.

Branch, W. T., & Barton, J. J. (2014). Approach to the patient with dizziness. In J. L. Wilterdink (Ed.), *UpToDate.* Retrieved from https://www.uptodate.com/contents/approach-to-the-patient-with-dizziness

Bulechek, G. M., Butcher, H. K., Dochterman, J. M., & Wagner, C. (2013). *Nursing Intervention Classification (NIC).* St. Louis, MO: Elsevier Mosby.

Chandrasekhar, S. S. (2013). The assessment of balance and dizziness in the TBI patient. *Neurorehabilitation, 32*(3), 445–454. doi:10.3233/NRE-130867

Collie, M. H., & Ramsey, A. R. (2014). Differentiating benign paroxysmal positional vertigo from other causes of dizziness. *Journal for Nurse Practitioners, 10*(6), 393–400. doi:10.1016/j.nurpra.2014.03.008

Desai, S. P. (2009). *Clinician's guide to laboratory medicine* (3rd ed.). Houston, TX: MD2B.

Furman, J. M. (2017). Pathophysiology, etiology, and differential diagnosis of vertigo. In J. L. Wilterdink (Ed.), *UpToDate.* Retrieved from https://www.uptodate.com/contents/pathophysiology-etiology-and-differential-diagnosis-of-vertigo

Furman, J. M., & Barton, J. J. (2015a). Evaluation of the patient with vertigo. In J. L. Wilterdink (Ed.), *UpToDate.* https://www.uptodate.com/contents/evaluation-of-the-patient-with-vertigo

Furman, J. M., & Barton, J. J. (2015b). Treatment of vertigo. In J. L. Wilterdink (Ed.), *UpToDate.* Retrieved from https://www.uptodate.com /contents/treatment-of-vertigo?search=vertigo&source=search_result &selectedTitle=2~150&usage_type=default&display_rank=2

Hale, A., & Hovey, M. J. (2014). *Fluid, electrolyte and acid-base imbalances.* Philadelphia, PA: F.A. Davis Company.

Honda, S., Inatomi, Y., Yonehara, T., Hashimoto, Y., Hirano, T., Ando, Y., & Uchino, M. (2014). Discrimination of acute ischemic stroke from nonischemic vertigo in patients presenting with only imbalance. *Journal of Stroke & Cerebrovascular Diseases, 23*(5), 888–895. doi:10.1016/j .jstrokecerebrovasdis.2013.07.029

Jarvis, C. (2015). *Physical examination & health assessment.* St. Louis, MO: Elsevier.

Kaufmann, H. (2015). Mechanisms, causes, and evaluation of orthostatic hypotension. In J. L. Wilterdink (Ed.), *UpToDate.* Retrieved from https:// www.uptodate.com/contents/mechanisms-causes-and-evaluation-of -orthostatic-hypotension

LeBlond, R. F., Brown, D. D., Suneja, M., & Szot, J. F. (2015). *DeGowin's diagnostic examination* (10th ed.). New York, NY: McGraw-Hill.

Lin, E., & Aligene, K. (2013). Pharmacology of balance and dizziness. *Neurorehabilitation, 32*(3), 529–542. doi:10.3233/NRE-130875

McCance, K. L., Huether, S. E., Brashers, V. L., & Rote, N. S. (2014). *Pathophysiology: The biologic basis for disease in adults and children* (7th ed.). St. Louis, MO: Elsevier.

Moskowitz, H. S., & Dinces, E. A. (2017). Meniere disease. In D. J. Sullivan (Ed.), *UpToDate.* Retrieved from https://www.uptodate.com /contents/meniere-disease

Muncie, H. L., & James, E. (2017). Dizziness: Approach to evaluation and management. *American Family Physician, 95*(3), 154–162.

Ozono, Y., Kitahara, T., Fukushima, M., Michiba, T., Imai, R., Tomiyama, Y., ... Morita, H. (2014). Differential diagnosis of vertigo and dizziness in the emergency department. *Acta Oto-Laryngologica, 134*(2), 140–145. doi:10.3109/00016489.2013.832377

Papadakis, M. A., & McPhee, S. J. (2017). *Current medical diagnosis and treatment* (56th ed.). New York, NY: McGraw-Hill.

Raftery, A. T., Lim, E., & Ostor, A. J. (2014). *Differential diagnosis* (4th ed.). London, UK: Elsevier.

Seller, R. H., & Symons, A. B. (2012). *Differential diagnosis of common complaints* (6th ed.). Philadelphia, PA: Elsevier.

Smoulia, E. (2013). Inner ear disorders *Neurorehabilitation, 32*(3), 455–462. doi:10.3233/NRE- 130868

Susanto, M. (2014). Dizziness: If not vertigo could it be cardiac disease? *Australian Family Physician, 43*(5), 264–269. Retrieved from http://www.racgp.org.au/afp/2014/may/dizziness/

Tepper, D. (2015). Migraine associated vertigo. *Headache: The Journal of Head & Face Pain, 55*(10), 1475–1476. doi:10.1111/head.12704

Uphold, C. R., & Graham, M. V. (2013). *Clinical guidelines in family practice* (5th ed.). Gainesville, FL: Barmarrae Books.

CHAPTER 11

Dyspepsia

Dyspepsia, also known as "indigestion," is characterized by symptoms such as upper abdominal/epigastric pain, bloating, heartburn, nausea, and postprandial fullness. Patients may also complain of early satiation or inability to finish a meal due to the discomfort. Dyspepsia is typically caused by a functional etiology, GERD, PUD, or NSAID use. It can also be a sign of GI malignancy. Initial treatment with lifestyle management and PPIs is recommended for dyspepsia, GERD, and PUD. The use of NSAIDs should also be avoided. It is important for the nurse to monitor for red flag symptoms such as signs of GI bleeding, severe abdominal pain, weight loss, vomiting, and swallowing difficulties. If these symptoms are present, a workup by the provider is urgent and may require a GI referral and endoscopy. The nurse should also assess for PPI treatment failure and educate the patient on helpful dietary changes.

Differential Diagnosis Considerations

Common: food/lactose intolerance or allergy, functional dyspepsia, gastritis, gastroenteritis, GERD, *Helicobacter pylori* infection, hiatal hernia, medication induced, PUD

Consider: angina, biliary colic, cholecystitis, cholelithiasis, esophageal spasm, esophagitis, gastroparesis, hypercalcemia, hyperkalemia, IBD, IBS, intestinal parasites, ischemic bowel disease, pancreatitis, SIBO, upper GI malignancy

Questions to Ask the Patient/ Family/Witness/Yourself

- When did the symptoms (pain, bloating, heartburn, nausea, fullness) start? Did it start gradually or suddenly?
- Are you having abdominal pain? If so, where is the pain exactly? Can you point to it?

- Is the pain constant, or does it come and go? If intermittent, how long does it last? How often is it happening per hour/day?
- Can you describe the pain (pressure, sharp, cramping, dull, achy, ripping, burning, heavy)?
- What makes the pain better (bowel/bladder elimination, certain positions, eating, medication, rest)?
- What triggers the pain or makes it worse (activity, bearing down, bowel/bladder elimination, eating, certain positions, coughing, touching)?
- Does the pain radiate to the back, chest, or flank?
- How severe is your pain? Can you rate it on a scale from 0 to 10? Is it waxing and waning in severity? Does it wake you from your sleep?
- How is your appetite? Are you able to keep down food and/ or fluids?
- Do you have a hard time finishing meals because of the discomfort?
- How much fluid are you drinking on a daily basis?
- When was your last bowel movement? What did it look like (consistency, amount, color)?
- Do you have a history of lactose intolerance? If so, have you recently ingested any milk, cheese, yogurt, ice cream, or other dairy products?
- Do you have a history of dyspepsia? If so, what have you done or used to treat it?
- Have you had any recent: GI/GU illness? dietary changes or eaten anything out of the ordinary? exposure to a GI infection, contaminated drinking water, or been around anyone who is sick? travel outside of the United States?
- Have you taken any new prescribed or over-the-counter medications? Have there been any recent changes to your current medication?
- Have you taken any NSAIDs (ASA, ibuprofen, naproxen)?
- What are you allergic to? Have you been exposed to a known allergen?
- Do you smoke? How much (ppd)? How long have you been smoking? (If applicable)

- Do you drink alcohol? How many drinks per day/week? What kind and amount of alcohol do you drink? When was your last drink? (If applicable)

Associated Signs/Symptoms: PAIN: pain anywhere else; GENERAL: fatigue, chills, fever, weight loss; EENT: sore throat; CARDIOVASCULAR: chest pain/tightness; RESPIRATORY: cough, dyspnea; GASTROINTESTINAL: belching, bloating, constipation, diarrhea, heartburn, nausea, signs of GI bleeding, swallowing difficulties, vomiting

Recommended Assessments

- Vital signs
- Temperature
- Weight and nutritional status
- I/O
- Pain scale (if applicable)
  - Tolerable pain level
- General
  - Inspect: signs of acute distress, acute illness, affect, restlessness
- Skin
  - Inspect: dryness, jaundice, pallor
  - Palpate: temperature, turgor
- Mouth
  - Inspect: mucous membrane moisture level
- Cardiovascular
  - Auscultate: heart sounds, rate, rhythm
- Respiratory
  - Inspect: respiratory effort
  - Auscultate: lung sounds
- Gastrointestinal
  - Inspect: distention
  - Auscultate: bowel sounds
  - Palpate: guarding, hernias, masses, organomegaly, (rebound) tenderness

Past Medical History Considerations
- Allergies

Puts the patient at risk for differential considerations
- Alcohol abuse/use
- Diabetes
- Nicotine use

Reoccurrence/exacerbation should be considered
- Angina
- Esophageal spasm
- *H. pylori* infection

Chronic conditions that can cause dyspepsia
- Cholelithiasis
- Esophagitis
- Gastroparesis
- GI malignancy
- GERD
- Hiatal hernia
- IBD
- IBS
- Pancreatitis
- PUD

Medication Evaluation
Most common causative/exacerbating medication
- Alpha adrenergic blockers
- Antibiotics
- Anticholinergics
- Beta blockers
- Bisphosphonates
- CCBs
- Corticosteroids

- Digoxin
- Iron supplements
- Metformin
- Niacin
- Nitrates
- NSAIDs
- Opioids
- Orlistat
- Potassium supplements
- Theophylline
- Tricyclic antidepressants

Used to treat dyspepsia

- Antacids
- H2 antagonist
- PPIs

Lab Evaluation and Trends

- CBC

Nursing Intervention Considerations

- Medications (if ordered or protocol allows)
  - Hold suspected causative medication until discussion with the provider
  - Hold all oral medication if NPO status is anticipated
  - PRN antiemetic for nausea, IV/IM if vomiting
- Diet
  - NPO if procedure or surgery is anticipated
  - Offer bland, simple foods that the patient can tolerate
  - Avoid late meals
  - Avoid foods that trigger symptoms
- Positioning
  - HOB raised for 2–3 hours after meals or at night
  - Supine or side lying position with knees flexed to chest to take tension off the abdominal wall if the patient has active abdominal pain

- Collect
  - Stool sample for diarrhea or signs of GI bleeding
- Monitor
  - Pain levels
  - Temperature trends
  - I/O
  - Weight trends
  - Agitation levels
  - Signs of dehydration such as lethargy, decreased skin turgor, dry mucous membranes, tachycardia, and (orthostatic) hypotension
  - Signs and symptoms of GI bleeding such as fatigue, dizziness, dyspnea, melena, hematochezia, hematemesis, pallor, ecchymosis, altered mental status, hypotension, tachycardia, and tachypnea
  - Emesis output color, consistency, frequency, and volume
  - Stool output color, consistency, frequency, and volume
- Environment
  - Provide a calm, quiet environment and reduce stimulation
  - Avoid bothersome odors in the room
  - Maintain a comfortable room temperature
- Supportive care
  - Maintain effective communication between yourself, patient, and family
  - Provide emotional support and reassurance to the patient and family
  - Maintain a calm manner during patient interactions
  - Discuss plan of care with the patient and decide reasonable goals together
  - Notify the patient and family of changes in the plan of care
  - **Educational topics (as applicable to the patient):**
    - General information regarding the patient's dyspepsia and differential diagnosis considerations
    - Explanation regarding referrals and specialist who may see them for this issue

- New medication education including reason, side effects, and administration needs
- Medication changes
- Pain scale and pain goals
- Trigger avoidance
- Avoidance of food/fluid that trigger symptoms
- Increased fluid intake
- BRAT diet, clear liquid diet, NPO diet
- Smoking cessation
- Alcohol cessation and support
- When to notify the nurse or provider
- Signs and symptoms of GI bleeding
- Dehydration prevention

ISBARR Recommendation Considerations

- Ask the provider to come assess the patient STAT if red flag symptoms are present
- Medication
  - Hold oral medications if the patient is unable to tolerate or NPO
  - Discuss changing medication routes with the provider (and pharmacy) if the patient is NPO
  - Discontinue/change suspected causative medication
  - Add PPI, H2 antagonist, or antacid
  - Add PRN antiemetic for nausea
- IV fluid needs if oral intake is poor, there are signs of dehydration, and the patient is NPO or hypotensive
- Labs (depending on the suspected cause)
  - Amylase, lipase
  - BMP/CMP
  - CBC
  - *H. pylori* breath/stool/serum
  - Occult stool
- Monitoring needs
  - Daily weights
  - Strict I/O

- Change diet to (depending on the suspected cause)
  - NPO
  - BRAT or bland
  - Clear liquid diet
- Referrals
  - Gastroenterology
- Ask if the provider wants anything else done
- Read back orders; ask that they enter all orders into the electronic medical record

ISBARR Template	
I **Introduction**	**Introduce Yourself and the Patient** • "Hello, Dr. Schedler, this is Lindsay Doherty. I am the nurse for Ms. Melissa Janson in Room 19 at Milwaukee Rehabilitation Center. She was admitted a week ago after a hip replacement."
S **Situation**	**Sign/Symptom You Are Concerned About** • "Ms. Janson has had intermittent symptoms of dyspepsia since yesterday evening at dinner time. Symptoms occur a few hours after eating." **Associated Signs/Symptoms** • "She is complaining of heartburn, abdominal bloating, and postprandial fullness. However, she has not had any severe abdominal pain, diarrhea, constipation, or signs of GI bleeding."
B **Background**	**Vitals** • "Today her blood pressure is 110/70, heart rate is 70, O_2 sat is 98% on room air, and temperature is 97.6." **Exam** • "When I did an exam, there was no abdominal distention, tenderness, or masses." **Past Medical History** • "She denied a history of GERD or PUD." **Labs and Medications** • "I noticed she is taking 800mg Ibuprofen twice a day for her hip pain and did not have a PPI ordered on admission."

ISBARR Template	
A **Assessment**	**Assessment** • "I am suspicious that her dyspepsia is related to her NSAID use."
R **Recommendations** **R** **Read Back**	**Nurse's Recommendations, Interventions, and Read Back** • "Can we start a PPI? Can we take her off Ibuprofen and try Tylenol instead? Is there anything else you want done at this time?" • "Thank you, Dr. Schedler. I would just like to read those orders back to you. You would like to start Protonix 40mg PO daily. Discontinue Ibuprofen and start Tylenol 500mg TID PRN for mild to moderate pain. Is that correct?"

Disclaimer: This dialogue is factitious and any resemblance to actual persons, living or dead, or actual events is purely coincidental.

In order to avoid order discrepancies, it is recommended that all orders be entered by the provider in the electronic medical record.

Select Differential Diagnosis Presentations

Angina (Stable)

Overview: chest pain caused by a decrease in myocardial oxygen supply that is improved with rest

Patient may complain of: fatigue, chest pain/tightness/heaviness that is worse with activity, better with rest or NTG, radiation of the pain to the left arm/neck/jaw, palpitations, dyspnea, activity intolerance, nausea, dyspepsia, dizziness, feelings of impending doom, anxiety; symptoms have a short duration

Objective findings: signs of acute distress, lethargy, diaphoresis, hypertension, tachycardia, murmur, weak pulses, sluggish capillary refill, tachypnea

PMH considerations/risk factors: hx of angina, CAD, HTN, heart failure, hyperlipidemia, diabetes, cardiac valve disorders, obesity, increased psychological stress, nicotine use, family hx of heart disease

Diagnostics: cardiac enzymes, ECG, stress test, coronary angiography

Angina (Unstable)

Overview: chest pain caused by a decrease in myocardial oxygen supply that is not improved with rest

Patient may complain of: fatigue, chest pain/tightness/heaviness that is worse with activity, not improved with rest or NTG, radiation of the pain to the left arm/neck/jaw, palpitations, dyspnea, activity intolerance, nausea, dyspepsia, dizziness, feelings of impending doom, anxiety; symptoms have a longer duration than stable angina

Objective findings: signs of acute distress, lethargy, diaphoresis, hypertension, tachycardia, murmur, weak pulses, sluggish capillary refill, tachypnea

PMH considerations/risk factors: hx of angina, CAD, HTN, heart failure, hyperlipidemia, diabetes, cardiac valve disorders, obesity, increased psychological stress, nicotine use, family hx of heart disease

Diagnostics: cardiac enzymes, ECG, stress test, coronary angiography

Cholecystitis

Overview: inflammation of the gallbladder

Patient may complain of: fever, chills, fatigue, RUQ/epigastric pain, right shoulder pain, nausea, vomiting, anorexia, dyspepsia

Objective findings: signs of acute distress/illness, lethargy, fever, diaphoresis, jaundice, tachycardia, RUQ/epigastric tenderness with guarding, positive Murphy's sign, palpable gallbladder

PMH considerations/risk factors: hx of cholelithiasis, obesity, female gender

Diagnostics: CBC, CMP, abdominal CT/US, HIDA scan

Esophagitis (Various Types)

Overview: inflammation of the esophagus

Patient may complain of: painful swallowing, dysphagia, chest pain, heartburn, upper abdominal/epigastric pain, dyspepsia, nausea, vomiting, signs of GI bleeding, dry coughing

Objective findings: oral herpes or thrush (depending on etiology), poor dentition, cough; exam is typically unremarkable

PMH considerations/risk factors: hx of esophagitis, GERD, hiatal hernia, cancer, immunosuppression, allergic diseases (food allergies, asthma, eczema), obesity, radiation therapy of the head, neck, and chest, alcohol abuse/use, nicotine use, NSAID use

Diagnostics: endoscopy with biopsy

Gastritis

Overview: inflammation of the stomach

Patient may complain of: anorexia, nausea, vomiting, dyspepsia, epigastric pain, signs of GI bleeding

Objective findings: nonspecific epigastric tenderness; exam is typically unremarkable

PMH considerations/risk factors: hx of PUD, *H. pylori* infection, NSAID use, alcohol abuse/use, recent travel outside of the United States, older age

Diagnostics: *H. pylori* serum/breath/stool testing, endoscopy with biopsy

Gastroenteritis

Overview: broad term for infection (typically viral) of the stomach and intestines

Patient may complain of: chills, fever, fatigue, anorexia, nausea, vomiting, diarrhea, generalized abdominal pain, dyspepsia

Objective findings: fever, lethargy, decreased skin turgor, dry mucous membranes, generalized abdominal tenderness without guarding

PMH considerations/risk factors: ingestion of undercooked food/contaminated water, hx of immunosuppression, recent antibiotic use, older age

Diagnostics: clinical diagnosis; stool cultures may be considered if symptoms are severe or prolonged

Gastroesophageal Reflux Disease

Overview: abnormal reflux of acid from the stomach back into the esophagus

Patient may complain of: sore throat, sour taste in mouth, dysphagia, chest pain or heartburn that may be worse lying flat or after meals, nausea, dyspepsia, epigastric pain, chronic coughing, insomnia

Objective findings: epigastric tenderness; exam is typically unremarkable

PMH considerations/risk factors: hx of GERD, hiatal hernia, obesity, diabetes, pregnancy, nicotine use, alcohol abuse/use

Diagnostics: clinical diagnosis

Helicobacter Pylori Infection

Overview: gram-negative bacterial infection in the stomach that disrupts the gastric mucosal lining making it vulnerable to peptic damage

Patient may complain of: abdominal pain, bloating, nausea, anorexia, dyspepsia, signs of GI bleeding

Objective findings: nonspecific epigastric tenderness; exam is typically unremarkable

PMH considerations/risk factors: hx of PUD, immunosuppression, recent travel outside of the United States, low socioeconomic status, ingestion of contaminated drinking water, NSAID use

Diagnostics: H. pylori serum/breath/stool testing, endoscopy with biopsy

Inflammatory Bowel Disease

Overview: chronic inflammation of all or different parts of the gastrointestinal tract

Patient may complain of: chills, fever, fatigue, weight loss, anorexia, abdominal pain/cramping, nausea, vomiting, dyspepsia, constipation/diarrhea, change in bowel habits, signs of GI bleeding

Objective findings: signs of acute distress/illness, lethargy, fever, signs of malnourishment, diaphoresis, pallor, tachycardia, abdominal tenderness, hematochezia

PMH considerations/risk factors: hx of Crohn's disease or ulcerative colitis, food intolerance/allergies, bleeding/clotting disorders, NSAID use, recent travel outside of the United States, nicotine use, family hx of IBS, younger age

Diagnostics: occult stool, CRP, CBC, endoscopy with biopsy

Irritable Bowel Syndrome

Overview: recurrent benign intestinal pain syndrome with associated bowel habit changes

Patient may complain of: abdominal pain and cramping, constipation/diarrhea, bloating, dyspepsia, heartburn, nausea, sensation of incomplete bowel movements

Objective findings: irritable, mild abdominal bloating, and generalized tenderness; exam is typically unremarkable

PMH considerations/risk factors: hx of IBS, IBD, depression, anxiety, family hx of IBS, female gender, younger age

Diagnostics: may not require any diagnostic testing; colonoscopy with biopsy, stool cultures, and CRP may be considered

Pancreatitis

Overview: inflammation of the pancreas

Patient may complain of: fatigue, chills, fever, epigastric/upper abdominal pain, radiation of the pain to the back, worse with movement, nausea, vomiting, dyspepsia, diarrhea

Objective findings: signs of acute distress/illness, lethargy, fever, diaphoresis, pallor, jaundice, tachycardia, hypotension, upper abdominal/epigastric tenderness, abdominal distention, positive Cullen's sign or Grey Turner sign (abdominal ecchymosis)

PMH considerations/risk factors: hx of chronic pancreatitis, hypertriglyceridemia, cholelithiasis, GI cancer, recent GI surgery or trauma to the abdomen, nicotine use, alcohol abuse/use

Diagnostics: amylase, lipase, abdominal CT/US

Peptic Ulcer Disease

    Overview: ulcers that develop in the lining of a stomach and/
or duodenum

    Patient may complain of: chest pain, dyspepsia, epigastric pain,
heartburn, pain relief with food or antacids, nausea, signs
of GI bleeding

    Objective findings: nonspecific epigastric tenderness; exam is
typically unremarkable

    PMH considerations/risk factors: hx of PUD, *H. pylori* infec-
tion, NSAID use, recent travel outside of the United States,
nicotine use, alcohol abuse/use

    Diagnostics: CBC, *H. pylori* serum/breath/stool testing, occult
stool, endoscopy with biopsy

References

Camilleri, M., Parkman, H. P., Shafi, M. A., Abell, T. L., & Gerson, L.
(2013). Clinical guideline: Management of gastroparesis. *American
Journal of Gastroenterology, 108*(1), 18–37.

Desai, S. P. (2009). *Clinician's guide to laboratory medicine* (3rd ed.).
Houston, TX: MD2B.

Elliot, D. (2013). Common causes of dyspepsia and the difficulties of
diagnosis. *Nursing & Residential Care, 15*(7), 481–483.

Fashner, J., & Gitu, A. C. (2015). Diagnosis and treatment of peptic ulcer
disease and *H. pylori* infection. *American Family Physician, 91*(4), 236–242.

Gulanick, M., & Myers, J. L. (2017). *Nursing care plans: Diagnosis, interventions, & outcomes* (9th ed.). St. Louis, MO: Elsevier.

Hale, A., & Hovey, M. J. (2014). *Fluid, electrolyte and acid-base imbalances.*
Philadelphia, PA: F.A. Davis Company.

Jarvis, C. (2015). *Physical examination & health assessment.* St. Louis, MO:
Elsevier.

Kahrilas, P. J. (2018). Clinical manifestations and diagnosis of gastroesophageal reflux in adults. In S. Grover (Ed.), *UpToDate.* Retrieved from https://
www.uptodate.com/contents/clinical-manifestations-and-diagnosis-of
-gastroesophageal-reflux-in-adults

Katz, P. O., Gerson, L. B., & Vela, M. F. (2013). Guidelines for the diagnosis
and management of gastroesophageal reflux disease. *American Journal
of Gastroenterology, 108*(3), 308–328.

LeBlond, R. F., Brown, D. D., Suneja, M., & Szot, J. F. (2015). *DeGowin's
diagnostic examination* (10th ed.). New York, NY: McGraw-Hill.

Longstreth, G. F., & Lacy, B. E. (2017a). Approach to the adult with dyspepsia. In S. Grover (Ed.), *UpToDate*. Retrieved from Retrieved from https://www.uptodate.com/contents/approach-to-the-adult-with-dyspepsia

Longstreth, G. F., & Lacy, B. E. (2017b). Functional dyspepsia in adults. In S. Grover (Ed.), *UpToDate*. Retrieved from https://www.uptodate.com/contents/functional-dyspepsia-in-adults

McCance, K. L., Huether, S. E., Brashers, V. L., & Rote, N. S. (2014). *Pathophysiology: The biologic basis for disease in adults and children* (7th ed.). St. Louis, MO: Elsevier.

Miwa, H., Kusano, M., Arisawa, T., Oshima, T., Kato, M., Joh, T., & . . . Sugano, K. (2015). Evidence-based clinical practice guidelines for functional dyspepsia. *Journal of Gastroenterology, 50*(2), 125–139. doi:10.1007/s00535-014-1022-3

Moayyedi, P. M., Lacy, B. E., Andrews, C. N., Enns, R. A., Howden, C. W., & Vakil, N. (2017). ACG and CAG clinical guideline: Management of dyspepsia. *The American Journal of Gastroenterology*. Retrieved from http://gi.org/wp-content/uploads/2017/06/ajg2017154a.pdf

National Institute for Health and Care Excellence (NICE). (2014). *Dyspepsia and gastroesophageal reflux disease: Investigation and management of dyspepsia, symptoms suggestive of gastroesophageal reflux disease, or both*. Retrieved from https://www.nice.org.uk/guidance/cg184/resources/gastrooesophageal-reflux-disease-and-dyspepsia-in-adults-investigation-and-management-pdf-35109812699845

O'Shea, L. (2010). Diagnosing indigestion. *Practice Nurse, 40*(10), 17–25.

Papadakis, M. A., & McPhee, S. J. (2017). *Current medical diagnosis and treatment* (56th ed.). New York, NY: McGraw-Hill.

Pimentel, M. (2016). Small intestinal bacterial overgrowth. In S. Grover (Ed.), *UpToDate*. Retrieved from https://www.uptodate.com/contents/small-intestinal-bacterial-overgrowth-management

Raftery, A. T., Lim, E., & Ostor, A. J. (2014). *Differential diagnosis* (4th ed.). London, UK: Elsevier.

Seller, R. H., & Symons, A. B. (2012). *Differential diagnosis of common complaints* (6th ed.). Philadelphia, PA: Elsevier.

Uphold, C. R., & Graham, M. V. (2013). *Clinical guidelines in family practice* (5th ed.). Gainesville, FL: Barmarrae Books.

Yang, Y. X., Brill, J., Krishnan, P., & Leontiadis, G. (2015). American gastroenterological association institute guideline on the role of upper gastrointestinal biopsy to evaluate dyspepsia in the adult patient in the absence of visible mucosal lesions. *Gastroenterology, 149*(4), 1082–1087.

CHAPTER 12

Dysphagia

Dysphagia is a subjective sensation of difficulty swallowing or inability to swallow. Other signs and symptoms indicative of dysphagia include eating habit changes, drooling, weight loss, throat clearing, voice changes, choking, and cough. The mechanics of swallowing are complex, and dysphagia can originate in either the oropharynx or the esophagus. Patients with oropharyngeal dysphagia have difficulty initiating a swallow, while patients with esophageal dysphagia have a sensation of food sticking in their throat or esophagus seconds after the initial swallow has occurred. In the acute care setting, dysphagia is a common issue for patients after a CVA. It is also commonly found in the general elderly population, but it cannot be attributed to the normal aging process. New complaints of dysphagia need to be evaluated urgently by the provider.

A multi-disciplinary evaluation and treatment approach is used that includes recommendations from speech pathology, because dysphagia puts the patient at risk for aspiration, choking, pneumonia, and dehydration. It is important for the nurse to be able to identify the signs and symptoms of dysphagia, protect the patient's airway, reduce their risk for aspiration, and report these symptoms immediately to the provider. If the dysphagia is not a new issue, but appears to have worsened, a reevaluation by the provider and/or speech pathologist needs to be completed and may include more invasive testing.

Differential Diagnosis Considerations

Common: CVA/TIA, dementia, dentition issues, eosinophilic esophagitis, esophageal ring/web, food impaction, foreign body, functional dysphagia, GERD, goiter, infectious esophagitis, nonspecific motility disorder, peptic stricture, pill esophagitis, post-surgical (laryngeal, esophageal, gastric) stricture, xerostomia

Consider: achalasia, ALS, cerebral palsy, cervical osteophytes, Chagas disease, esophageal spasm, globus sensation, Guillain-Barré syndrome, hiatal hernia, lymphocytic esophagitis, malignancy (mouth/throat/esophageal/gastric), mediastinal mass, medication induced, MS, muscular dystrophy, myasthenia gravis, Parkinson's disease, radiation therapy, scleroderma, Sjogren's syndrome, spinal cord injury, TBI, Zenker diverticulum

Questions to Ask the Patient/ Family/Witness/Yourself

- When did the swallowing issues start? Did it start gradually or suddenly?
- Is it every time you swallow or does it come and go? If intermittent, how often is it happening per hour/day?
- What makes the swallowing difficulties better or worse (certain food or positions)?
- Do you have problems starting to swallow or is it a feeling of food getting stuck in your throat or esophagus? Where does it feel like it is getting stuck (point to the area if able)?
- Do you have problems swallowing food, fluids, or both? Is it more difficult to swallow food or fluids?
- Is it easier to swallow smaller pieces/amounts of fluid versus large?
- Do you feel like you are choking or do you cough up/regurgitate food?
- Is your swallowing painful?
- How is your appetite?
- Do you have a history of swallowing difficulties? If so, what has been done or used to treat it?
- Have you had any recent: ENT, GI, or neck surgery? trauma to the head or neck?
- Have you taken any new prescribed or over-the-counter medications? Have there been any recent changes to your current medication?

- Do you drink alcohol? How many drinks per day/week? What kind and amount of alcohol do you drink? When was your last drink? (if applicable)

Associated Signs/Symptoms: PAIN: pain anywhere; GENERAL: chills, fatigue, fever, weakness, weight loss; EENT: drooling, frequent throat clearing, voice changes (hoarseness, wetness); NECK: lumps, stiffness, swollen glands; CARDIOVASCULAR: chest pain/tightness; RESPIRATORY: cough (before/after/during eating or drinking), dyspnea; GASTROINTESTINAL: heartburn, nausea, signs of GI bleeding, vomiting; NEUROLOGICAL: headache, numbness/tingling, dizziness

Recommended Assessments

- Vital signs
- Temperature
- Weight and nutritional status
- I/O
- Pain scale (if applicable)
  - Tolerable pain level
- General
  - Level of consciousness and orientation
  - Inspect: signs of acute distress, acute illness, affect, restlessness
  - Speech changes, wet or gurgling voice, hoarseness
- Skin
  - Inspect: cyanosis, diaphoresis, dryness, pallor
  - Palpate: turgor
- Mouth
  - Inspect: dentition, drooling, food pocketing, halitosis, lesions, swelling or erythema of the lips, posterior pharynx and/or tongue, mucous membrane moisture level
  - Gag reflex
- Head/face/neck
  - Inspect: goiter, signs of trauma
  - Palpate: lymphadenopathy, swelling, tenderness

- Cardiovascular
  - Auscultate: heart sounds, rate, rhythm
- Respiratory
  - Inspect: respiratory effort, depth, pattern, use of accessory muscles
  - Auscultate: lung sounds
- Gastrointestinal
  - Auscultate: bowel sounds
  - Palpate: guarding, (rebound) tenderness
- Neurological
  - Inspect: facial droop, tremors
  - Palpate: extremity strength, sensation
  - Cranial nerve exam
- Extremities
  - Inspect: IV site
  - Palpate: capillary refill, pulses

Past Medical History Considerations
Puts the patient at risk for differential considerations

- AIDS/HIV
- Alcohol abuse/use
- Diabetes
- GI/head/neck surgery
- Nicotine use
- Radiation therapy to the head/neck/thoracic cavity
- Thyroid disease

Chronic conditions that can cause dysphagia

- ALS
- Alzheimer's disease/dementia
- Cerebral palsy
- CVA/TIA
- Eosinophilic esophagitis

- GERD
- Guillain-Barré syndrome
- Hiatal hernia
- MS
- Muscular dystrophy
- Myasthenia gravis
- Parkinson's disease
- Scleroderma
- Sjogren's syndrome
- Spinal cord injury
- TBI
- Throat/esophagus/GI/thoracic cavity malignancy
- Xerostomia

Medication Evaluation

Most common causative/exacerbating medication

- Anticonvulsants
- Antipsychotics
- Benzodiazepines
- Opioids

Has GI tract inflammation as a side effect

- Ascorbic acid
- Bisphosphonates
- Chemotherapy
- Iron supplements
- NSAIDs
- Potassium supplements

Has xerostomia as a side effect

- ACE inhibitors
- Antiarrhythmics
- Anticholinergics

- Antiemetics
- Antihistamines
- CCBs
- Diuretics
- SSRIs

Lab Evaluation and Trends

- CBC

Nursing Intervention Considerations

- Call for help or rapid response/code team if vital signs are unstable or there are signs of urgent distress
- Maintain a patent airway
  - Apply oxygen if hypoxic
  - Encourage cough and deep breathing
  - Chest splinting with a pillow to promote more effective coughing
  - Suction as needed
  - Provide oral care throughout the day (q2–4hrs)
  - Call respiratory therapy for signs of respiratory distress
- Verify patent IV if IVF or IV medication treatment is anticipated
  - Flush according to facility protocol; watch for swelling, erythema, pain, and other signs of infiltration
- Medications (if ordered or protocol allows)
  - Hold oral medication if NPO status is anticipated
  - PRN bronchodilator treatment per respiratory therapy if the patient is coughing or short of breath
- Diet
  - NPO until cleared by speech pathologist and provider
- Positioning
  - HOB raised to comfort for respiratory distress
  - HOB raised to 90 degrees during eating attempts
  - HOB raised for 2–3 hours after meals or at night

- Reposition every 2–4 hours or establish an individualized turning schedule
- Monitor
  - Stay with the patient until stable
  - Vital signs and trends
  - Pain levels
  - Oxygen saturation/pulse oximetry
  - Temperature trends
  - I/O
  - Weight trends
  - Orientation status changes
  - Agitation levels
  - Neurological exam
  - Skin assessment every 8–24 hours
  - Signs of respiratory distress such as cyanosis, tachypnea, hypoxia, use of accessory muscles, diaphoresis, and adventitious lung sounds
  - Signs of dehydration such as lethargy, decreased skin turgor, dry mucous membranes, tachycardia, and (orthostatic) hypotension
  - Signs and symptoms of aspiration, such as coughing, throat clearing, dyspnea, drooling, and voice changes
- Safety
  - Perform a fall risk assessment and implement the appropriate strategies
- Environment
  - Maintain a well-lit environment
  - Remove distractions during eating and drinking attempts
- Supportive care
  - Maintain effective communication between yourself, patient, and family
  - Provide emotional support and reassurance to the patient and family
  - Maintain a calm manner during patient interactions

- Discuss plan of care with the patient and decide reasonable goals together
- Notify the patient and family of changes in the plan of care
- Identify barriers to care and compliance
- Promote skin care and integrity
- **Educational topics (as applicable to the patient):**
  - General information regarding the patient's dysphagia and differential diagnosis considerations
  - Procedure and intervention explanation and justification
  - Explanation regarding referrals and specialist who may see them for this issue
  - Medication changes
  - Pain scale and pain goals
  - Cough and deep-breathing techniques
  - Oxygen therapy and maintenance
  - Skin care
  - Proper positioning and turning schedule
  - Safety needs and fall risk
  - NPO diet, dysphagia diet
  - Swallow precautions
  - Alcohol cessation and support
  - Smoking cessation
  - When to notify the nurse or provider
  - Signs and symptoms of aspiration
  - Signs and symptoms of respiratory emergencies
  - Dehydration prevention
  - Pressure injury prevention

ISBARR Recommendation Considerations

- Ask the provider to come assess the patient STAT if there is suspicion for CVA or aspiration

- Medication
  - Hold oral medications if the patient is unable to tolerate or NPO
  - Discuss changing medication routes with the provider (and pharmacy) if the patient is NPO
  - Discontinue/change suspected causative medication
  - Discuss (with pharmacy) medications that can be crushed (if applicable)
  - Add PPI, H2 antagonist or antacid for dyspepsia, heartburn, or other signs/symptoms of GERD
  - Add PRN and/or scheduled bronchodilator nebulizer treatments per respiratory therapy for coughing, dyspnea, or other signs of respiratory distress
- IV fluid needs if oral intake is poor, there are signs of dehydration, and the patient is NPO or hypotensive
- Imaging (depending on the suspected cause)
  - Chest X-ray, swallow study
- Safety
  - 1:1 monitoring during eating
  - Aspiration precautions
  - Fall risk protocol
- Monitoring needs
  - Continuous O_2 monitoring
  - Daily weights
  - Strict I/O
- Change diet to
  - NPO
  - Dysphagia diet per speech pathology's recommendations
- Referrals
  - ENT
  - Gastroenterology
  - Speech pathology
- Ask if the provider wants anything else done
- Read back orders; ask that they enter all orders into the electronic medical record

Dysphagia

ISBARR Template	
I **Introduction**	**Introduce Yourself and the Patient** • "Hello, Dr. Wakeham, this is Jules Vann. I am the nurse for Mrs. Erin Sass in Room 301. She is your patient that was admitted two days ago for a right-sided CVA."
S **Situation**	**Sign/Symptom You Are Concerned About** • "Mrs. Sass seems to be having more issues with dysphagia today. She was evaluated yesterday by speech therapy and cleared without a special diet, but I noticed she has been coughing with attempts to swallow food and fluid." **Associated Signs/Symptoms** • "She is also pocketing small amounts of food on her left side and is clearing her throat frequently."
B **Background**	**Vitals** • "Her vitals are stable but I noticed her oxygen sat has been between 90–92% on room air. That is lower than her averages yesterday which were between 96–100%." **Exam** • "She continues to have a left-sided facial droop and weakness. She also has some mild drooling. I did not hear any abnormal lung sounds." **Past Medical History** • "She denies any history of swallowing difficulties prior to her CVA." **Labs and Medications** • N/A in this situation
A **Assessment**	**Assessment** • "I am concerned she may be at risk or has already aspirated."

ISBARR Template	
R **Recommendations** **R** **Read Back**	**Nurse's Recommendations, Interventions, and Read Back** • "I have placed her on 2 liters nasal cannula and her O_2 sat is now 96%. I wanted to hold her PO meds and intake until I discussed this situation with you. I have paged speech therapy to come reevaluate her. Should I continue her NPO status? Did you want to start IV fluids because she is NPO? Did you want a chest X-ray to evaluate for aspiration? Do you want anything else done at this time?" • "Thank you, Dr. Wakeham. I just want to read those orders back to you. You would like a chest X-ray now, and a chest X-ray, CBC, and CMP in the morning. Keep the patient NPO until evaluated by speech therapy and have speech therapy page you when they are done with their assessment. Is this correct?"

Disclaimer: This dialogue is factitious and any resemblance to actual persons, living or dead, or actual events is purely coincidental.

In order to avoid order discrepancies, it is recommended that all orders be entered by the provider in the electronic medical record.

Select Differential Diagnosis Presentations

Cerebral Vascular Accident

Overview: partial or complete obstruction of blood flow to the brain due to ischemia or hemorrhage causing brain tissue death

Patient may complain of: vision changes, nausea, vomiting, dysphagia, headache, dizziness, seizures, insomnia, difficulty with memory, speaking, focusing, and understanding; unilateral paralysis of the face, arms, and legs

Objective findings: signs of acute distress, altered mental status, ptosis, dysarthria, hypertension, carotid bruit(s), facial droop, seizures, unilateral weakness and sensation disturbances, immobility, gait disturbances

PMH considerations/risk factors: hx of HTN, CAD, heart failure, hyperlipidemia, arrhythmia, cardiac valve disease, diabetes, obesity, nicotine use, substance abuse, family hx of heart disease

Diagnostics: Head CT/MRI

Esophagitis (Various Types)

Overview: inflammation of the esophagus

Patient may complain of: painful swallowing, dysphagia, chest pain, heartburn, upper abdominal/epigastric pain, dyspepsia, nausea, vomiting, signs of GI bleeding, dry coughing

Objective findings: oral herpes or thrush (depending on etiology), poor dentition, cough; exam is typically unremarkable

PMH considerations/risk factors: hx of esophagitis, GERD, hiatal hernia, cancer, immunosuppression, allergic diseases (food allergies, asthma, eczema), obesity, radiation therapy of the head, neck, and chest, alcohol abuse/use, nicotine use, NSAID use

Diagnostics: endoscopy with biopsy

Gastroesophageal Reflux Disease

Overview: abnormal reflux of acid from the stomach back into the esophagus

Patient may complain of: sore throat, sour taste in mouth, dysphagia, chest pain or heartburn that may be worse lying flat or after meals, nausea, dyspepsia, epigastric pain, chronic coughing, insomnia

Objective findings: epigastric tenderness; exam is typically unremarkable

PMH considerations/risk factors: hx of GERD, hiatal hernia, obesity, diabetes, pregnancy, nicotine use, alcohol abuse/use

Diagnostics: clinical diagnosis

Goiter

Overview: abnormal enlargement of the thyroid gland

Patient may complain of: dysphagia, neck pain/swelling, dyspnea, coughing; patient is typically asymptomatic unless hyper/hypothyroidism is present

Objective findings: enlarged thyroid with or without tenderness and nodules

PMH considerations/risk factors: hx of goiter, hyper/hypothyroidism, pregnancy, diet low in iodine

Diagnostics: TSH, T3, T4, thyroid US, radioactive iodine uptake scan, fine needle biopsy

Parkinson's Disease

Overview: progressive movement disorder of the CNS

Patient may complain of: fatigue, generalized weakness, vision changes, dysphagia, constipation, urinary retention, gait instability, joint rigidity, tremors, confusion, hallucinations, insomnia; symptoms are progressive in nature

Objective findings: altered mental status, lethargy, flat affect, dysarthria, (orthostatic) hypotension, bradykinesia, generalized muscle and joint rigidity, postural instability, resting tremor, psychosis

PMH considerations/risk factors: hx of Parkinson's disease, trauma to the head, family hx of Parkinson's, male gender, older age

Diagnostics: clinical diagnosis; head MRI may be ordered initially

Transient Ischemic Attack

Overview: transient obstruction of blood flow to the brain mimicking a CVA

Patient may complain of: vision changes, nausea, vomiting, dysphagia, headache, dizziness, seizures, difficulty with memory, speaking, focusing, and understanding; unilateral paralysis of face, arms, and legs; signs and symptoms are transient in nature

Objective findings: signs of acute distress, altered mental status, ptosis, dysarthria, hypertension, carotid bruit(s), facial droop, seizures, unilateral weakness and sensation disturbances, immobility, gait disturbances; may not have abnormal exam findings due to transient nature of the issue

PMH considerations/risk factors: hx of HTN, CAD, heart failure, hyperlipidemia, arrhythmia, cardiac valve disease, diabetes, obesity, nicotine use, substance abuse, family hx of heart disease

Diagnostics: Head CT/MRI

Xerostomia

Overview: dryness of the mouth

Patient may complain of: dry mouth, dysphagia, sore throat, mouth sores, tongue pain, thirst

Objective findings: halitosis, cheilitis, dry mucous membranes, poor dentition, mouth breathing, hoarseness

PMH considerations/risk factors: dehydration, hx of diabetes, Sjogren's syndrome, AIDS/HIV, rheumatoid arthritis, SLE, medication (various), radiation therapy of the head and neck, chemotherapy, nicotine use, alcohol use

Diagnostics: clinical diagnosis

References

American Medical Directors Association. (2010). *Know-it-all before you call: Data collection system.* Columbia, MD: Author.

Bulechek, G. M., Butcher, H. K., Dochterman, J. M., & Wagner, C. (2013). *Nursing intervention classification (NIC).* St. Louis, MO: Elsevier Mosby.

Carucci, L. R., Lalani, T., Rosen, M. P., Cash, B. D., Katz, D. S., Kim, D. H., . . . Yee J. (2013). *Expert panel on gastrointestinal imaging: ACR appropriateness criteria dysphagia.* Retrieved from https://guideline.gov/summaries /summary/47651/acr-appropriateness-criteria--dysphagia?q=Cytology

Cummings, J., Soomans, D., O'Laughlin, J., Snapp, V., Jodoin, A., Proco, H., . . . Rood, D. (2015). Sensitivity and specificity of a nurse dysphagia screen in stroke patients. *MEDSURG Nursing, 24*(4), 219–222.

Desai, S. P. (2009). *Clinician's guide to laboratory medicine* (3rd ed.). Houston, TX: MD2B.

Fass, R. (2016). Overview of dysphagia in adults. In K. M. Robson (Ed.), *UpToDate.* Retrieved from https://www.uptodate.com/contents/approach -to-the-evaluation-of-dysphagia-in-adults

Fletcher, J. (2015). Dealing with dysphagia: A multidisciplinary approach. *Nursing & Residential Care, 17*(8), 430–432.

Goldsmith, T., & Cohen, A. K. (2017). Swallowing disorders and aspiration in palliative care: Definition, consequences, pathophysiology, and etiology. In D. M. Savarese (Ed.), *UpToDate*. Retrieved from https://www.uptodate.com/contents/swallowing-disorders-and-aspiration-in-palliative-care-definition-consequences-pathophysiology-and-etiology

Goldsmith, T., & Cohen, A. K. (2018). Swallowing disorders and aspiration in palliative care: Assessment and strategies for management. In D. M. Savarese (Ed.), *UpToDate*. Retrieved from https://www.uptodate.com/contents/swallowing-disorders-and-aspiration-in-palliative-care-assessment-and-strategies-for-management

Griffith, R. (2016). District nurses' role in managing medication dysphagia. *British Journal of Community Nursing, 21*(8), 411–415.

Hale, A., & Hovey, M. J. (2014). *Fluid, electrolyte and acid-base imbalances.* Philadelphia, PA: F.A. Davis Company.

Heijnen, B. J., Speyer, R., Kertscher, B., Cordier, R., Koetsenruijter, K. J., Swan, K., & Bogaardt, H. (2016). Dysphagia, speech, voice, and trismus following radiotherapy and/or chemotherapy in patients with head and neck carcinoma: Review of the literature. *Biomed Research International, 2016,* 1–24. doi:10.1155/2016/6086894

Jarvis, C. (2015). *Physical examination & health assessment.* St. Louis, MO: Elsevier.

Jiang, J. L., Fu, S. Y., Wang, W. H., & Ma, Y. C. (2016). Validity and reliability of swallow screening tools used by nurses for dysphagia: A systematic review. *Tzu Chi Medical Journal, 28,* 41–48.

Kenny, B. (2015). Food culture, preferences and ethics in dysphagia management. *Bioethics, 29*(9), 646–652. doi:10.1111/bioe.12189

Lancaster, J. (2015). Dysphagia: Its nature, assessment and management. *British Journal of Community Nursing, 20*(7), S28–32.

LeBlond, R. F., Brown, D. D., Suneja, M., & Szot, J. F. (2015). *DeGowin's diagnostic examination* (10th ed.). New York, NY: McGraw-Hill.

Lembo, A. J. (2017). Oropharyngeal dysphagia: Clinical features, diagnosis, and management. In K. M. Robson (Ed.), *UpToDate*. Retrieved from https://www.uptodate.com/contents/oropharyngeal-dysphagia-clinical-features-diagnosis-and-management

Lohmann, K., Ferber, J., Haefeli, M. F., Störzinger, D., Schwald, M., Haefeli, W. E., & Seidling, H. M. (2015). Knowledge and training needs of nurses and physicians on unsuitable drugs for patients with dysphagia or feeding tubes. *Journal of Clinical Nursing, 24*(19/20), 3016–3019. doi:10.1111/jocn.12910

Malhi, H. (2016). Dysphagia: Warning signs and management. *British Journal of Nursing, 25*(10), 546–549.

McCance, K. L., Huether, S. E., Brashers, V. L., & Rote, N. S. (2014). *Pathophysiology: The biologic basis for disease in adults and children* (7th ed.). St. Louis, MO: Elsevier.

Nazarko, L. (2016). Considering the difficulties with dysphagia: An overview for community nurses. *British Journal of Community Nursing, 21*(5), 226–230.

Papadakis, M. A., & McPhee, S. J. (2017). *Current medical diagnosis and treatment* (56th ed.). New York, NY: McGraw-Hill.

Raftery, A. T., Lim, E., & Ostor, A. J. (2014). *Differential diagnosis* (4th ed.). London: Elsevier.

Scottish Intercollegiate Guidelines Network. (2010). *Management of patients with stroke: Identification and management of dysphagia.* Retrieved from http://www.sign.ac.uk/assets/sign119.pdf

Seller, R. H., & Symons, A. B. (2012). *Differential diagnosis of common complaints* (6th ed.). Philadelphia, PA: Elsevier.

Thompson, R. (2016a). Identifying and managing dysphagia in the community. *Journal of Community Nursing, 30*(6), 42–47.

Thompson, R. (2016b). Treating and preventing dysphagia in the community. *British Journal of Community Nursing, 21*(7), 10–13.

Uphold, C. R., & Graham, M. V. (2013). *Clinical guidelines in family practice* (5th ed.). Gainesville, FL: Barmarrae Books.

World Gastroenterology Organization. (2014). *World Gastroenterology Organization Global Guidelines: Dysphagia.* Retrieved from http://www.worldgastroenterology.org/UserFiles/file/guidelines/dysphagia-english-2014.pdf

CHAPTER 13

Dyspnea

Dyspnea is a stressful subjective experience of difficulty breathing that can cause the patient fear and anxiety. It can vary in intensity and may not always present with objective findings like hypoxia or use of accessory muscles. Measuring dyspnea can be difficult, because there is no specific scale recommended for clinical use. It is important to understand the patient's experience with dyspnea and the impact it is having on them. A thorough history and physical examination can help identify the cause. Dyspnea can be associated with a worsening underlying disease such as COPD or CHF, or be triggered by a new issue entirely. The nurse's top priority is to maintain the patient's airway, breathing, and circulation; prevent hypoxia; monitor for signs of infection; and provide pharmacological and non-pharmacological comfort measures. It will also be important to give the patient education on infection prevention and chronic disease management (if applicable). In this chapter, nursing intervention considerations and plan of care recommendations should reflect whatever the suspected cause is.

Differential Diagnosis Considerations

Common acute (minutes–1week) causes: airway trauma, anxiety, arrhythmia, aspiration, asthma exacerbation, bronchitis, COPD exacerbation, heart failure exacerbation, hypercapnia, hypoxia, MI, PE, pleural effusion, pneumonia, pneumothorax, sepsis, stable angina, unstable angina

Common chronic (>4 weeks) causes: asthma, cardiomyopathy, COPD, heart failure, interstitial lung disease

Consider: acute chest syndrome, ALS, anaphylaxis, anemia, angioedema, aortic dissection, ARDS, ascites, cardiac tamponade, cardiac valve disorder, cystic fibrosis, diaphragmatic paralysis, DKA, epiglottitis, flail chest, foreign body, goiter, Guillain-Barré syndrome, interstitial fibrosis, kyphoscoliosis, metabolic acidosis, myasthenia gravis, neck mass, obesity, pericarditis, poisoning (CO, organophosphate, salicylate), pregnancy, pulmonary edema, pulmonary HTN, pulmonary malignancy, pulmonary tumor, renal failure, rib fracture, superior vena cava obstruction, upper airway obstruction, vocal cord paralysis

Questions to Ask the Patient/ Family/Witness/Yourself

- When did the shortness of breath start? Did it start gradually or suddenly?
- What were you doing before/when the symptoms started?
- How does it feel (gasping, inability to get enough air, hurts to breathe, tightness)?
- Is the shortness of breath constant or does it come and go? If intermittent, how long does it last? How often is it happening per hour/day?
- What makes the shortness of breath better (certain positions, medication, rest)?
- What triggers or makes the shortness of breath worse (activity, certain positions, certain times of the day, coughing, eating, psychological stress)?
- How severe is your shortness of breath (mild/moderate/severe)?
- How is it affecting your daily living (difficulty getting dressed, eating, ambulation)?
- Do you have a history of shortness of breath issues? If so, what have you done or used to treat it?
- Do you use any inhalers? If so, have you been taking them as prescribed?
- Have you had any recent: respiratory illness? vigorous exercise? exposure to respiratory infection or have been around anyone who is sick? exposure to CO, chemicals, smoke, or toxins? insect bite/sting? immobilization such as prolonged time spent in bed or sitting? immunization? CV/thoracic surgery? trauma to the back, chest, or neck?

- Have you had any recent invasive interventions such as intubation?
- Have you taken any new prescribed or over-the-counter medications? Have there been any recent changes to your current medication?
- What are you allergic to? Have you been exposed to a known allergen?
- Do you smoke? How much (ppd)? How long have you been smoking? (if applicable)

Associated Signs/Symptoms: PAIN: pain anywhere; GENERAL: chills, fatigue, fever, weakness, weight changes; EENT: nasal congestion, sore throat; CARDIOVASCULAR: chest pain/tightness, edema, palpitations, PND, orthopnea; RESPIRATORY: cough, hemoptysis, painful breathing/coughing, sputum production, wheezing; GASTROINTESTINAL: heartburn, nausea, signs of GI bleeding, swallowing difficulties, vomiting; NEUROLOGICAL: dizziness; PSYCH: anxiety, confusion, feelings of impending doom

Recommended Assessments

- Vital signs
- Temperature
- Weight and nutritional status
- I/O
- Pain scale (if applicable)
  - Tolerable pain level
- General
  - Level of consciousness and orientation
  - Inspect: signs of acute distress, acute illness, affect, restlessness
  - Difficulty speaking due to breathlessness
- Skin
  - Inspect: cyanosis, diaphoresis, mottling, pallor, urticarial rash
  - Palpate: temperature

- Mouth
  - Inspect: swelling or erythema of the lips, posterior pharynx and/or tongue
- Head/face/neck
  - Inspect: JVD, goiter, signs of trauma, tracheal deviation
  - Palpate: lymphadenopathy, swelling, tenderness
- Cardiovascular
  - Auscultate: heart sounds, rate, rhythm
  - Palpate: heaves, thrills
- Respiratory
  - Inspect: chest asymmetry, respiratory effort, depth, pattern, use of accessory muscles
  - Auscultate: lung sounds, stridor
- Gastrointestinal
  - Inspect: distention
  - Palpate: ascites, organomegaly
- Extremities
  - Inspect: clubbing, IV site
  - Palpate: capillary refill, edema, pulses

Past Medical History Considerations

- Allergies
- Immunization status: influenza, pertussis, pneumonia

Puts the patient at risk for differential considerations

- Bleeding/clotting disorder
- CAD
- CKD
- Diabetes
- DVT
- Dysphagia
- HTN
- Immobilization
- Liver disease
- Nicotine use

- Radiation therapy to the thoracic cavity
- Sickle cell anemia
- Thyroid disease

Reoccurrence/exacerbation should be considered

- Anaphylaxis
- Arrhythmias (various)
- Asthma
- COPD
- Heart failure
- MI
- PE

Chronic conditions that can cause dyspnea

- ALS
- Anemia
- Anxiety
- Arrhythmias (various)
- Asthma
- Cardiac valve disorders
- COPD
- CVA/TIA
- Cystic fibrosis
- ENT/pulmonary malignancy
- Guillain-Barré syndrome
- Heart failure
- Interstitial lung disease
- Myasthenia gravis
- Obesity

Medication Evaluation
Used to treat common differential considerations

- Antibiotics → various respiratory infections
- Benzodiazepines → acute anxiety

- Corticosteroids → airway inflammation
- Diuretics → fluid overload
- ICS, LABA, LAMA, SABA, SAMA, and combination inhalers → chronic lung disease
- Opioids → dyspnea in palliative care

Lab Evaluation and Trends

- ABG
- BMP/CMP
- BNP
- Cardiac enzymes
- CBC

Nursing Intervention Considerations

- Call for help or rapid response/code team if vital signs are unstable or there are signs of urgent distress
- Maintain a patent airway
  - Apply oxygen if hypoxic
  - Encourage cough and deep breathing
  - Encourage pursed lip breathing
  - Encourage slow relaxed deep breathing if hyperventilating
  - Suction as needed
  - Provide oral care throughout the day (q2–4hrs)
  - Call respiratory therapy for signs of respiratory distress
- Verify patent IV if IVF or IV medication treatment is anticipated
  - Flush according to facility protocol; watch for swelling, erythema, pain, and other signs of infiltration
- ECG if cardiac etiology is suspected
- Medications (if ordered or protocol allows)
  - PRN bronchodilator treatment per respiratory therapy
- Diet
  - NPO until discussion with the provider if aspiration is suspected

- Restrict fluids until discussion with the provider, if there are signs of fluid overload
- Encourage heart healthy, low-sodium food choices
- Activity
  - Keep the patient in bed until discussion with the provider
- Positioning
  - HOB raised to comfort for respiratory distress
  - Tripod positioning
  - Reposition every 2–4 hours or establish an individualized turning schedule
- Collect
  - Sputum sample (if applicable)
- Monitor
  - Stay with the patient until stable
  - Vital signs and trends
  - Pain levels
  - Oxygen saturation/pulse oximetry
  - Temperature trends
  - I/O
  - Telemetry/cardiac monitor
  - Weight trends
  - Orientation status changes
  - Agitation levels
  - Peripheral pulses
  - Skin assessment every 8–24 hours
  - Signs of decreased cardiac output such as weak pulses, cool skin, altered mental status, hypotension, oliguria, and mottling
  - Signs of respiratory distress such as cyanosis, tachypnea, hypoxia, use of accessory muscles, diaphoresis, and adventitious lung sounds
  - Signs and symptoms of aspiration such as coughing, throat clearing, dyspnea, drooling, and voice changes

- Signs and symptoms of fluid overload such as cough, adventitious lung sounds, dyspnea, tachypnea, weight gain, edema, JVD, and ascites
- Signs and symptoms of sepsis such as fever, chills, hypotension, altered mental status, hypoxia, cool clammy skin, dyspnea, oliguria, tachycardia, and tachypnea
- Signs and symptoms of blood loss such as fatigue, dizziness, dyspnea, melena, hematochezia, hematemesis, hematuria, epistaxis, pallor, ecchymosis, altered mental status, hypotension, tachycardia, tachypnea, and hemoptysis
- Sputum output color, consistency, frequency, and volume
- Safety
  - Perform a fall risk assessment and implement the appropriate strategies
- Environment
  - Provide a calm, quiet environment and reduce stimulation
  - Maintain a well-lit environment
  - Provide distractions
  - Maintain a comfortable room temperature
  - Initiate isolation precautions: droplet, airborne
  - Offer aromatherapy and/or music therapy (if appropriate)
  - Utilize a fan (if appropriate)
- Supportive care
  - Maintain effective communication between yourself, patient, and family
  - Provide emotional support and reassurance to the patient and family
  - Maintain calm manner during patient interactions
  - Discuss plan of care with the patient and decide reasonable goals together
  - Notify the patient and family of changes in the plan of care
  - Identify barriers to care and compliance

- Promote skin care and integrity
- Provide light clothing and bed linen
- **Educational topics (as applicable to the patient):**
  - General information regarding the patient's dyspnea and differential diagnosis considerations
  - Explanation regarding referrals and specialist who may see them for this issue
  - Procedure and intervention explanation and justification
  - New medication education including reason, side effects, and administration needs
  - Medication compliance
  - MDI administration techniques
  - Pain scale and pain goals
  - Relaxation techniques and breathing exercises
  - Pursed lip breathing
  - Oxygen therapy and maintenance
  - Cough and deep-breathing techniques
  - Trigger avoidance
  - Energy conservation techniques: placing items within reach, sitting to do tasks, taking breaks in between activities, sliding rather than lifting, pushing rather than pulling
  - Telemetry
  - Proper positioning and turning schedule
  - Skin care
  - Safety needs and fall risk
  - Handwashing and infection control measures
  - Isolation precaution needs
  - Fluid restriction
  - DASH diet, NPO diet, dysphagia diet
  - Swallow precautions
  - Stress reduction and management
  - Weight loss, physical activity, and exercise needs
  - Immunization needs

- Smoking cessation
- When to notify the nurse or provider
- Signs and symptoms of aspiration
- Signs and symptoms of cardiac emergencies
- Signs and symptoms of respiratory emergencies
- Signs and symptoms of fluid overload
- Signs and symptoms of abnormal bleeding
- Pressure injury prevention

ISBARR Recommendation Considerations

- Ask the provider to come assess the patient STAT if they are unstable
- Transfer to the ICU if hemodynamically unstable, advanced medication management is required, or closer monitoring is needed
- Medication
  - Hold oral medications if the patient is unable to tolerate or NPO
  - Discuss changing medication routes with the provider (and pharmacy) if the patient is NPO
  - Add corticosteroids for airway inflammation
  - Add/change diuretics for signs of fluid overload
  - Add PRN and/or scheduled medication for anxiety or irritability
  - Add PRN and/or scheduled bronchodilator nebulizer treatments per respiratory therapy for coughing, dyspnea, or other signs of respiratory distress
  - Add PRN opioids for palliative care patients
- IV fluid needs if oral intake is poor, there are signs of dehydration, and the patient is NPO or hypotensive
- ECG if not already done or repeat testing is needed
- Imaging (depending on the suspected cause)
  - Chest CT scan, chest X-ray

- Labs (depending on the suspected cause)
  - ABG
  - Blood culture
  - BMP/CMP
  - BNP
  - Cardiac enzymes
  - CBC
  - D-dimer
  - Sputum culture
- Safety
  - Activity level changes
  - Fall risk protocol
  - Aspiration precautions
  - Isolation precautions: airborne, droplet
- Monitoring needs
  - Continuous O_2 monitoring
  - Daily weights
  - Telemetry/continuous cardiac monitoring
  - Strict I/O
  - Vital signs including frequency and parameters to call the provider
- Supportive cares
  - Compression stockings or SCDs
- Change diet to (depending on the suspected cause)
  - DASH, low sodium
  - Dysphagia diet per speech pathology's recommendations
  - Fluid restriction
  - NPO
- Referrals
  - Pulmonology
  - Respiratory therapy
  - Speech pathology
- Ask if the provider wants anything else done
- Read back orders, ask that they enter all orders into the electronic medical record

Dyspnea

ISBARR Template	
I **Introduction**	**Introduce Yourself and the Patient** • "Hello, Dr. Stark. This is Tara Cochart. I am the nurse for your patient Rachel Dworak in Room 817. I know you are covering for Dr. Tate, so just as a brief background: She is a 70-year-old that was admitted for CHF exacerbation yesterday."
S **Situation**	**Sign/Symptom You Are Concerned About** • "She has been complaining of worsening shortness of breath for the past hour or so. It is mild at rest but more severe with activity." **Associated Signs/Symptoms** • "She also has chest tightness with coughing. Coughing is dry and persistent."
B **Background**	**Vitals** • "She was at 89% on 2 liters nasal cannula, but is now at 95% on 4 liters nasal cannula. BP is 150/87, heart rate is 74, and her temperature is 98.2." **Exam** • "Crackles in her bases have not changed and are still persistent. She is tachypnic with ambulation and has +3 pitting edema in her lower extremities. I also noticed she has gained 2lbs since yesterday." **Past Medical History** • "Her past medical history includes CHF, COPD, and hypertension," **Labs and Medications** • "and she is on 40mg IV push furosemide BID. She got her morning dose already at 0800. Her CMP this morning was unremarkable and had a potassium of 4.3."
A **Assessment**	**Assessment** • "I'm concerned about worsening fluid overload from her CHF."

ISBARR Template	
R Recommendations R Read Back	**Nurse's Recommendations, Interventions, and Read Back** • "I have respiratory therapy giving her a PRN breathing treatment. Did you want me to do an ECG? Can we put her on a fluid restriction and continuous pulse ox monitor? Did you want to change her furosemide dose? Did you want another chest X-ray or labs? Did you want anything else done at this time? • "Thank you, Dr. Ali Stark, let me read those orders back to you. Give another 40mg IV push furosemide now and then start 80mg IV push furosemide BID, with that dose starting this evening. Put her on a 1500cc fluid restriction and low-sodium diet. Keep her on a continuous pulse ox monitor. Maintain oxygen levels above 92%, and a CMP and chest X-ray PA/Lat in the AM?"

Disclaimer: This dialogue is factitious and any resemblance to actual persons, living or dead, or actual events is purely coincidental.

In order to avoid order discrepancies, it is recommended that all orders be entered by the provider in the electronic medical record.

Select Differential Diagnosis Presentations

Acute Chest Syndrome

Overview: vaso-occlusive crisis of the pulmonary vasculature in patients with sickle cell anemia

Patient may complain of: chills, fever, fatigue, chest pain, dyspnea, wheezing, coughing, sputum production

Objective findings: signs of acute distress/illness, fever, lethargy, warm skin, hypoxia, tachypnea, cough, sputum, use of accessory muscles, adventitious breath sounds

PMH considerations/risk factors: hx of sickle cell anemia, asthma, recent respiratory illness

Diagnostics: CBC, ECG, chest X-ray, chest CT

Angina (Stable)

Overview: chest pain caused by a decrease in myocardial oxygen supply that is improved with rest

Patient may complain of: fatigue, chest pain/tightness/heaviness that is worse with activity, better with rest or NTG, radiation of the pain to the left arm/neck/jaw, palpitations, dyspnea, activity intolerance, nausea, dyspepsia, dizziness, feelings of impending doom, anxiety; symptoms have a short duration

Objective findings: signs of acute distress, lethargy, diaphoresis, hypertension, tachycardia, murmur, weak pulses, sluggish capillary refill, tachypnea

PMH considerations/risk factors: hx of angina, CAD, HTN, heart failure, hyperlipidemia, diabetes, cardiac valve disorders, obesity, increased psychological stress, nicotine use, family hx of heart disease

Diagnostics: cardiac enzymes, ECG, stress test, coronary angiography

Angina (Unstable)

Overview: chest pain caused by a decrease in myocardial oxygen supply that is not improved with rest

Patient may complain of: fatigue, chest pain/tightness/heaviness that is worse with activity, not improved with rest or NTG, radiation of the pain to the left arm/neck/jaw, palpitations, dyspnea, activity intolerance, nausea, dyspepsia, dizziness, feelings of impending doom, anxiety; symptoms have a longer duration than stable angina

Objective findings: signs of acute distress, lethargy, diaphoresis, hypertension, tachycardia, murmur, weak pulses, sluggish capillary refill, tachypnea

PMH considerations/risk factors: hx of angina, CAD, HTN, heart failure, hyperlipidemia, diabetes, cardiac valve disorders, obesity, increased psychological stress, nicotine use, family hx of heart disease

Diagnostics: cardiac enzymes, ECG, stress test, coronary angiography

Anxiety

Overview: psychiatric disorder that can cause intense fear and worry

Patient may complain of: fatigue, chest pain, palpitations, dyspnea, nausea, vomiting, abdominal pain, constipation/diarrhea, paresthesias, tremors, headache, insomnia, dizziness, mind racing, feelings of impending doom

Objective findings: signs of acute distress, irritability, inability to focus, diaphoresis, tachycardia, hypertension, tachypnea, muscle tension

PMH considerations/risk factors: hx of anxiety, depression, PTSD, insomnia, substance abuse, physical abuse, recent physical or emotional trauma, family hx of psychiatric diseases

Diagnostics: clinical diagnosis; workup to rule out more emergent causes may be indicated

Aortic Dissection

Overview: a tear in the intima layer of the aorta

Patient may complain of: severe chest/back pain described as ripping or tearing, abdominal pain, flank pain, dyspnea, nausea, dizziness, (pre)syncope, paresthesias, feelings of impending doom

Objective findings: signs of acute distress, altered mental status, diaphoresis, cool clammy skin, syncope, JVD, murmur, hypotension/hypertension, weak pulses or pulse deficit, sluggish capillary refill, tachypnea

PMH considerations/risk factors: hx of HTN, heart failure, cardiac valve disorders, connective tissue disorders, diabetes, substance abuse, pregnancy, nicotine use, male gender, older age

Diagnostics: ECG, TEE, chest X-ray, chest CT, aortography

Arrhythmia

Overview: any irregular heart rhythm

Patient may complain of: fatigue, generalized weakness, (pre)syncope, palpitations, chest pain, dyspnea, dizziness, seizures, anxiety

Objective findings: signs of acute distress, lethargy, irritability, diaphoresis, irregular heart rhythm, bradycardia/tachycardia, murmur, hypertension/hypotension, tachypnea, seizures

PMH considerations/risk factors: hx of arrhythmia, CAD, HTN, heart failure, MI, cardiac valve disorders, diabetes, previous CV surgery, substance abuse, increased psychological stress, nicotine use, family hx of heart disease

Diagnostics: BMP/CMP, CBC, TSH, ECG, ECHO, Holter monitor/loop recorder/event recorder

Aspiration

Overview: inhalation of foreign object, food, or liquid into the airway

Patient may complain of: fever, fatigue, inability/difficulty swallowing, chest pain, coughing, dyspnea, wheezing, sputum production, heartburn, nausea, vomiting

Objective findings: signs of acute distress, fever, irritability, diaphoresis, cyanosis, drooling, hoarseness, choking, hypoxia, cough, tachypnea, adventitious lung sounds, sputum

PMH considerations/risk factors: hx of dysphagia, myasthenia gravis, Parkinson's disease, CVA, esophageal stricture, GERD, asthma, ENT/GI cancer, dementia, trauma to the neck, dentition issues, radiation therapy to the head and neck, intubation, NG tube, immobility, nicotine use, alcohol abuse/use

Diagnostics: CBC, swallow study, chest X-ray

Asthma Exacerbation

Overview: acute inflammation and swelling of the airway, progressively worsening asthma symptomology

Patient may complain of: activity intolerance, chest pain/tightness, coughing, dyspnea, wheezing, sputum production, insomnia

Objective findings: signs of acute distress, irritability, diaphoresis, cyanosis, breathlessness, hypoxia, tachypnea, cough, sputum, use of accessory muscles, adventitious breath sounds

PMH considerations/risk factors: hx of asthma, allergies, obesity, eczema, recent respiratory illness, nicotine use

Diagnostics: clinical diagnosis; chest X-ray, spirometry, PEF may be considered

Bronchitis

Overview: inflammation of the bronchioles typically due to an infection

Patient may complain of: fever, chills, fatigue, sore throat, nasal congestion, chest pain/tightness, coughing, dyspnea, wheezing, sputum production, hemoptysis

Objective findings: signs of acute illness, lethargy, low-grade fever, rhinorrhea, pharyngeal erythema, cough, sputum, adventitious breath sounds, tachypnea

PMH considerations/risk factors: hx of asthma, COPD, allergies, GERD, exposure to lung irritants, nicotine use, older age

Diagnostics: clinical diagnosis; ABG, chest X-ray, spirometry may be considered

COPD Exacerbation

Overview: acute inflammation and swelling of the airway, progressively worsening COPD symptomology

Patient may complain of: worsening fatigue, activity intolerance, and sputum production from baseline, chest pain/tightness, coughing, dyspnea, wheezing, hemoptysis, insomnia

Objective findings: signs of acute distress, lethargy, cyanosis, diaphoresis, hypoxia, breathlessness, cough, adventitious breath sounds, sputum, prolonged expirations, use of accessory muscles, barrel chest, digital clubbing

PMH considerations/risk factors: hx of COPD, asthma, allergies, GERD, recent respiratory illness, nicotine use

Diagnostics: clinical diagnosis; chest X-ray, spirometry may be considered

Goiter

Overview: abnormal enlargement of the thyroid gland

Patient may complain of: dysphagia, neck pain/swelling, dyspnea, coughing; patient is typically asymptomatic unless hyper/hypothyroidism is present

Objective findings: enlarged thyroid with or without tenderness and nodules

PMH considerations/risk factors: hx of goiter, hyper/hypothyroidism, pregnancy, diet low in iodine

Diagnostics: TSH, T3, T4, thyroid US, radioactive iodine uptake scan, fine needle biopsy

Heart Failure

Overview: broad term to describe pumping malfunction of the heart

Patient may complain of: fatigue, activity intolerance, chest pain, palpitations, dyspnea, orthopnea, PND, coughing, sputum production, weight gain/loss, anorexia, nausea, nocturia, insomnia

Objective findings: signs of acute distress, lethargy, diaphoresis, cyanosis, JVD, bradycardia/tachycardia, hypertension/hypotension, displaced PMI, murmur, gallop, weak pulses, sluggish capillary refill, digital clubbing, edema, breathlessness, tachypnea, cough, adventitious lung sounds, sputum, hepatomegaly, ascites

PMH considerations/risk factors: hx of heart failure, HTN, CAD, cardiac valve disorders, MI, diabetes, arrhythmias, hyper/hypothyroidism, obesity, nicotine use, substance abuse, family hx of heart disease

Diagnostics: BNP, BMP/CMP, TSH, ECG, I/O, chest X-ray, ECHO, cardiac catheterization

Myocardial Infarction

Overview: decreased or no blood flow through the coronary arteries causing cardiac muscle death

Patient may complain of: fatigue, chest pain not improved with rest, radiation of the pain to the left arm/neck/jaw, palpitations, dyspnea, activity intolerance, abdominal pain, nausea, dizziness, anxiety, feelings of impending doom; symptoms have longer duration than stable angina

Objective findings: signs of acute distress, lethargy, irritability, altered mental status, diaphoresis, cool clammy skin, hypertension/hypotension, tachycardia/bradycardia, arrhythmia, murmur, ST elevations, pathologic Q waves, weak pulses, sluggish capillary refill, tachypnea

PMH considerations/risk factors: hx of MI, CAD, HTN, heart failure, hyperlipidemia, diabetes, cardiac valve disorders, sedentary lifestyle, NSAID use, nicotine use, substance abuse, family hx of heart disease, older age

Diagnostics: cardiac enzymes, ECG, stress test, coronary angiography

Pneumonia

Overview: infection of the air sacs in one or both lungs causing inflammation and fluid accumulation

Patient may complain of: chills, fever, fatigue, chest pain/tightness, dyspnea, wheezing, coughing, sputum production, hemoptysis, activity intolerance, anorexia, nausea, vomiting, headache

Objective findings: signs of acute distress/illness, lethargy, altered mental status (elderly), fever, tachycardia, tachypnea, use of accessory muscles, cough, sputum, hypoxia, adventitious breath sounds, dullness to percussion over consolidation, pleural friction rub

PMH considerations/risk factors: hx of COPD, asthma, immunosuppression, dysphagia, immunization status, recent/current hospitalization, intubation, nicotine use, alcohol abuse, older/younger age

Diagnostics: CBC, sputum culture, chest X-ray

Pneumothorax

Overview: abnormal air or fluid in the pleural cavity causing lung collapse

Patient may complain of: sudden onset of chest pain, palpitations, dyspnea, coughing, anxiety, feelings of impending doom

Objective findings: signs of acute distress, tachycardia, hypotension, tachypnea, diminished/absent unilateral breath sounds, uneven chest excursion, tracheal deviation, hypoxia, cough

PMH considerations/risk factors: hx of Marfan syndrome, COPD, cystic fibrosis, asthma, TB, trauma to the chest/back, thin body habitus, recent thoracentesis or pulmonary biopsy, family hx of pneumothorax, nicotine use, male gender

Diagnostics: chest X-ray

Pulmonary Embolism

Overview: a blood clot in the pulmonary vasculature

Patient may complain of: chills, fever, chest pain, pain with deep breaths, palpitations, activity intolerance, dyspnea, coughing, hemoptysis, abdominal pain, dizziness

Objective findings: signs of acute distress, fever, pallor, cyanosis, diaphoresis, tachycardia, hypotension, S3/S4 heart sounds, tachypnea, hypoxia, cough, signs of DVT

PMH considerations/risk factors: hx of DVT, PE, or CVA, bleeding/clotting disorder, cancer, pregnancy, HRT/birth control use, IV drug use, recent surgery, immobility, nicotine use

Diagnostics: D-dimer, chest CT, V/Q scan, chest X-ray

Sepsis

Overview: severe inflammatory response due to an infection causing organ dysfunction

Patient may complain of: chills, fever, fatigue, generalized weakness, palpitations, (pre)syncope, dyspnea, oliguria; symptoms of whatever infection is suspected (i.e., appendicitis, diverticulitis, cholecystitis, pneumonia, cellulitis, meningitis, UTI)

Objective findings: signs of acute distress/illness, lethargy, fever, altered mental status, cyanosis, cool clammy skin or warm to the touch, tachycardia, hypotension, tachypnea, hypoxia, oliguria; signs of whatever infection is suspected

PMH considerations/risk factors: hx of immunosuppression, diabetes, cancer, recent infection, or hospitalization, older/younger age

Diagnostics: blood culture, lactate, CBC, BMP/CMP, PT/INR; workup may also relate to whatever infection is suspected

References

Ahmed, A., & Graber, M. A. (2017). Evaluation of the adult with dyspnea in the emergency department. In J. Grayzel (Ed.), *UpToDate*. Retrieved from https://www.uptodate.com/contents/evaluation -of-the-adult-with-dyspnea-in-the-emergency-department

Albertson, T., Schivo, M., Zeki, A., Louie, S., Sutter, M., Avdalovic, M., & Chan, A. (2013). The pharmacological approach to the elderly COPD patient. *Drugs & Aging, 30*(7), 479–502. doi:10.1007/s40266-013-0080-1

American Medical Directors Association. (2010). *Know-it-all before you call: Data collection system.* Columbia, MD: Author.

BC Cancer Agency. (2013). *Symptom management guidelines: Dyspnea.* Retrieved from http://www.bccancer.bc.ca/nursing-site/Documents/4.% 20Dyspnea.pdf

Coviello, J., & Chyun, D. (2012). Fluid overload: Identifying and managing heart failure patients at risk for hospital readmission. In M. Boltz, E. Capezuti, T. Fulmer, & D. Zwicker (Eds.), *Evidence-based geriatric nursing protocols for best practice* (4th ed.). New York, NY: Springer Publishing Company.

Criner, G. J., Bourbeau, J., Diekemper, R. L., Ouellette, D. R., Goodridge, D., Hernandez, P., . . . Mularski, R. A. (2015). Prevention of acute exacerbations of COPD: American College of Chest Physicians and Canadian Thoracic Society guideline. *Chest, 147*(4), 894–942. doi:10.1378/chest .14-1676

Doran, D., Lefebre, N., O'Brien-Pallas, L., Estabrook, C. A., White, P., Carryer, J., . . . Li, M. (2014). The relationship among evidence-based practice and client dyspnea, pain, falls, and pressure ulcer outcomes in the community setting. *Worldviews on Evidence-Based Nursing, 11*(5), 274–283. doi:10.1111/wvn.12051

Duck, A. (2015). Recognizing and managing patients with interstitial lung disease. *Journal of Community Nursing, 29*(1), 48–52.

Dudgeon, D., & Shadd, J. (2018). Assessment and management of dyspnea in palliative care. In D. M. Savarese (Ed.), *UpToDate*. Retrieved from https://www.uptodate.com/contents/assessment-and-management-of-dyspnea-in-palliative-care

Gulanick, M., & Myers, J. L. (2017). *Nursing care plans: Diagnosis, interventions, & outcomes* (9th ed.). St. Louis, MO: Elsevier.

Harrison, G., Evans, M. M., Shaffer, A., & Romero, L. (2016). Treating a patient experiencing an acute exacerbation of chronic heart failure. *Med-Surg Matters, 25*(4), 8–10.

Kloke, M., & Cherny, N. (2015). Treatment of dyspnea in advanced cancer patients: ESMO clinical practice guidelines. *Annals of Oncology, 26*(5), 169–173.

Mahler, D. A., & O'Donnell, D. E. (2015). Recent advances in dyspnea. *Chest, 147*(1), 232–241.

Mularski, R. A., Reinke, L. F., Carrieri-Kohlman, V., Fischer, M. D., Campbell, M. L., Rocker, G., . . . White, D. B. (2013). An official American thoracic society workshop report: Assessment and palliative management of dyspnea crisis. *AnnalsATS, 10*(5), 98–106.

Parshall, M. B., Schwartzstein, R. M., Adams, L., Banzett, R. B., Manning, H. L., Bourbeau, J., . . . O'Donnell, D. E. (2012). An official American thoracic society statement: Update on the mechanisms, assessment, and management of dyspnea. *American Journal of Respiratory and Critical Care Medicine, 185*(4), 435–452.

Pickstock, S. (2015). Managing and preventing acute exacerbations of COPD in the community. *Journal of Community Nursing, 29*(3), 39–44.

Raftery, A. T., Lim, E., & Ostor, A. J. (2014). *Differential diagnosis* (4th ed.). London: Elsevier.

Rohde, J., Hartley, S. E., Hanigan, S., Lin, J., Morganstern, L. B., Seagull, F. J., . . . Crawford, T.C. (2014). *Management of acute atrial fibrillation and atrial flutter in non-pregnant hospitalized adults*. Retrieved from www.med.umich.edu/1info/IHP/practiveguides/Afib/afibfinal.pdf

Schwartzstein, R. M. (2017a). Approach to the patient with dyspnea. In H. Hollingsworth (Ed.), *UpToDate*. Retrieved from https://www.uptodate.com/contents/approach-to-the-patient-with-dyspnea

Schwartzstein, R. M. (2017b). Physiology of dyspnea. In H. Hollingsworth (Ed.), *UpToDate*. Retrieved from https://www.uptodate.com/contents/physiology-of-dyspnea

Strickland, S. L., Rubin, B. K., Drescher, G. S., Haas, C. F., O'Malley, C. A., Volsko, T. A., . . . Hess, D. R. (2013). AARC clinical practice

guideline: Effectiveness of nonpharmacologic airway clearance therapies in hospitalized patients. *Respiratory Care, 58*(12), 2187–2193.

United States Preventive Services Task Force. Siu, A. L., Bibbins-Domingo,
K., Grossman, D. C., Davidson, K. W., Epling, J. W., Garcia, F. A.,. . .
Pignone, M. P. (2016). Screening for chronic obstructive pulmonary
disease: U.S. preventive services task force recommendation statement.
JAMA, 315(13), 1372–1377.

Yancy, C. W., Jessup, M., Bozkurt, B., Butler, J., Casey, D. E., Drazner,
M. H., . . . Wilkoff, B. L. (2013). 2013 ACCF/AHA guideline for the
management of heart failure: A report of the American college of cardiology foundation/American heart association task force on practice
guidelines. *Journal of American College of Cardiology, 62*(16), 147–239.

Edema of the Lower Extremities

Edema is a palpable swelling caused by increased capillary permeability or lymphatic obstruction, leading to an increase in interstitial fluid volume. It can occur anywhere in the body, but this chapter will focus on edema of the lower extremities. When a patient's edema is acute (<72 hours) and unilateral, the nurse's top priority is to help rule out a DVT or an infectious process. Finding and treating the underlying cause and utilizing compression stockings (contraindicated in PAD) are the cornerstones to edema management.

Differential Diagnosis Considerations

Common:
- Unilateral: cellulitis, DVT, venous insufficiency
- Bilateral: dependent edema, fluid overload, heart failure, idiopathic edema, liver disease, lymphedema, medication induced, obesity, pregnancy, premenstrual edema, PVD, renal disease/failure, venous insufficiency, venous stenosis

Consider:
- Unilateral: compartment syndrome, congenital venous malformations, lymphedema, May-Thurner syndrome, pelvic tumor, reflex sympathetic dystrophy, ruptured Baker's cyst, ruptured gastrocnemius
- Bilateral: diuretic induced, DVT, filariasis, hypoproteinemia, iliac vein obstruction, lipedema, malignant ascites, malnutrition, myxedema, nephrotic syndrome, pelvic tumor, preeclampsia, pulmonary HTN, restrictive cardiomyopathy, sepsis, sleep apnea, thyroid disease

Questions to Ask the Patient/ Family/Witness/Yourself

- When did the swelling in your leg(s) start? Did it start gradu- ally or suddenly?
- Is the swelling constant, or does it come and go? If intermit- tent, how long does it last? How often is it happening per hour/day?
- What makes the swelling better (certain positions, certain times of the day, elevation of the legs, medication)?
- What makes the swelling worse (activity, certain positions, certain times of the day, rest)?
- Are you having pain in your leg(s)?
- Do you have swelling anywhere else?
- How is it affecting your daily living (difficulty getting dressed, ambulation)?
- How much fluid are you drinking on a daily basis?
- Do you have a diet high in salt?
- Do you have a history of edema in your leg(s)? If so, what have you done or used to treat it?
- Have you had any recent: GI/GU/GYN/vascular surgery? immobilization such as prolonged time spent in bed or sit- ting? pregnancy? trauma to the abdomen, pelvis, or lower extremities?
- Have you taken any new prescribed or over-the-counter medi- cations? Have there been any recent changes to your current medication?

Associated Signs/Symptoms: PAIN: pain anywhere; GEN- ERAL: chills, fever, fatigue, weight changes; CARDIOVASCU- LAR: chest pain/tightness, PND, orthopnea; RESPIRATORY: cough, painful breathing/coughing, dyspnea; GENITOURINARY: oliguria; MUSCULOSKELETAL: hip, knee, ankle erythema, pain, stiffness, swelling; NEUROLOGICAL: numbness/tingling

Recommended Assessments

- Vital signs
- Temperature
- Weight and nutritional status
- I/O
- Pain scale (if applicable)
  - Tolerable pain level
- General
  - Inspect: signs of acute distress, acute illness, affect, restlessness
- Skin
  - Inspect: diaphoresis, jaundice, pallor
  - Palpate: temperature
- Head/face/neck
  - Inspect: JVD
- Cardiovascular
  - Auscultate: heart sounds, rate, rhythm
- Respiratory
  - Inspect: respiratory effort, depth
  - Auscultate: lung sounds
- Gastrointestinal
  - Inspect: distention
  - Palpate: ascites, masses, organomegaly
- Musculoskeletal
  - Inspect: hips, knees, ankles erythema
  - Palpate: hips, knees, ankles swelling, tenderness, warmth
  - Passive and active ROM examinations of the hips, knees, and ankles
- Neurological
  - Palpate: lower extremity sensation, strength
- Extremities
  - Inspect: clubbing, discoloration, erythema, hair distribution, varicose veins, wounds

- Palpate: capillary refill, pitting, pulses, temperature, tenderness, texture
- Measure leg circumference

Past Medical History Considerations
Puts the patient at risk for differential considerations

- Abdominal/groin/lower extremity surgery
- Alcohol abuse/use
- Diabetes
- GI/GU/GYN malignancy
- HTN
- Immobilization
- Nicotine use

Reoccurrence/exacerbation should be considered

- DVT

Chronic conditions that can cause edema

- Cardiomyopathy
- CKD
- Heart failure
- Liver disease
- Lymphedema
- Obesity
- Pregnancy
- PVD
- Sleep apnea
- Thyroid disease
- Venous insufficiency

Medication Evaluation
Most common causative/exacerbating medication

- Beta blockers
- Birth control/HRT

- CCBs
- Chemotherapy
- Corticosteroids
- Diuretics
- Gabapentin
- NSAIDs
- Pregabalin
- TZDs
- Vasodilators

Used to treat common differential considerations

- Antibiotics → soft tissue infection
- Anticoagulants → DVT
- Diuretics → fluid overload

Lab Evaluation and Trends

- BMP/CMP
- CBC

Nursing Intervention Considerations

- Call for help or rapid response/code team if vital signs are unstable or there are signs of urgent distress
- Maintain a patent airway
  - Apply oxygen if hypoxic
- Verify patent IV if IVF or IV medication treatment is anticipated
  - Flush according to facility protocol; watch for swelling, erythema, pain, and other signs of infiltration
- Diet
  - Restrict fluids until discussion with the provider if there are signs of fluid overload
  - Encourage heart healthy, low-sodium food choices
- Activity
  - Encourage activity and ambulation if safety permits

- Positioning
  - Elevate effected extremity
  - Reposition every 2–4 hours or establish an individualized turning schedule
- Collect
  - Wound drainage sample (if applicable)
- Monitor
  - Pain levels
  - Temperature trends
  - I/O
  - Weight trends
  - Edema and leg circumference
  - Sensation changes
  - Peripheral pulses
  - Skin assessment every 8–24 hours
  - Wound healing progression (if applicable)
  - Signs of decreased cardiac output such as weak pulses, cool skin, altered mental status, hypotension, oliguria, and mottling
  - Signs of respiratory distress such as cyanosis, tachypnea, hypoxia, use of accessory muscles, diaphoresis, and adventitious lung sounds
  - Signs and symptoms of skin infection such as fever, erythema, swelling, warmth, pain, and purulent drainage
  - Signs and symptoms of fluid overload such as cough, adventitious lung sounds, dyspnea, tachypnea, weight gain, edema, JVD, and ascites
- Safety
  - Perform a fall risk assessment and implement the appropriate strategies
- Supportive care
  - Maintain effective communication between yourself, patient, and family

- Provide emotional support and reassurance to the patient and family
- Maintain a calm manner during patient interactions
- Discuss plan of care with the patient and decide reasonable goals together
- Notify the patient and family of changes in the plan of care
- Promote skin care and integrity
- Identify barriers to care and compliance
- **Educational topics (as applicable to the patient):**
  - General information regarding the patient's edema and differential diagnosis considerations
  - Procedure and intervention explanation and justification
  - New medication education including reason, side effects, and administration needs
  - Medication compliance
  - Medication changes
  - Pain scale and pain goals
  - Skin care
  - Dressing changes
  - Proper positioning and turning schedule
  - Safety needs and fall risk
  - Handwashing and infection control measures
  - DASH diet
  - Fluid restriction
  - Weight loss, physical activity, and exercise needs
  - Increased physical activity
  - When to notify the nurse or provider
  - Signs and symptoms of skin infection
  - Signs and symptoms of cardiac emergencies
  - Signs and symptoms of respiratory emergencies
  - Signs and symptoms of fluid overload
  - Pressure injury prevention

ISBARR Recommendation Considerations

- Medication
  - Discontinue/change suspected causative medication
  - Add/change diuretics for signs of fluid overload
  - If antibiotics appear to be warranted (signs of skin infection), the provider needs to examine the patient
- Imaging (depending on the suspected cause)
  - Venous doppler US
- Labs (depending on the suspected cause)
  - BMP/CMP
  - BNP
  - CBC
  - D-dimer
  - Wound culture
- Safety
  - Activity level changes
  - Fall risk protocol
- Monitoring needs
  - Leg/calf circumference
  - Continuous O_2 monitoring
  - Daily weights
  - Strict I/O
- Supportive cares
  - Compression stockings or SCDs
- Change diet to
  - DASH, low sodium
  - Fluid restriction
- Ask if the provider wants anything else done
- Read back orders; ask that they enter all orders into the electronic medical record

Edema of the Lower Extremities

ISBARR Template	
I **Introduction**	**Introduce Yourself and the Patient** • "Hello, Dr. Schindler. This is Rachel Senk. I am the nurse for your patient Jennifer Williams in Room 208, who is post-op day two after her right ankle repair."
S **Situation**	**Sign/Symptom You Are Concerned About** • "Ms. Williams developed acute right lower calf pain and swelling this morning. The swelling and pain has been constant and severe. It is different than the surgical pain she has been having in her right ankle, which she also describes as constant and severe." **Associated Signs/Symptoms** • "She is denying numbness and tingling."
B **Background**	**Vitals** • "Vitals are stable. Blood pressure is 130/82, heart rate is 90, respirations are 14, and her temperature is 99.0." **Exam** • "Her right calf is warm, red, and has moderate non-pitting edema present. Pedal pulses are +2 bilaterally. Her surgical incision is clean, dry, and intact." **Past Medical History** • "She has rarely been out of bed the past two days unless it is with PT or when she gets up to go to the bathroom. As you know, yesterday she was refusing physical therapy." **Labs and Medications** • "and her Lovenox injections."
A **Assessment**	**Assessment** • "I am concerned about DVT."

(continues)

ISBARR Template	
R **Recommendations** **R** **Read Back**	**Nurse's Recommendations, Interventions, and Read Back** • "I have elevated her leg on pillows. She is currently in bed. Did you want a D-dimer or venous Doppler? What would you like her activity level to be? Would you like anything else done at this time? • "Thank you, Dr. Schindler, I just want to verify your orders. You would like a STAT venous Doppler of the right leg, and then to call you with the results. Is that correct?"

Disclaimer: This dialogue is factitious and any resemblance to actual persons, living or dead, or actual events is purely coincidental.

In order to avoid order discrepancies, it is recommended that all orders be entered by the provider in the electronic medical record.

Select Differential Diagnosis Presentations

Cellulitis

Overview: bacterial infection of the skin

Patient may complain of: fever, chills, localized skin erythema, swelling, and pain; symptoms are progressive in nature

Objective findings: fever, localized skin erythema, swelling, warmth, tenderness, drainage, open wound(s)

PMH considerations/risk factors: hx of diabetes, PVD, (lymph) edema, preexisting skin condition, obesity, immunosuppression, trauma to the area, IV drug use, older age

Diagnostics: clinical diagnosis; CBC and wound culture may be considered

Deep Vein Thrombosis

Overview: a blood clot in a deep vein, typically in the legs

Patient may complain of: chills, fever, extremity erythema, pain and swelling (typically unilateral but can be bilateral); symptoms are acute in nature

Objective findings: fever, extremity swelling, erythema, tenderness, weak pulses, sluggish capillary refill, difference in calf circumference

PMH considerations/risk factors: hx of DVT, PE or CVA, clotting/bleeding disorders, venous insufficiency, cancer, pregnancy, obesity, immobility, recent surgery, use of HRT/birth control, older age

Diagnostics: D-dimer, US of effected extremity

Heart Failure

Overview: broad term to describe pumping malfunction of the heart

Patient may complain of: fatigue, activity intolerance, chest pain, palpitations, dyspnea, orthopnea, PND, coughing, sputum production, weight gain/loss, anorexia, nausea, nocturia, insomnia

Objective findings: signs of acute distress, lethargy, diaphoresis, cyanosis, JVD, bradycardia/tachycardia, hypertension/hypotension, displaced PMI, murmur, gallop, weak pulses, sluggish capillary refill, digital clubbing, edema, breathlessness, tachypnea, cough, adventitious lung sounds, sputum, hepatomegaly, ascites

PMH considerations/risk factors: hx of heart failure, HTN, CAD, cardiac valve disorders, MI, diabetes, arrhythmias, hyper/hypothyroidism, obesity, nicotine use, substance abuse, family hx of heart disease

Diagnostics: BNP, BMP/CMP, TSH, ECG, I/O, chest X-ray, ECHO, cardiac catheterization

Liver Disease/Failure

Overview: broad term to describe damage and malfunction of the liver

Patient may complain of: fatigue, itching, anorexia, nausea, vomiting, RUQ abdominal pain, bloating, signs of GI bleeding

Objective findings: altered mental status, lethargy, jaundice, hypertension/hypotension, edema, ascites, abdominal distention, hepatomegaly, spider angiomas; exam may be unremarkable

PMH considerations/risk factors: hx of liver disease, hepatitis, diabetes, sepsis, obesity, cancer, Wilson's disease, IV drug use, alcohol abuse

Diagnostics: CMP, hepatitis panel, ammonia, PT/INR, abdominal US/CT, biopsy

Lymphedema

Overview: swelling caused by lymph node dysfunction and inadequate drainage

Patient may complain of: pain, swelling, aching, and heaviness of the extremity (typically unilateral but can be bilateral); symptoms are progressive in nature

Objective findings: swelling with hard thickened skin of effected limb, difference in limb circumference, weak pulses

PMH considerations/risk factors: hx of cancer, obesity, previous lymphadenectomy, radiation therapy, recent travel outside of the United States (subtropical infections), older age

Diagnostics: clinical diagnoses; limb CT/MRI/US may be considered initially

Renal Disease/Failure

Overview: broad term to describe damage and malfunction of the kidneys

Patient may complain of: fatigue, itching, dyspnea, anorexia, nausea, vomiting, oliguria, confusion

Objective findings: lethargy, altered mental status, arrhythmia, edema, hypertension/hypotension, pericardial rub, adventitious lung sounds, oliguria or anuria; exam is typically unremarkable unless severe

PMH considerations/risk factors: hx of CKD, diabetes, HTN, CAD, sepsis, BPH, burn injury, heart failure, dehydration, GI/blood loss, NSAID use, ACE inhibitor use, diuretic use, older age

Diagnostics: BMP/CMP, anion gap, urinalysis, renal US

Venous Insufficiency

Overview: dysfunction of the valves in the veins of the lower extremities causing inadequate blood flow and venous congestion

Patient may complain of: pain, swelling, aching, and heaviness in the extremities

Objective findings: varicose veins, edema, skin dryness and thickening, hyperpigmentation, wounds/ulceration, weak pedal pulses

PMH considerations: hx of PVD, diabetes, pregnancy, obesity, standing for long periods of time, sedentary lifestyle, trauma to the extremities, nicotine use, family hx of PVD, older age

Diagnostics: clinical diagnosis; venous doppler US may be considered initially

References

American Medical Directors Association. (2010). *Know-it-all before you call: Data collection system.* Columbia, MD: Author.

Bulechek, G. M., Butcher, H. K., Dochterman, J. M., & Wagner, C. (2013). *Nursing intervention classification (NIC).* St. Louis, MO: Elsevier Mosby.

Cooper, G. (2016). Chronic edema: Its prevalence, effects and management. *British Journal of Community Nursing, 21*(10), 32–36.

Desai, S. P. (2009). *Clinician's guide to laboratory medicine* (3rd ed.). Houston, TX: MD2B.

Elwell, R. (2016). An overview of the use of compression in lower-limb chronic edema. *British Journal of Community Nursing, 21*(1), 36–42.

Gulanick, M., & Myers, J. L. (2017). *Nursing care plans: Diagnosis, interventions, & outcomes* (9th ed.). St. Louis, MO: Elsevier.

Hale, A., & Hovey, M. J. (2014). *Fluid, electrolyte and acid-base imbalances.* Philadelphia, PA: F.A. Davis Company.

Jarvis, C. (2015). *Physical examination & health assessment.* St. Louis, MO: Elsevier.

Kataoka, H. (2013). Clinical characteristics of lower-extremity edema in stage A cardiovascular disease status defined by the ACC/AHA 2001 chronic heart failure guidelines. *Clinical Cardiology, 36*(9), 555–559.

Kelechi, T. J., & Johnson, J. J. (2012). Guideline for the management of wounds in patients with lower extremity venous disease: An executive summary. *Journal of Wound, Ostomy, & Continence Nursing, 39*(6), 598–606.

LeBlond, R. F., Brown, D. D., Suneja, M., & Szot, J. F. (2015). *DeGowin's diagnostic examination* (10th ed.). New York, NY: McGraw-Hill.

McCance, K. L., Huether, S. E., Brashers, V. L., & Rote, N. S. (2014). *Pathophysiology: The biologic basis for disease in adults and children* (7th ed.). St. Louis, MO: Elsevier.

Mehrara, B. (2017). Clinical staging and conservative management of peripheral lymphedema. In K. A. Collins and D. M. Savarese (Eds.), *UpToDate*. Retrieved from https://www.uptodate.com/contents/clinical-staging-and-conservative-management-of-peripheral-lymphedema

Papadakis, M. A., & McPhee, S. J. (2017). *Current medical diagnosis and treatment* (56th ed.). New York, NY: McGraw-Hill.

Ponikowski, P., Voors, A. A., Anker, S. D., Bueno, H., Cleland, J. G., Coats, A. J., . . . Van der Meer, P. (2016). 2016 ESC guidelines for the diagnosis and treatment of acute and chronic heart failure – Web addenda. *European Heart Journal,* 1–17. Retrieved from https://www.escardio.org/static_file/Escardio/Guidelines/ehw128_Addenda.pdf

Raftery, A. T., Lim, E., & Ostor, A. J. (2014). *Differential diagnosis* (4th ed.). London: Elsevier.

Seller, R. H., & Symons, A. B. (2012). *Differential diagnosis of common complaints* (6th ed.). Philadelphia, PA: Elsevier.

Simon, E. B. (2014). Leg edema assessment and management. *Medsurg Nursing,* 23(1), 44–53.

Smithson, C., Ham, J. C., & Juergens, A. (2015). Bilateral lower extremity swelling: Black pearl. *American Journal of Emergency Medicine,* 33(12), 1841.e3–1841.e4. doi:10.1016/j.ajem.2015.04.036

Sterns, R. H. (2016a). Clinical manifestations and diagnosis of edema in adults. In D. J., Sullivan, & J. P. Forman (Eds.), *UpToDate*. Retrieved from https://www.uptodate.com/contents/clinical-manifestations-and-diagnosis-of-edema-in-adults

Sterns, R. H. (2016b). Pathophysiology and etiology of edema in adults. In D. J., Sullivan, & J. P. Forman (Eds.), *UpToDate*. Retrieved from https://www.uptodate.com/contents/pathophysiology-and-etiology-of-edema-in-adults

Sterns, R. H. (2017). Idiopathic edema. In J. P. Forman (Ed.), *UpToDate*. Retrieved from https://www.uptodate.com/contents/idiopathic-edema

Sterns, R. H. (2018a). General principles of the treatment of edema in adults. In D. J. Sullivan (Ed.), *UpToDate*. Retrieved from https://www.uptodate.com/contents/general-principles-of-the-treatment-of-edema-in-adults

Stoll, B. C. (2014). *Practical approach to lower extremity edema.* Retrieved from http://anmedhealth.org/Portals/16/Services-Images/stoll2014.pdf

Trayes, K. P., Studdiford, J. S., Pickle, S., & Tully, A. S. (2013). Edema: Diagnosis and management. *American Family Physician,* 88(2), 102–110.

Uphold, C. R., & Graham, M. V. (2013). *Clinical guidelines in family practice* (5th ed.). Gainesville, FL: Barmarrae Books.

CHAPTER 15

Fever

Fever is not an illness itself, but rather a sign of an underlying issue. The terms fever and hyperthermia are commonly used interchangeably but need to be recognized as different physiological processes. Hyperthermia is an unregulated rise in body temperature, most commonly associated with heat stroke. Temperature levels are usually extreme (>105°F) and do not respond to antipyretics. If hyperthermia is suspected, the provider needs to be contacted immediately.

The American College of Critical Care Medicine and the Infectious Diseases Society of America define a fever as a temperature of >101°F. A fever increases the body's metabolic demands and can lead to dehydration, irritability, and seizures. A normal baseline temperature is 98.6 but can vary depending on a patient's age, gender, menstrual cycle status, and circadian rhythm. The elderly population has a lower baseline temperature and may not always meet the definition of a fever even when an infectious process occurs.

The pulmonary artery catheter core temperature reading is considered to be the most accurate, but is not available in most clinical situations. A rectal temperature is then the most ideal, but can be uncomfortable for the patient. If the patient is unable to tolerate rectal temperatures, oral temperatures are preferred over axillary methods. Although the differential for fever is broad, the majority are caused by infections, malignancies, and autoimmune diseases. Fever is also a common benign inflammatory event in the first 48 hours after surgery. When a fever is present, infection should be the first concern and ruled out before other considerations can be made. In order to avoid a costly workup, once the patient's fever has been recognized, it is important for the nurse to perform a thorough health history and physical exam in order to aid the provider in finding the etiology. It will also be important to give the patient education on infection prevention. In this chapter, nursing intervention considerations and recommendations should reflect whatever infectious process is suspected.

Differential Diagnosis Considerations

Common: bronchitis, cellulitis, gastroenteritis, influenza, IV catheter infection, otitis media, PID, pneumonia, post-operative fever, pyelonephritis, sepsis, sinusitis, SSI, URI, UTI

Consider: abdominal abscess, acalculous cholecystitis, acute chest syndrome, adrenal insufficiency, alcohol withdrawal, appendicitis, aspiration, blood transfusion reaction, cancer, cholangitis, cholecystitis, cocaine use, dehydration, dental abscess, diverticulitis, drug fever, DVT, ectopic pregnancy, empyema, endocarditis, epididymitis, fat embolism, foreign body infection, GCA, gout, heat stroke, hematoma, hepatitis, HSV, hyperthyroidism, IBD, immunizations, ischemic bowel disease, lymphomas, malignant hyperthermia, meningitis, mononucleosis, neuroleptic malignant syndrome, osteomyelitis, pancreatitis, parotitis, PE, pericarditis, peritonitis, polyarteritis nodosa, prostatitis, Q fever, rheumatic fever, rheumatoid arthritis, sarcoidosis, serotonin syndrome, SLE, syphilis, TB, thrombophlebitis, thyroid storm, toxoplasmosis, transplant rejection, typhoid fever, vasculitis, Zika virus

Questions to Ask the Patient/Family/Witness/Yourself

- When did the fever start? Is it constant, or does it come and go?
- When was your last menstrual period? (if applicable)
- Have you had any recent: illness/infection? exposure to any infection, contaminated drinking water, or been around anyone who is sick? hospitalization? immobilization such as prolonged time spent in bed or sitting? immunizations? surgery? trauma? travel outside of the United States?

- Have you had any recent invasive interventions such as a blood transfusion, central or peripheral IV, intubation, tube feeding, or urinary catheter?
- Have you taken any new prescribed or over-the-counter medications? Have there been any recent changes to your current medication?
- Have you taken any NSAIDs (ASA, ibuprofen, naproxen) or acetaminophen for the fever?
- Do you drink alcohol? How many drinks per day/week? What kind and amount of alcohol do you drink? When was your last drink? (if applicable)
- Do you have a history of drug use? What types and how much? Do you use on a daily basis? When was your last use? (if applicable)

Associated Signs/Symptoms: PAIN: pain anywhere; GENERAL: chills, fatigue, weakness; EENT: ear pain, eye pain, hearing changes, sore throat, tinnitus, vision changes; NECK: stiffness, swollen glands; CARDIOVASCULAR: chest pain/tightness, edema, palpitations; RESPIRATORY: cough, hemoptysis, painful breathing/coughing, dyspnea, sputum production, wheezing; GASTROINTESTINAL: appetite changes, constipation, diarrhea, heartburn, nausea, signs of GI bleeding, swallowing difficulties, vomiting; GENITOURINARY: dysuria, hematuria, incontinence, itching, nocturia, penile/vaginal discharge, urinary frequency, urinary urgency; MUSCULOSKEL-ETAL: joint erythema, pain, stiffness, swelling; NEUROLOGICAL: dizziness, headache, numbness/tingling, seizures, syncope, tremors; SKIN: erythema, rash, swelling, wounds; ENDOCRINE: hot/cold intolerance, sweating; PSYCHOLOGICAL: anxiety, confusion, hallucinations

Recommended Assessments

- Vital signs
- Temperature
- I/O
- Pain scale (if applicable)
  - Tolerable pain level

- General
  - Level of consciousness and orientation
  - Inspect: signs of acute distress, acute illness, affect, restlessness
- Skin
  - Inspect: cyanosis, diaphoresis, dryness, jaundice, pallor, rash, surgical site (if applicable), wounds
  - Palpate: temperature, turgor
- Eyes
  - Inspect: conjunctival erythema, lid erythema or swelling, periorbital edema
- Mouth
  - Inspect: dentition, halitosis, lesions, posterior pharynx erythema or swelling, tonsillar exudates, mucous membrane moisture level
- Ears
  - Inspect: erythema, external drainage
  - Palpate: external tenderness
- Nose
  - Inspect: drainage, turbinate erythema, or swelling
- Head/face/neck
  - Inspect: ROM of neck, signs of trauma, tracheal deviation
  - Palpate: lymphadenopathy, swelling, tenderness
- Cardiovascular
  - Auscultate: heart sounds, rate, rhythm
- Respiratory
  - Inspect: respiratory effort, depth, pattern, use of accessory muscles
  - Auscultate: lung sounds
- Gastrointestinal
  - Inspect: distention
  - Auscultate: bowel sounds
  - Palpate: guarding, masses, organomegaly, (rebound) tenderness

- Genitourinary
  - Inspect: external drainage, erythema, swelling, lesions
  - Palpate: bladder distention, CVAT
- Musculoskeletal
  - Inspect: joint erythema
  - Palpate: joint swelling, tenderness, warmth
  - Passive and active ROM examinations of effected joint (if applicable)
- Extremities
  - Inspect: discoloration, erythema, IV site
  - Palpate: capillary refill, edema, pulses, temperature, tenderness

Past Medical History Considerations

- Allergies
- Immunization status: influenza, meningitis, pertussis, pneumonia

Puts the patient at risk for differential considerations

- AIDS/HIV
- Alcohol abuse/use
- Asthma
- Cholelithiasis
- COPD
- Diabetes
- Drug abuse/use
- Dysphasia
- Immobilization
- Sickle cell anemia
- Surgery

Reoccurrence/exacerbation should be considered

- Diverticulitis
- DVT

- Gout
- HSV
- Otitis media
- PE
- Sinusitis
- UTI

Chronic conditions that can cause fever

- Addison's disease / adrenal insufficiency
- Cancer
- CVA/TIA
- Hepatitis
- IBD
- Pancreatitis
- Rheumatoid arthritis
- Sarcoidosis
- SLE
- Thyroid disease

Medication Evaluation

Have been reported to cause drug fever

- Allopurinol
- Antibiotics
- Anticonvulsants
- Antihistamines
- Antithyroid agents
- Atropine
- Captopril
- Cimetidine
- Furosemide
- Heparin
- Hydralazine
- Isoniazid
- Methyldopa

- Nifedipine
- NSAIDs
- SSRIs
- Tricyclic antidepressants
- Quinidine

Puts the patient at higher risk for infections

- Biologic/immunosuppressive agents
- Chemotherapy
- Corticosteroids

Used to treat fever

- Acetaminophen
- NSAIDs

Lab Evaluation and Trends

- CBC

Nursing Intervention Considerations

- Call for help or rapid response/code team if vital signs are unstable or there are signs of urgent distress
- Maintain a patent airway
  - Apply oxygen if hypoxic
  - Encourage cough and deep breathing
- Verify patent IV if IVF or IV medication treatment is anticipated
  - Flush according to facility protocol; watch for swelling, erythema, pain, and other signs of infiltration
- Medications (if ordered or protocol allows)
  - Hold suspected causative medication until discussion with the provider
  - PRN antipyretic (acetaminophen or NSAIDs)
- Diet
  - Push fluids if there are no contraindications (>2,000mL/day)

- Activity
  - Encourage activity and ambulation if safety permits
- Positioning
  - Supine or side lying position with knees flexed to chest to take tension off the abdominal wall if the patient has active abdominal pain
  - Lay supine with feet elevated if the patient has hypotension
  - HOB raised to comfort for respiratory distress
  - Reposition every 2–4 hours or establish an individualized turning schedule
- Collect
  - Urine sample for signs of UTI, ectopic pregnancy, or hematuria
  - Stool sample for diarrhea or signs of GI bleeding
  - Sputum sample for signs of respiratory infection or hemoptysis
  - Wound drainage sample if present
- Monitor
  - Stay with the patient until stable
  - Pain levels
  - Vital signs and trends
  - Oxygen saturation/pulse oximetry
  - Temperature trends
  - I/O
  - Orientation status changes
  - Agitation levels
  - Peripheral pulses
  - Skin assessment every 8–24 hours
  - Signs of decreased cardiac output such as weak pulses, cool skin, altered mental status, hypotension, oliguria, and mottling
  - Signs of respiratory distress such as cyanosis, tachypnea, hypoxia, use of accessory muscles, diaphoresis, and adventitious lung sounds

- Signs of dehydration such as lethargy, decreased skin turgor, dry mucous membranes, tachycardia, and (orthostatic) hypotension
- Signs and symptoms of GU infection such as fever, chills, dysuria, hematuria, increased urinary frequency and urgency, fatigue, altered mental status, and back/flank pain
- Signs of skin infection such as fever, pain, wounds, purulent drainage, localized erythema, swelling, heat, and pain
- Signs and symptoms of sepsis such as fever, chills, hypotension, altered mental status, hypoxia, cool clammy skin, dyspnea, oliguria, tachycardia, and tachypnea
- Safety
  - Perform a fall risk assessment and implement the appropriate strategies
- Environment
  - Provide a calm, quiet environment and reduce stimulation
  - Maintain a comfortable room temperature
  - Utilize a fan (if appropriate)
  - Initiate isolation precautions: standard, contact, droplet, airborne
- Supportive care
  - Maintain effective communication between yourself, patient, and family
  - Provide emotional support and reassurance to the patient and family
  - Maintain a calm manner during patient interactions
  - Discuss plan of care with the patient and decide reasonable goals together
  - Notify the patient and family of changes in the plan of care
  - Promote skin care and integrity

- Avoid application of heating devices
- Provide light clothing and bed linen
- **Educational topics (as applicable to the patient):**
  - General information regarding the patient's fever and differential diagnosis considerations
  - Procedure and intervention explanation and justification
  - Medication changes
  - Pain scale and pain goals
  - Relaxation techniques and breathing exercises
  - Cough and deep-breathing techniques
  - Oxygen therapy and maintenance
  - Proper positioning and turning schedule
  - Skin care
  - Peri-care and proper hygiene
  - Safety needs and fall risk
  - Handwashing and infection control measures
  - Isolation precaution needs
  - Increased fluid intake
  - Immunization needs
  - Increased physical activity
  - Alcohol and/or drug cessation and support
  - When to notify the nurse or provider
  - Signs and symptoms of various infections
  - Pressure injury prevention
  - Dehydration prevention

ISBARR Recommendation Considerations

- Ask the provider to come assess the patient STAT if they are unstable, showing signs of respiratory distress, or sepsis
- Transfer to the ICU if hemodynamically unstable, advanced medication management is required, or closer monitoring is needed

- Medication
  - Discontinue/change suspected causative medication
  - Add PRN antipyretic
- IV fluid needs if oral intake is poor, there are signs of dehydration, the patient is NPO or hypotensive
- Foley catheter discontinuation
- Imaging (depending on the suspected cause)
  - Abdominal or chest CT scan, chest X-ray
- Labs (depending on the suspected cause)
  - Amylase, lipase
  - Blood culture
  - BMP/CMP
  - CBC
  - D-dimer
  - Lactate
  - Sputum culture
  - Stool culture with *Clostridium difficile* testing
  - TSH
  - Urinalysis
  - Urine culture
  - Wound culture
- Safety
  - Activity level changes
  - Fall risk protocol
  - Isolation precautions: airborne, contact, droplet
- Monitoring needs
  - Continuous O_2 monitoring
  - Vital signs including frequency and parameters to call the provider
- Change diet to
  - Push oral fluids
- Protocols
  - CIWA-Ar if alcohol withdrawal is suspected
- Ask if the provider wants anything else done
- Read back orders; ask that they enter all orders into the electronic medical record

ISBARR Template	
I **Introduction**	**Introduce Yourself and the Patient** • "Hello, Dr. Kim. This is Susan Breakwell at Northwoods Long Term Care. I am the nurse for your resident Brittney Carr in Room 109."
S **Situation**	**Sign/Symptom You Are Concerned About** • "This morning, Ms. Carr had a temperature of 103.1." **Associated Signs/Symptoms** • "When I came to see her, she had no cough, shortness of breath, chest pain, or urinary complaints."
B **Background**	**Vitals** • "Her blood pressure is 86/40, pulse is 104, respirations are 20, and O_2 sat is 96% on room air." **Exam** • "She appeared more lethargic than usual but she's not acutely confused. I did a full head-to-toe assessment and found a small laceration on her left lateral shin. The surrounding skin is red, warm, and swollen. It is a large area that extends from the middle of her shin to the knee. I also saw a small amount of purulent drainage from the laceration when I was palpating the area. Pedal pulses were +2." **Past Medical History** • "She has a history of type 2 diabetes and peripheral vascular disease," **Labs and Medications** • "and has not had any recent labs."
A **Assessment**	**Assessment** • "I am concerned about cellulitis and sepsis."

ISBARR Template	
R **Recommendations** **R** **Read Back**	**Nurse's Recommendations, Interventions, and Read Back** • "I am recommending Ms. Carr be transferred to the hospital for a workup. Did you want to come evaluate her first? Did you want me to collect a wound culture?" • "Thank you, Dr. Kim, I would like to read those orders back to you. You would like me to call for an ambulance and transfer Ms. Carr to St. Joseph's hospital. You are going to call the emergency room to give a report, and I will notify Ms. Carr's daughter of the situation. Is all that correct?"

Disclaimer: This dialogue is factitious and any resemblance to actual persons, living or dead, or actual events is purely coincidental.

In order to avoid order discrepancies, it is recommended that all orders be entered by the provider in the electronic medical record.

Select Differential Diagnosis Presentations

Acute Chest Syndrome

Overview: vaso-occlusive crisis of the pulmonary vasculature in patients with sickle cell anemia

Patient may complain of: chills, fever, fatigue, chest pain, dyspnea, wheezing, coughing, sputum production

Objective findings: signs of acute distress/illness, fever, lethargy, warm skin, hypoxia, tachypnea, cough, sputum, use of accessory muscles, adventitious breath sounds

PMH considerations/risk factors: hx of sickle cell anemia, asthma, recent respiratory illness

Diagnostics: CBC, ECG, chest X-ray, chest CT

Appendicitis

Overview: inflammation of the appendix

Patient may complain of: chills, fever, fatigue, umbilical abdominal pain (initially), RLQ abdominal pain, anorexia, nausea, vomiting, diarrhea

Objective findings: signs of acute distress/illness, lethargy, low-grade fever, RLQ tenderness with guarding, positive McBurney's point tenderness, positive psoas, and obturator sign

PMH considerations/risk factors: hx of IBD, previous GI surgery, younger age (<30 years old)

Diagnostics: CBC, abdominal CT

Aspiration

Overview: inhalation of foreign object, food, or liquid into the airway

Patient may complain of: fever, fatigue, inability/difficulty swallowing, chest pain, coughing, dyspnea, wheezing, sputum production, heartburn, nausea, vomiting

Objective findings: signs of acute distress, fever, irritability, diaphoresis, cyanosis, drooling, hoarseness, choking, hypoxia, cough, tachypnea, adventitious lung sounds, sputum

PMH considerations/risk factors: hx of dysphagia, myasthenia gravis, Parkinson's disease, CVA, esophageal stricture, GERD, asthma, ENT/GI cancer, dementia, trauma to the neck, dentition issues, radiation therapy to the head and neck, intubation, NG tube, immobility, nicotine use, alcohol abuse/use

Diagnostics: CBC, swallow study, chest X-ray

Bronchitis

Overview: inflammation of the bronchioles typically due to an infection

Patient may complain of: fever, chills, fatigue, sore throat, nasal congestion, chest pain/tightness, coughing, dyspnea, wheezing, sputum production, hemoptysis

Objective findings: signs of acute illness, lethargy, low-grade fever, rhinorrhea, pharyngeal erythema, cough, sputum, adventitious breath sounds, tachypnea

PMH considerations/risk factors: hx of asthma, COPD, allergies, GERD, exposure to lung irritants, nicotine use, older age

Diagnostics: clinical diagnosis; ABG, chest X-ray, spirometry may be considered

Cellulitis

Overview: bacterial infection of the skin

Patient may complain of: fever, chills, localized skin erythema, swelling, and pain; symptoms are progressive in nature

Objective findings: fever, localized skin erythema, swelling, warmth, tenderness, drainage, open wound(s)

PMH considerations/risk factors: hx of diabetes, PVD, (lymph) edema, preexisting skin condition, obesity, immunosuppression, trauma to the area, IV drug use, older age

Diagnostics: clinical diagnosis; CBC and wound culture may be considered

Cholecystitis

Overview: inflammation of the gallbladder

Patient may complain of: fever, chills, fatigue, RUQ/epigastric pain, right shoulder pain, nausea, vomiting, anorexia, dyspepsia

Objective findings: signs of acute distress/illness, lethargy, fever, diaphoresis, jaundice, tachycardia, RUQ/epigastric tenderness with guarding, positive Murphy's sign, palpable gallbladder

PMH considerations/risk factors: hx of cholelithiasis, obesity, female gender

Diagnostics: CBC, CMP, abdominal CT/US, HIDA scan

Deep Vein Thrombosis

Overview: a blood clot in a deep vein, typically in the legs

Patient may complain of: chills, fever, extremity erythema, pain and swelling (typically unilateral but can be bilateral); symptoms are acute in nature

Objective findings: fever, extremity swelling, erythema, and tenderness, weak pulses, sluggish capillary refill, difference in calf circumference

PMH considerations/risk factors: hx of DVT, PE or CVA, clotting/bleeding disorders, venous insufficiency, cancer, pregnancy, obesity, immobility, recent surgery, use of HRT/birth control, older age

Diagnostics: D-dimer, US of effected extremity

Dehydration

Overview: abnormal loss of extracellular fluid volume

Patient may complain of: fatigue, thirst, dry mouth, palpitations, constipation, oliguria, muscle cramps, dizziness, headache

Objective findings: fever, altered mental status, lethargy, irritability, decreased skin turgor, generalized skin dryness, dry mucous membranes, (orthostatic) hypotension, tachycardia, oliguria

PMH considerations/risk factors: hx of liver or renal disease/failure, recent vomiting and/or diarrhea, GI bleeding, polyuria, diuretic use, burn injury, or intense physical activity

Diagnostics: BMP/CMP, CBC, urine Na, I/O

Diverticulitis

Overview: inflammation of diverticulum

Patient may complain of: fever, chills, LLQ abdominal pain (typically), constipation/diarrhea, nausea, vomiting

Objective findings: signs of acute distress/illness, fever, palpable abdominal mass, LLQ tenderness with guarding

PMH considerations/risk factors: hx of IBD, IBS, diverticulosis, GI cancer, obesity, nicotine use, older age

Diagnostics: CBC, occult stool, abdomen CT/US

Ectopic Pregnancy

Overview: fertilized egg implants outside of the uterus, typically in the fallopian tubes

Patient may complain of: chills, fever, breast tenderness, severe lower abdominal pain, nausea, vomiting, irregular vaginal bleeding, dizziness

Objective findings: signs of acute distress/illness, fever, hypotension, tachycardia, lower abdominal tenderness, vaginal bleeding

PMH considerations/risk factors: hx of infertility, IUD, previous GYN surgeries

Diagnostics: urine or serum Hcg, pelvic US, pelvic exam

Gastroenteritis

Overview: broad term for infection (typically viral) of the stomach and intestines

Patient may complain of: chills, fever, fatigue, anorexia, nausea, vomiting, diarrhea, generalized abdominal pain, dyspepsia

Objective findings: fever, lethargy, decreased skin turgor, dry mucous membranes, generalized abdominal tenderness without guarding

PMH considerations/risk factors: recent ingestion of undercooked food/contaminated water, hx of immunosuppression, recent antibiotic use, older age

Diagnostics: clinical diagnosis; stool cultures may be considered if symptoms are severe or prolonged

Inflammatory Bowel Disease

Overview: chronic inflammation of all or different parts of the gastrointestinal tract

Patient may complain of: chills, fever, fatigue, weight loss, anorexia, abdominal pain/cramping, nausea, vomiting, dyspepsia, constipation/diarrhea, change in bowel habits, signs of GI bleeding

Objective findings: signs of acute distress/illness, lethargy, fever, signs of malnourishment, diaphoresis, pallor, tachycardia, abdominal tenderness, hematochezia

PMH considerations/risk factors: hx of Crohn's disease or ulcerative colitis, food intolerance/allergies, bleeding/clotting disorders, NSAID use, recent travel outside of the United States, nicotine use, family hx of IBS, younger age

Diagnostics: occult stool, CRP, CBC, endoscopy with biopsy

Influenza

Overview: viral respiratory illness

Patient may complain of: chills, fever, fatigue, body aches, sore throat, nasal congestion, nasal drainage, dry coughing, headache

Objective findings: signs of acute distress/illness, lethargy, altered mental status (elderly), fever, tachycardia, pharyngeal erythema, conjunctival erythema, nasal turbinate swelling, rhinorrhea, lymphadenopathy, cough

PMH considerations/risk factors: recent exposure to influenza, pregnancy, hx of immunosuppression, older/younger age, influenza season, immunization status

Diagnostics: clinical diagnosis; rapid flu test and CBC may be considered

Meningitis

Overview: inflammation and infection of the meninges surrounding the brain and spinal cord

Patient may complain of: chills, fever, fatigue, photophobia, neck pain, anorexia, nausea, vomiting, headache, confusion, dizziness

Objective findings: signs of acute distress/illness, lethargy, fever, irritability, altered mental status, petechial rash, nuchal rigidity (positive Brudzinski, Kernig sign), seizures, signs of increased ICP

PMH considerations/risk factors: hx of TBI, immunosuppression, pregnancy, close quarter living situations, recent travel outside of the United States, alcohol abuse, older/younger age

Diagnostics: CBC, lumbar puncture, head CT

Otitis Media

Overview: infection or inflammation of the middle ear

Patient may complain of: chills, fever, fatigue, otalgia, hearing changes, tinnitus, nasal congestion, nasal drainage, coughing, anorexia, nausea, headache, dizziness

Objective findings: signs of acute distress/illness, lethargy, fever, irritability, erythematous bulging tympanic membrane with or without effusion, otorrhea (perforation)

PMH considerations/risk factors: hx of otitis media, eustachian tube dysfunction, younger age

Diagnostics: clinical diagnosis

Pancreatitis

Overview: inflammation of the pancreas

Patient may complain of: fatigue, chills, fever, epigastric/upper abdominal pain, radiation of the pain to the back, worse with movement, nausea, vomiting, dyspepsia, diarrhea

Objective findings: signs of acute distress/illness, lethargy, fever, diaphoresis, pallor, jaundice, tachycardia, hypotension, upper abdominal/epigastric tenderness, abdominal distention, positive Cullen's sign or Grey Turner sign (abdominal ecchymosis)

PMH considerations/risk factors: hx of chronic pancreatitis, hypertriglyceridemia, cholelithiasis, GI cancer, recent GI surgery or trauma to the abdomen, nicotine use, alcohol abuse/use

Diagnostics: amylase, lipase, abdominal CT/US

Pelvic Inflammatory Disease

Overview: broad term for inflammation and infection of the female reproductive organs

Patient may complain of: chills, fever, pelvic/abdominal pain, back pain, vaginal discharge, abnormal vaginal bleeding, pain with sexual intercourse, urinary frequency

Objective findings: signs of acute distress/illness, fever, abdominal/pelvic tenderness with guarding, mucopurulent vaginal discharge, cervical motion tenderness

PMH considerations/risk factors: multiple sexual partners, hx of STDs, nicotine use, younger age

Diagnostics: pelvic exam, STD testing, serum or urine Hcg, pelvic US

Pneumonia

Overview: infection of the air sacs in one or both lungs causing inflammation and fluid accumulation

Patient may complain of: chills, fever, fatigue, chest pain/tightness, dyspnea, wheezing, coughing, sputum production, hemoptysis, activity intolerance, anorexia, nausea, vomiting, headache

Objective findings: signs of acute distress/illness, lethargy, altered mental status (elderly), fever, tachycardia, tachypnea, use of accessory muscles, cough, sputum, hypoxia, adventitious breath sounds, dullness to percussion over consolidation, pleural friction rub

PMH considerations/risk factors: hx of COPD, asthma, immunosuppression, dysphagia, immunization status, recent/current hospitalization, intubation, nicotine use, alcohol abuse, older/younger age

Diagnostics: CBC, sputum culture, chest X-ray

Pulmonary Embolism

Overview: a blood clot in the pulmonary vasculature

Patient may complain of: chills, fever, chest pain, pain with deep breaths, palpitations, activity intolerance, dyspnea, coughing, hemoptysis, abdominal pain, dizziness

Objective findings: signs of acute distress, fever, pallor, cyanosis, diaphoresis, tachycardia, hypotension, S3/S4 heart sounds, tachypnea, hypoxia, cough, signs of DVT

PMH considerations/risk factors: hx of DVT, PE or CVA, bleeding/clotting disorder, cancer, pregnancy, HRT/birth control use, IV drug use, recent surgery, immobility, nicotine use

Diagnostics: D-dimer, chest CT, V/Q scan, chest X-ray

Pyelonephritis

Overview: bacterial infection of the kidney

Patient may complain of: fever, chills, nausea, vomiting, abdominal/back/flank pain, increased urinary frequency, retention, and urgency, dysuria, hematuria, urine odor, confusion (elderly)

Objective findings: signs of acute distress/illness, altered mental status (elderly), fever, tachycardia, CVAT, abdominal tenderness, bladder distention

PMH considerations: hx of frequent UTIs, diabetes, urolithiasis, urinary retention, immunosuppression, pregnancy, poor fluid intake, immobility, recent catheter use or GU surgery, female gender

Diagnostics: CBC, urinalysis, urine culture, renal US

Sepsis

Overview: severe inflammatory response due to an infection causing organ dysfunction

Patient may complain of: chills, fever, fatigue, generalized weakness, palpitations, (pre)syncope, dyspnea, oliguria; symptoms of whatever infection is suspected (i.e., appendicitis, diverticulitis, cholecystitis, pneumonia, cellulitis, meningitis, UTI)

Objective findings: signs of acute distress/illness, lethargy, fever, altered mental status, cyanosis, cool clammy skin or warm to the touch, tachycardia, hypotension, tachypnea, hypoxia, oliguria; signs of whatever infection is suspected

PMH considerations/risk factors: hx of immunosuppression, diabetes, cancer, recent infection or hospitalization, older/younger age

Diagnostics: blood culture, lactate, CBC, BMP/CMP, PT/INR; workup may also relate to whatever infection is suspected

Sinusitis

Overview: inflammation of the sinuses typically due to an infection

Patient may complain of: chills, fever, fatigue, facial pain, nasal congestion, nasal drainage, ear pain, dental pain, sore throat, coughing, sputum production, nausea, headache; acute symptoms last <4 weeks

Objective findings: signs of acute illness, low-grade fever, lethargy, frontal/maxillary tenderness, nasal turbinate swelling, rhinorrhea (purulent can indicate bacterial infection), halitosis, pharyngeal erythema, cough, sputum; signs and symptoms are more severe with a bacterial infection

PMH considerations/risk factors: hx of chronic sinusitis, allergies, asthma, immunosuppression, nicotine use

Diagnostics: clinical diagnosis; workup to rule out more emergent causes may be indicated

Upper Respiratory Infection

Overview: broad term for infection of the upper respiratory tract including the nose, throat, and upper airway

Patient may complain of: chills, fever, fatigue, nasal congestion, nasal drainage, sore throat, coughing, sputum production, nausea, vomiting, headache; symptoms have a short duration (<10 days)

Objective findings: signs of acute illness, low-grade fever, lethargy, conjunctival erythema, nasal turbinate swelling, rhinorrhea, halitosis, pharyngeal erythema, cough, sputum; signs and symptoms are typically mild in nature

PMH considerations/risk factors: hx of asthma, COPD, immunosuppression, allergies, nicotine use

Diagnostics: clinical diagnosis; workup to rule out more emergent causes may be indicated

Urinary Tract Infection

Overview: broad term for infection of the urinary tract including the urethra, bladder, ureters, and kidneys

Patient may complain of: fever, chills, abdominal/back/flank/pelvic pain, nausea, vomiting, dysuria, increased urinary frequency, retention and urgency, hematuria, incontinence, urine odor, confusion (elderly)

Objective findings: fever, altered mental status (elderly), pelvic tenderness, bladder distention; exam is typically unremarkable

PMH considerations/risk factors: hx of frequent UTIs, diabetes, interstitial cystitis, urinary retention, immunosuppression, dehydration, pregnancy, incontinence, recent catheter use, GU surgery or sexual activity, immobility, female gender

Diagnostics: urinalysis/urine dipstick, urine culture

Withdrawal (Alcohol)

Overview: rapid or abrupt decrease in alcohol intake causing physical and psychological disturbances

Patient may complain of: fever, chills, palpitations, anorexia, nausea, vomiting, diarrhea, seizures, headache, alcohol craving, insomnia, anxiety

Objective findings: signs of acute distress, fever, irritability, altered mental status, diaphoresis, tachycardia, hypertension, hepatomegaly, ascites, seizures, tremors, hallucinations/delirium

PMH considerations: hx of alcohol abuse, longer cessation (>48 hrs) since last drink, other substance abuse

Diagnostics: toxicology screen; workup to rule out more emergent causes may be indicated

Withdrawal (Opioids)

Overview: rapid or abrupt decrease in opioid intake causing physical and psychological disturbances

Patient may complain of: fever, body aches, nasal congestion, nasal drainage, anorexia, abdominal cramping, diarrhea, nausea, vomiting, tremors, opioid craving, anxiety, insomnia

Objective findings: signs of acute distress, fever, irritability, altered mental status, diaphoresis, piloerection, frequent yawning, pupil dilatation, rhinorrhea, hypertension, tachycardia, hyperactive bowel sounds

PMH considerations/risk factors: hx of daily opioid use, chronic pain, other substance abuse

Diagnostics: toxicology screen; workup to rule out more emergent causes may be indicated

References

American Medical Directors Association. (2010). *Know-it-all before you call: Data collection system.* Columbia, MD: Author.

Blum, F. C., & Biros, M. H. (2014). Fever in the adult patient. In *Principles and practice of infectious diseases* (pp. 119–125). London: Churchill Livingstone.

Bor, D .H. (2016). Etiologies of fever of unknown origin in adults. In A. R. Thorner (Ed.), *UpToDate.* Retrieved from https://www.uptodate.com/contents/etiologies-of-fever-of-unknown-origin-in-adults

Bor, D. H. (2018). Approach to the adult with fever of unknown origin. In A. R. Thorner (Ed.), *UpToDate.* Retrieved from https://www.uptodate.com/contents/approach-to-the-adult-with-fever-of-unknown-origin

Bulechek, G. M., Butcher, H. K., Dochterman, J. M., & Wagner, C. (2013). *Nursing intervention classification (NIC).* St. Louis, MO: Elsevier Mosby.

Desai, S. P. (2009). *Clinician's guide to laboratory medicine* (3rd ed.). Houston, TX: MD2B.

Flowers, C. R., Seidenfeld, J., Bow, E. J., Karten, C., Gleason, C., Hawley, D. K., . . . Ramsey, S. D. (2013). Antimicrobial prophylaxis and outpatient management of fever and neutropenia in adults treated for malignancy: American society of clinical oncology clinical practice guideline. *Journal of Clinical Oncology, 31*(6), 794–810.

Hale, A., & Hovey, M. J. (2014). *Fluid, electrolyte and acid-base imbalances.* Philadelphia, PA: F. A. Davis Company.

High, K. P., Bradley, S. F., Gravenstein, S., Mehr, D. R., Quagliarello, V. J., Richards, C., & Yoshikawa, T. T. (2009). Clinical practice guideline for the evaluation of fever and infection in older adult residents of long-term care facilities: 2008 update by the infectious diseases society of America. *Clinical Infectious Diseases, 48,* 149–171.

Jarvis, C. (2015). *Physical examination & health assessment.* St. Louis, MO: Elsevier.

Krzyzanowska, M. K., Walker-Dilks, C., Atzema, C. L., Morris, A., Gupta, R., Halligan, R., . . . McCann, K. (2015). *Fever assessment expert panel: Approach to fever assessment in ambulatory cancer patients receiving chemotherapy.* Retrieved from https://www.ncbi.nlm.nih.gov/pmc/articles/PMC4974036/pdf/conc-23-280.pdf

LeBlond, R. F., Brown, D. D., Suneja, M., & Szot, J. F. (2015). *DeGowin's diagnostic examination* (10th ed.). New York, NY: McGraw-Hill.

MacLaren, G., & Spelman, D. (2016). Fever in the intensive care unit. In G. Finlay (Ed.), *UpToDate.* Retrieved from https://www.uptodate.com/contents/fever-in-the-intensive-care-unit

McCance, K. L., Huether, S. E., Brashers, V. L., & Rote, N. S. (2014). *Pathophysiology: The biologic basis for disease in adults and children* (7th ed.). St. Louis, MO: Elsevier.

McDonald, M., & Sexton, D. J. (2017). Drug fever. In A. R. Thorner (Ed.), *UpToDate.* Retrieved from https://www.uptodate.com/contents/drug-fever

National Institute for Health Care Excellence. (2016). *Sepsis: Recognition, diagnosis and early management.* Retrieved from https://www.nice.org.uk/guidance/ng51

Niven, D. J., Gaudet, J. E., Laupland, K. B., Mrklas, K. J., Roberts, D. J., & Stelfox, H. T. (2015). Accuracy of peripheral thermometers for estimating temperature: A systematic review and meta-analysis. *Annals of Internal Medicine, 163*(10), 768–777.

Papadakis, M. A., & McPhee, S. J. (2017). *Current medical diagnosis and treatment* (56th ed.). New York, NY: McGraw-Hill.

Porat, R., & Dinarello, C. A. (2016). Pathophysiology and treatment of fever in adults. In A. R. Thorner (Ed.), *UpToDate*. Retrieved from https://www.uptodate.com/contents/pathophysiology-and-treatment-of-fever-in-adults

Raftery, A. T., Lim, E., & Ostor, A. J. (2014). *Differential diagnosis* (4th ed.). London: Elsevier.

Russo, P. R., Landon, M., Burkard, J. F., Andicochea, C. T., & Hannon, M. (2014). Fever evaluation cost and time to treatment in the general surgery patient can be reduced by using a fever practice guideline. *Military Medicine, 179*(10), 1166–2014.

Seller, R. H., & Symons, A. B. (2012). *Differential diagnosis of common complaints* (6th ed.). Philadelphia, PA: Elsevier.

Tinegate, H., Birchall, J., Gray, A., Haggas, R., Massey, E., Norfolk, D., . . . Allard, S. (2012). Guideline on the investigation and management of acute transfusion reactions: Prepared by the BCSH blood transfusion task force. *British Journal of Haematology, 159*(2), 143–153.

Uphold, C. R., & Graham, M. V. (2013). *Clinical guidelines in family practice* (5th ed.). Gainesville, FL: Barmarrae Books.

Weed, H. G, & Baddour, L. M. (2018). Postoperative fever. In K. A. Collins (Ed.), *UpToDate*. Retrieved from https://www.uptodate.com/contents/postoperative-fever

World Health Organization. (2013). *WHO informal consultation on fever management in peripheral health care settings: A global review of evidence and practice*. Retrieved from http://apps.who.int/iris/bitstream/10665/95116/1/9789241506489_eng.pdf

Yates, E., Mitchell, S. L., Habtemariam, D., Dufour, A. B., & Givens, J. L. (2015). Interventions associated with the management of suspected infections in advanced dementia. *Journal of Pain & Symptom Management, 50*(6), 806–813. doi:10.1016/j.jpainsymman.2015.06.011

CHAPTER 16

Gastrointestinal Bleeding

The term *GI bleeding* can refer to melena, hematochezia, and/or hematemesis. Melena and hematemesis are usually associated with upper GI bleeding, while hematochezia is a common sign of lower GI bleeding. However, the appearance of blood cannot exclusively determine the location of the bleeding, and an endoscopy is required to make a definitive diagnosis. Small intestinal bleeding is uncommon and most lower GI bleeds take place in the large intestines and rectum.

When the nurse identifies signs of GI bleeding, their top priority is to determine if there is any hemodynamic instability, and if found, IVF and blood product resuscitation are needed quickly. Signs and symptoms of hemodynamic instability include hypotension, tachypnea, altered mental status, weak pulses, and cool clammy skin. A gastroenterology consult will be needed if endoscopy is required.

Differential Diagnosis Considerations
Upper Gastrointestinal Tract

Common: anticoagulant use, duodenitis, esophagitis, gastritis, *Helicobacter pylori* infection, medication induced, PUD

Consider: angiodysplasia, aortoenteric fistula, benign GI tumors (lipoma, polyp), bleeding/clotting disorders, Boerhaave's syndrome, epistaxis, esophageal varices, foreign body ingestion, Mallory-Weiss tear, portal HTN gastropathy, upper GI malignancy

Lower Gastrointestinal Tract

Common: anal fissure, angiodysplasia, anticoagulant use, AV malformation, diverticulosis, hemorrhoid

Consider: aortoenteric fistula, bleb nevus syndrome, bleeding/clotting disorders, Dieulafoy's lesion, diverticulitis, IBD, infectious colitis, ischemic bowel disease, lower GI malignancy, Meckel's diverticulum, medication induced, polyp, post-biopsy/polypectomy, proctitis, radiation colitis, rectal ulcers

Questions to Ask the Patient/Family/Witness/Yourself

- When did you notice the blood in the stool/vomit?
- Is there blood with every bowel movement/vomiting episode?
- When was your last bowel movement/vomiting episode?
- Was there blood within the stool? Streaked on the side of the stool? On toilet paper with wiping?
- What color is the blood? Bright red? Black? Maroon?
- Have you seen any blood clots?
- How easy is it to have a bowel movement? Do you have any straining or pain?
- How is your appetite? Are you able to keep down food and/or fluids?
- Any recent intake of red wine, beets, blueberries, bismuth preparations, or licorice?
- Do you have any other bowel habit changes?
- Do you have a history of blood in your stool/vomit? If so, what was done or used to treat it?
- Have you had any recent: dietary changes or eaten anything out of the ordinary? GI illness? GI surgery? radiation therapy? trauma to the abdomen, chest, face, or throat? travel outside of the United States?
- Have you had any recent invasive interventions such as endoscopy or GI biopsy?

- Do you take any anticoagulants or NSAIDs (ASA, ibuprofen, naproxen)?
- Have you taken any new prescribed or over-the-counter medications? Have there been any recent changes to your current medication?
- Do you smoke? How much (ppd)? How long have you been smoking? (if applicable)
- Do you drink alcohol? How many drinks per day/week? What kind and amount of alcohol do you drink? When was your last drink? (if applicable)

Associated Signs/Symptoms: PAIN: pain anywhere; GENERAL: chills, fatigue, fever, weakness, weight changes; CARDIOVASCULAR: chest pain/tightness, palpitations; RESPIRATORY: hemoptysis, dyspnea; GASTROINTESTINAL: constipation, diarrhea, heartburn, nausea, swallowing difficulties; GENITOURINARY: hematuria; NEUROLOGICAL: dizziness, syncope; SKIN: ecchymosis

Recommended Assessments

- Vital signs
- Temperature
- Weight and nutritional status
- I/O
- Pain scale (if applicable)
  - Tolerable pain level
- General
  - Level of consciousness and orientation
  - Inspect: signs of acute distress, acute illness, affect, restlessness
- Skin
  - Inspect: cyanosis, diaphoresis, dryness, ecchymosis, pallor, wounds
  - Palpate: temperature, turgor
- Mouth
  - Inspect: bleeding, mucous membrane moisture level

- Nose
  - Inspect: bleeding
- Head/face/neck
  - Inspect: signs of trauma
- Cardiovascular
  - Auscultate: heart sounds, rate, rhythm
- Respiratory
  - Inspect: respiratory effort
  - Auscultate: lung sounds
- Gastrointestinal
  - Inspect: distention
  - Auscultate: bowel sounds, bruits
  - Palpate: guarding, (rebound) tenderness
- Rectal
  - Inspect: bleeding, erythema, fissures, hemorrhoids, open lesions, swelling
  - Palpate: masses, tenderness
- Extremities
  - Inspect: IV site
  - Palpate: capillary refill, pulses

Past Medical History Considerations
Puts the patient at risk for differential considerations

- Abdominal surgery
- AIDS/HIV
- Alcohol abuse/use
- CKD
- Constipation
- Hiatal hernia
- Liver disease
- Nicotine use
- Radiation therapy to the abdomen/pelvis

Reoccurrence/exacerbation should be considered

- Anal fissure
- Diverticulitis
- *H. pylori* infection

Chronic conditions that can cause GI bleeding

- Bleeding/clotting disorder
- Esophageal varices
- GI malignancy
- Diverticulosis
- Hemorrhoids
- IBD
- LVAD use
- PUD

Medication Evaluation

Used to treat common differential considerations

- Antibiotics → various GI infections
- PPIs, H2 antagonists, antacids → upper GI tract inflammation
- Topical analgesic and steroid agents → hemorrhoids

Puts the patient at higher risk for GI bleeding

- Anticoagulants
- Antiplatelet agents
- Bisphosphonates
- Chemotherapy
- Corticosteroids
- Iron supplements
- NSAIDs
- Potassium supplements

Lab Evaluation and Trends

- CBC
- PT/INR

Nursing Intervention Considerations

- Call for help or rapid response/code team if vital signs are unstable or there are signs of urgent distress
- Maintain a patent airway
  - Apply oxygen if hypoxic
  - Suction as needed
  - Provide oral care throughout the day (q2–4hrs)
  - Call respiratory therapy for signs of respiratory distress
- Verify patent IV if IVF or IV medication treatment is anticipated
  - Flush according to facility protocol; watch for swelling, erythema, pain, and signs of infiltration
  - Large bore IV is preferred
- Medications (if ordered or protocol allows)
  - Hold suspected causative medication until discussion with the provider
  - Hold oral medication if NPO status is anticipated
- Diet
  - NPO until discussion with the provider
  - Avoid foods/fluids that can darken stool such as beets, red wine, blueberries, and black licorice
  - Encourage high-fiber food choices
- Activity
  - Keep the patient in bed until discussion with the provider
- Positioning
  - Lay supine with feet elevated if the patient is hypotensive
  - Side lying position if there is a decrease in LOC or the patient is vomiting
  - Reposition every 2–4 hours or establish an individualized turning schedule
- Collect
  - Stool sample

- Monitor
  - Stay with the patient until stable
  - Pain levels
  - Vital signs and trends
  - Oxygen saturation/pulse oximetry
  - I/O
  - Weight trends
  - Orientation status changes
  - Agitation levels
  - Peripheral pulses
  - Skin assessment every 8–24 hours
  - Signs of decreased cardiac output such as weak pulses, cool skin, altered mental status, hypotension, oliguria, and mottling
  - Signs of respiratory distress such as cyanosis, tachypnea, hypoxia, use of accessory muscles, diaphoresis, and adventitious lung sounds
  - Signs and symptoms of blood loss such as fatigue, dizziness, dyspnea, melena, hematochezia, hematemesis, hematuria, epistaxis, pallor, ecchymosis, altered mental status, hypotension, tachycardia, tachypnea, and hemoptysis
  - Stool output color, consistency, frequency, and volume
  - Emesis output color, consistency, frequency, and volume
- Safety
  - Perform a fall risk assessment and implement the appropriate strategies
- Environment
  - Provide a calm, quiet environment, and reduce stimulation
  - Maintain a well-lit environment
  - Maintain a comfortable room temperature
- Supportive care
  - Maintain effective communication between yourself, patient, and family
  - Provide emotional support and reassurance to the patient and family

- Maintain a calm manner during patient interactions
- Discuss plan of care with the patient and decide reasonable goals together
- Notify the patient and family of changes in the plan of care
- Identify barriers to care and compliance
- Discuss any religious restrictions that may affect their care (blood transfusion)
- Promote skin care and integrity
- **Educational topics (as applicable to the patient):**
  - General information regarding the patient's GI bleeding and differential diagnosis considerations
  - Procedure and intervention explanation and justification
  - Explanation regarding referrals and specialist who may see them for this issue
  - New medication education including reason, side effects, and administration needs
  - Medication changes
  - Laboratory monitoring needs
  - Occult stool test
  - Blood transfusion needs
  - Pain scale and pain goals
  - Oxygen therapy and maintenance
  - Proper positioning and turning schedule
  - Skin care
  - Safety needs and fall risk
  - NPO diet, high-fiber diet
  - Avoidance of food/fluid that can discolor the stool
  - Sitz baths
  - Alcohol cessation and support
  - Smoking cessation
  - Age appropriate colonoscopy screening recommendations
  - When to notify the nurse or provider
  - Signs and symptoms of abnormal bleeding

- Pressure injury prevention
- Constipation prevention

ISBARR Recommendation Considerations

- Ask the provider to come assess the patient STAT if they are unstable
- Transfer to the ICU if hemodynamically unstable, advanced medication management is required, or closer monitoring is needed
- Medication
  - Hold oral medications if the patient is unable to tolerate or NPO
  - Discuss changing medication routes with the provider (and pharmacy) if the patient is NPO
  - Discontinue/change suspected causative medication
  - Add PPI, H2 antagonist, or antacid for dyspepsia, heartburn, or other signs/symptoms of GERD
  - Add PRN and/or scheduled enema, fiber supplement, stool softener, laxative, or suppository for constipation
- IV fluid needs if oral intake is poor, there are signs of dehydration, the patient is NPO or hypotensive
- Labs (depending on the suspected cause)
  - BMP/CMP
  - CBC
  - *H. pylori* breath/stool/serum
  - Occult stool
  - PT/INR
  - Type and cross match
- Safety
  - Activity-level changes
  - Fall risk protocol
- Monitoring needs
  - Daily weights
  - Continuous O_2 monitoring

- Strict I/O
- Vital signs including frequency and parameters to call the provider
- Change diet to
  - NPO
  - High-fiber
- Protocols
  - Blood transfusion
- Referrals
  - Gastroenterology
- Ask if the provider wants anything else done
- Read back orders; ask that they enter all orders into the electronic medical record

ISBARR Template	
I **Introduction**	**Introduce Yourself and the Patient** • "Hello, Dr. Shaw, this is Laura Nigh. I am the nurse for Theresa Schnable in Room 304. She is your patient who was admitted for pulmonary embolism four days ago."
S **Situation**	**Sign/Symptom You Are Concerned About** • "I am calling because Ms. Schnable called me into the room this morning concerned over the color of her stool. I saw that there was a moderate amount of black loose stool in the toilet." **Associated Signs/Symptoms** • "Her only other symptom is she is feeling mildly fatigued. She denies any abdominal pain, shortness of breath, or dizziness."
B **Background**	**Vitals** • "Blood pressure is 122/65, heart rate is 60, respirations are 14, and temperature is 98.2."

ISBARR Template

	Exam • "She does not appear pale, her lungs are clear, and she didn't have any abdominal distention or tenderness with palpation." **Past Medical History** • "She denies any previous GI bleeds or ulcers, but she is on daily Protonix for GERD." **Labs and Medications** • "I know she was started on Warfarin this week. Her PT/INR yesterday was 2.9 and this morning it was 3.8. Her last CBC was done three days ago; hemoglobin was 12.0."
A **Assessment**	**Assessment** • "I am concerned about an upper GI bleed."
R **Recommendations** **R** **Read Back**	**Nurse's Recommendations, Interventions, and Read Back** • "I collected a stool sample. Did you want to see the stool or send it for any testing? Did you want an updated CBC? Did you want me to hold her Warfarin?" • "Thanks, Dr. Shaw. If I could just read those orders back to you. You want a CBC with type and cross match now. A CBC and PT/INR in the AM. You also want me to consult the GI on call to come evaluate the patient. I will call you with CBC results as soon as they are available, and will hold tonight's warfarin dose until further notice. Is all that correct?"

Disclaimer: This dialogue is factitious and any resemblance to actual persons, living or dead, or actual events is purely coincidental.

In order to avoid order discrepancies, it is recommended that all orders be entered by the provider in the electronic medical record.

Select Differential Diagnosis Presentations

Anal Fissure

Overview: a tear in the lining of the anal canal

Patient may complain of: pain with defecation, rectal bleeding, and itching

Objective findings: crack(fissure)-like lesion within the anal sphincter, hematochezia, anal skin tags, erythema, swelling, tenderness

PMH considerations/risk factors: hx of constipation, chronic diarrhea, IBD, recent vaginal delivery, hx of anal intercourse

Diagnostics: clinical diagnosis

Diverticulitis

Overview: inflammation of diverticulum

Patient may complain of: fever, chills, LLQ abdominal pain (typically), constipation/diarrhea, nausea, vomiting

Objective findings: signs of acute distress/illness, fever, palpable abdominal mass, LLQ tenderness with guarding

PMH considerations/risk factors: hx of IBD, IBS, diverticulosis, GI cancer, obesity, nicotine use, older age

Diagnostics: CBC, occult stool, abdomen CT/US

Diverticulosis

Overview: abnormal out hx of pouchings or sacs that develop in the GI tract wall

Patient may complain of: constipation, abdominal pain, and rectal bleeding if diverticular bleeding is present; patient is typically asymptomatic

Objective findings: vague abdominal tenderness, hematochezia if diverticular bleeding is present; exam is typically unremarkable

PMH considerations/risk factors: hx of diverticulosis, obesity, low-fiber diet, nicotine use

Diagnostics: occult stool, colonoscopy

Esophagitis (Various Types)

Overview: inflammation of the esophagus

Patient may complain of: painful swallowing, dysphagia, chest pain, heartburn, upper abdominal/epigastric pain, dyspepsia, nausea, vomiting, signs of GI bleeding, dry coughing

Objective findings: oral herpes or thrush (depending on etiology), poor dentition, cough; exam is typically unremarkable

PMH considerations/risk factors: hx of esophagitis; GERD; hiatal hernia; cancer; immunosuppression; allergic diseases (food allergies, asthma, eczema); obesity; radiation therapy of the head, neck, and chest; alcohol abuse/use; nicotine use; NSAID use

Diagnostics: endoscopy with biopsy

Gastritis

Overview: inflammation of the stomach

Patient may complain of: anorexia, nausea, vomiting, dyspepsia, epigastric pain, signs of GI bleeding

Objective findings: nonspecific epigastric tenderness; exam is typically unremarkable

PMH considerations/risk factors: hx of PUD, *H. pylori* infection, NSAID use, alcohol abuse/use, recent travel outside of the United States, older age

Diagnostics: *H. pylori* serum/breath/stool testing, endoscopy with biopsy

Helicobacter pylori Infection

Overview: gram-negative bacterial infection in the stomach that disrupts the gastric mucosal lining, making it vulnerable to peptic damage

Patient may complain of: abdominal pain, bloating, nausea, anorexia, dyspepsia, signs of GI bleeding

Objective findings: nonspecific epigastric tenderness; exam is typically unremarkable

PMH considerations/risk factors: hx of PUD, immunosuppression, recent travel outside of the United States, low socioeconomic status, ingestion of contaminated drinking water, NSAID use

Diagnostics: H. *pylori* serum/breath/stool testing, endoscopy with biopsy

Hemorrhoid

Overview: swollen veins that occur in the anal and/or rectal canal

Patient may complain of: blood streaked in stool or with wiping (small amount), anorectal pain and pruritis

Objective findings: external hemorrhoids are visible on exam; internal hemorrhoids may not be visualized or palpated

PMH considerations/risk factors: hx of constipation, pregnancy, obesity, straining during defecation, immobility

Diagnostics: clinical diagnosis; occult stool may be considered

Inflammatory Bowel Disease

Overview: chronic inflammation of all or different parts of the GI tract

Patient may complain of: chills, fever, fatigue, weight loss, anorexia, abdominal pain/cramping, nausea, vomiting, dyspepsia, constipation/diarrhea, change in bowel habits, signs of GI bleeding

Objective findings: signs of acute distress/illness, lethargy, fever, signs of malnourishment, diaphoresis, pallor, tachycardia, abdominal tenderness, hematochezia

PMH considerations/risk factors: hx of Crohn's disease or ulcerative colitis, food intolerance/allergies, bleeding/clotting disorders, NSAID use, recent travel outside of the United States, nicotine use, family hx of IBS, younger age

Diagnostics: occult stool, CRP, CBC, endoscopy with biopsy

Peptic Ulcer Disease

Overview: ulcers that develop in the lining of a stomach and/or duodenum

Patient may complain of: chest pain, dyspepsia, epigastric pain, heartburn, pain relief with food or antacids, nausea, signs of GI bleeding

Objective findings: nonspecific epigastric tenderness; exam is typically unremarkable

PMH considerations/risk factors: hx of PUD, *H. pylori* infection, NSAID use, recent travel outside of the United States, nicotine use, alcohol abuse/use

Diagnostics: CBC, *H. pylori* serum/breath/stool testing, occult stool, endoscopy with biopsy

References

American Medical Directors Association. (2010). *Know-it-all before you call: Data collection system.* Columbia, MD: Author.

Ballew, C. C., Surratt, J. F., Collins, T. L., & Shah, N. (2013). Gastrointestinal bleeding in patients with ventricular assist devices: What every cardiac nurse should know. *Progress in Transplantation, 23,* 229–234.

Bulechek, G. M., Butcher, H. K., Dochterman, J. M., & Wagner, C. (2013). *Nursing intervention classification (NIC).* St. Louis, MO: Elsevier Mosby.

Cave, D. (2015). Evaluation of suspected small bowel bleeding (formerly obscure gastrointestinal bleeding). In A. C. Travis (Ed.), *UpToDate.* Retrieved from https://www.uptodate.com/contents/evaluation-of-suspected-small-bowel-bleeding-formerly-obscure-gastrointestinal-bleeding

Darcy, M. D., Cash, B. D., Feig, B. W., Fidelman, N., Hara, A. K., Kapoor, B. S., . . . Lorenz, J. M. (2014). *Expert panel on interventional radiology: ACR appropriateness criteria radiologic management of lower gastrointestinal tract bleeding.* Retrieved from https://acsearch.acr.org/docs/69457/Narrative

Desai, S. P. (2009). *Clinician's guide to laboratory medicine* (3rd ed.). Houston, TX: MD2B.

Gerson, L. B., Fidler, J. L., Cave, D. R., & Leighton, J. A. (2015). ACG clinical guideline: Diagnosis and management of small bowel bleeding. *American Journal of Gastroenterology, 110,* 1265–1286.

Gralnek, I. M., Dumonceau, J. M., Kuipers, E. J., Lanas, A., Sanders, D. S., Kurien, M., . . . Hassan, C. (2015). Diagnosis and management of nonvariceal upper gastrointestinal hemorrhage: European society of gastrointestinal endoscopy (ESGE) guideline. *Endoscopy, 47,* 1–46.

Gulanick, M., & Myers, J. L. (2017). *Nursing care plans: Diagnosis, interventions, & outcomes* (9th ed.). St. Louis, MO: Elsevier.

Hale, A., & Hovey, M. J. (2014). *Fluid, electrolyte and acid-base imbalances.* Philadelphia, PA: F.A. Davis Company.

Jarvis, C. (2015). *Physical examination & health assessment*. St. Louis, MO: Elsevier.

Kim, B., Li, B. T., Engel, A., Samra, J. S., Clarke, S., Norton, I. D., & Li, A. E. (2014). Diagnosis of gastrointestinal bleeding: A practical guide for clinicians. *World Journal of Gastrointestinal Pathophysiology, 5*(4), 467–478.

Kyaw, M. H., & Chan, F. K. (2014). Pharmacologic options in the management of upper gastrointestinal bleeding: Focus on the elderly. *Drugs Aging, 31,* 349–361.

LeBlond, R. F., Brown, D. D., Suneja, M., & Szot, J. F. (2015). *DeGowin's diagnostic examination* (10th ed.). New York, NY: McGraw-Hill.

McCance, K. L., Huether, S. E., Brashers, V. L., & Rote, N. S. (2014). *Pathophysiology: The biologic basis for disease in adults and children* (7th ed.). St. Louis, MO: Elsevier.

Papadakis, M. A., & McPhee, S. J. (2017). *Current medical diagnosis and treatment* (56th ed.). New York, NY: McGraw-Hill.

Penner, R. M., & Majumdar, S. R. (2016). Approach to minimal bright red blood per rectum in adults. In D. J. Sullivan (Ed.), *UpToDate*. Retrieved from https://0-www.uptodate.com.libus.csd.mu.edu/contents/approach-to-minimal-bright-red-blood-per-rectum-in-adults?source=search_result&search=GI%20bleed&selectedTitle=12~150

Raftery, A. T., Lim, E., & Ostor, A. J. (2014). *Differential diagnosis* (4th ed.). London: Elsevier.

Rockey, D. C. (2016). Causes of upper gastrointestinal bleeding in adults. In A. Travis (Ed.), *UpToDate*. Retrieved from https://www.uptodate.com/contents/causes-of-upper-gastrointestinal-bleeding-in-adults

Salzman, J. R. (2018). Approach to acute upper gastrointestinal bleeding in adults. In A. C. Travis (Ed.), *UpToDate*. Retrieved from https://www.uptodate.com/contents/approach-to-acute-upper-gastrointestinal-bleeding-in-adults

Seller, R. H., & Symons, A. B. (2012). *Differential diagnosis of common complaints* (6th ed.). Philadelphia, PA: Elsevier.

Strate, L. (2016). Approach to acute lower gastrointestinal bleeding in adults. In S. Grover (Ed.), *UpToDate*. Retrieved from https://www.uptodate.com/contents/approach-to-acute-lower-gastrointestinal-bleeding-in-adults

Strate, L. (2017). Etiology of lower gastrointestinal bleeding. In S. Grover (Ed.), *UpToDate*. Retrieved from https://www.uptodate.com/contents/etiology-of-lower-gastrointestinal-bleeding-in-adults

Strate, L. L., & Gralnek, I. M. (2016). ACG clinical guideline: Management of patients with acute lower gastrointestinal bleeding. *The American Journal of Gastroenterology, 111,* 459–474.

Travis, A. C., & Salzman, J. R. (2016). Evaluation of occult gastrointestinal bleeding. In S. Grover (Ed.), *UpToDate*. Retrieved from https://www.uptodate.com/contents/evaluation-of-occult-gastrointestinal-bleeding

Uphold, C. R., & Graham, M. V. (2013). *Clinical guidelines in family practice* (5th ed.). Gainesville, FL: Barmarrae Books.

CHAPTER 17

Headache

Headache is a very common patient complaint with primary and secondary etiologies. Primary etiologies are benign and include migraine, tension, and cluster headaches. Typically, headaches from a secondary etiology can be differentiated with a quality history and assessment, but an immediate workup to rule out emergent issues, such as subdural hemorrhage, may be required if red flag signs and symptoms are present. Red flag signs and symptoms include neurological deficits, fever, neck stiffness, vision changes, vomiting, altered mental status, and new onset of a severe headache. Headache symptoms are more concerning when the patient is age 50 and older, immunocompromised, or pregnant. When the patient has a history of chronic headaches, it is important to ask if there has been a change in the quality or frequency. It is the nurse's priority to frequently assess for red flags and manage the patient's discomfort.

Differential Diagnosis Considerations

Common: asthenopia, dehydration, dental infection, hypoglycemia, hypoxia, influenza, medication induced, migraine headache, otitis media, rebound headache, sinusitis, TBI, TMJ dysfunction, tension headache, UACS, URI

Consider: alcohol withdrawal, anemia, anxiety, caffeine withdrawal, carotid dissection, cerebral aneurysm, cervical disc disease, closed angle glaucoma, cluster headache, CO poisoning, CVA/TIA, depression, digoxin toxicity, encephalitis, GCA, herpes zoster, hypermagnesemia, hypertensive emergency, hyponatremia, hypothyroidism, intracranial hemorrhage, intracranial malignancy, intracranial mass, lumbar puncture, Lyme's disease, meningitis, optic neuritis, pheochromocytoma, post-herpetic neuralgia, preeclampsia, sickle cell crisis, sleep apnea, spontaneous intracranial hypotension, substance abuse, trigeminal neuralgia

Questions to Ask the Patient/ Family/Witness/Yourself

- When did the headache start? Did it start gradually or suddenly?
- Where is the pain exactly? Can you point to it?
- Is the pain constant or does it come and go? If intermittent, how long does it last? How often is it happening per hour/day?
- Can you describe the pain (pressure, sharp, dull, achy, tightness, stabbing, throbbing)?
- What makes the pain better (certain positions, eating, dark room, medication, sleeping)?
- What triggers the headache or makes the pain worse (activity, bearing down, certain positions, coughing, head movements, light/sound, menstrual cycle, psychological stress, smells)?
- Does the pain radiate into your arms, jaw, neck?
- How severe is your headache? Can you rate it on a scale from 0 to 10? If severe, would you consider it the worst headache of your life?
- Can you tell when you are going to have a headache (aura)? If so, what symptoms do you have?
- Do you have a history of headaches? If so, is this headache different? What have you done or used to treat it in the past? How often are you using as needed medication for your headaches?
- Have you had any recent: dietary changes? exposure to CO? ENT infection? sleep habit changes? trauma to the head?
- Have you had any recent invasive interventions such as a lumbar puncture?
- Have you taken any new prescribed or over-the-counter medications? Have there been any recent changes to your current medication?
- Do you have a family history of headaches (or migraines)?
- Do you drink caffeine? How many drinks in a day? When was the last time you had any?
- Do you drink alcohol? How many drinks per day/week? What kind and amount of alcohol do you drink? When was your last drink? (if applicable)

- Do you have a history of drug use? What types and how much? Do you use on a daily basis? When was your last use? (if applicable)

Associated Signs/Symptoms: PAIN: pain anywhere else; GENERAL: chills, fatigue, fever, weakness, weight loss; EENT: dental pain, ear pain, eye pain, nasal congestion, sneezing, sore throat, tinnitus, vision changes; NECK: stiffness, swollen glands; RESPIRATORY: dyspnea, cough; GASTROINTESTINAL: nausea, vomiting; NEUROLOGICAL: dizziness, numbness/tingling, seizures, (pre)syncope; PSYCHOLOGICAL: anxiety, confusion, depression, hallucinations

Recommended Assessments

- Vital signs
- Temperature
- I/O
- Pain scale
  - Tolerable pain level
- General
  - Level of consciousness and orientation
  - Inspect: signs of acute distress, acute illness, affect, restlessness
  - Speech changes
  - GCS
- Skin
  - Inspect: cyanosis, diaphoresis, dryness, pallor, vesicular rash
  - Palpate: temperature, turgor
- Eyes
  - Inspect: conjunctival erythema, nystagmus, lid swelling, peri-orbital edema, ptosis, pupillary response
- Mouth
  - Inspect: dentition, exudates, lesions, mucous membrane moisture level, swelling or erythema of the posterior pharynx

- Ears
  - Inspect: erythema, external drainage
  - Palpate: external tenderness
- Head/face/neck
  - Inspect: ROM of neck, signs of trauma
  - Auscultate: carotid bruits
  - Palpate: goiter, lymphadenopathy, swelling, tenderness, TMJ popping
- Respiratory
  - Inspect: respiratory effort, depth, use of accessory muscles
  - Auscultate: lung sounds
- Neurological
  - Inspect: facial droop, gait, tremors
  - Palpate: extremity strength, sensation
  - Cranial nerve exam
- Extremities
  - Inspect: IV site (if applicable)

Past Medical History Considerations
Puts the patient at risk for differential considerations

- AIDS/HIV
- Alcohol abuse/use
- Bleeding/clotting disorder
- COPD
- Diabetes
- Drug abuse/use
- HTN
- Obesity
- Pregnancy
- Sickle cell disease

Reoccurrence/exacerbation should be considered

- Cluster headache

- Herpes zoster
- Migraines
- Rebound headache
- Sinusitis
- Tension headache

Chronic conditions that can cause headache

- AIDS/HIV
- Allergies
- Anemia
- Anxiety
- Brain malignancy
- Cervical DDD
- CVA/TIA
- Depression
- Glaucoma
- Insomnia
- Sleep apnea
- TBI
- Thyroid disease
- TMJ dysfunction
- Trigeminal neuralgia

Medication Evaluation

Puts the patient at risk for intracranial bleeding

- Anticoagulants
- Antiplatelet agents
- Corticosteroids
- NSAIDs

Most common causative/exacerbating medication

- Birth control/HRT
- Nitrates

Overuse can cause rebound headaches

- Acetaminophen
- Butalbital
- NSAIDs
- Opioids
- Triptans

Used to treat chronic headaches

- Acetaminophen
- Anticonvulsants
- Beta blockers
- CCBs
- NSAIDs
- Tricyclic antidepressants
- Triptans

Lab Evaluation and Trends

- Bedside capillary glucose trends
- BMP/CMP
- CBC

Nursing Intervention Considerations

- Call for help or rapid response/code team if vital signs are unstable or there are signs of urgent distress
- Maintain a patent airway
  - Apply oxygen if hypoxic
- Verify patent IV if IVF or IV medication treatment is anticipated
  - Flush according to facility protocol; watch for swelling, erythema, pain, and other signs of infiltration
- Blood sugar if hypoglycemia is suspected
- Medications (if ordered or protocol allows)
  - PRN anti-emetic for nausea, IV/IM if vomiting
  - PRN acetaminophen or NSAIDs

- If hypoglycemic and has altered mental status or unable to swallow, give 1mg IV/IM/SQ glucagon, and/or 25–50mL IV 50% dextrose, or follow your facility's hypoglycemia protocol (goal is >100)
- Diet
  - Push fluids if there are no contraindications (>2,000mL/day)
  - Offer caffeinated beverages
  - If hypoglycemic, alert, and can swallow, give a fast-acting carbohydrate like a glucose tablet, 4oz of fruit juice, 8oz of milk, 4oz of non-diet soda, hard candy, or teaspoon of honey/sugar. Repeat until sugar is normalized (goal is >100)
- Positioning
  - HOB raised to comfort
  - Supine position may improve headache post-lumbar puncture
  - Side lying position if there is a decrease in LOC or the patient is vomiting
  - Reposition every 2–4 hours or establish an individualized turning schedule
- Monitor
  - Stay with the patient until stable
  - Pain levels
  - Vital signs and trends
  - Temperature trends
  - Oxygen saturation/pulse oximetry
  - Blood sugar trends (if applicable)
  - Orientation status changes, GCS
  - Neurological exam
  - Agitation levels
  - Sensation changes
  - Skin assessment every 8–24 hours
  - Signs of dehydration such as lethargy, decreased skin turgor, dry mucous membranes, tachycardia, and (orthostatic) hypotension

- Signs and symptoms of increased ICP such as worsening headache, nausea, vomiting, hypertension, bradypnea, altered mental status, vision changes, fixed or sluggish pupillary response, and GCS changes
- Signs of respiratory distress such as cyanosis, tachypnea, hypoxia, use of accessory muscles, diaphoresis, and adventitious lung sounds
- Safety
  - Perform a fall risk assessment and implement the appropriate strategies
- Environment
  - Provide a calm, quiet environment and reduce stimulation
  - Maintain a dimly lit environment if safety permits
  - Avoid bothersome odors in the room
  - Maintain a comfortable room temperature
  - Offer aromatherapy and/or music therapy (if appropriate)
  - Utilize a fan (if appropriate)
- Supportive care
  - Maintain effective communication between yourself, patient, and family
  - Provide emotional support and reassurance to the patient and family
  - Maintain a calm manner during patient interactions
  - Discuss plan of care with the patient and decide reasonable goals together
  - Notify the patient and family of changes in the plan of care
  - Promote skin care and integrity
  - Provide light clothing and bed linen
  - Offer heat or ice therapy
  - Encourage the use of glasses (if applicable)
  - **Educational topics (as applicable to the patient):**
    - General information regarding the patient's headache and differential diagnosis considerations
    - Procedure and intervention explanation and justification

- Explanation regarding referrals and specialist who may see them for this issue
- New medication education including reason, side effects, and administration needs
- Medication changes
- Pain scale and pain goals
- Oxygen therapy and maintenance
- Relaxation techniques and breathing exercises
- Trigger avoidance
- Proper positioning and turning schedule
- Skin care
- Safety needs and fall risk
- Increased fluid intake
- Stress reduction and management
- Sleep hygiene
- Alcohol and/or drug cessation and support
- Blood glucose measurement techniques and frequency
- When to notify the nurse or provider
- Signs and symptoms of hypoglycemia
- Dehydration prevention
- Pressure injury prevention

ISBARR Recommendation Considerations

- Ask the provider to come assess the patient STAT if they are unstable or red flag signs and symptoms are present
- Transfer to the ICU if hemodynamically unstable, advanced medication management is required, or closer monitoring is needed
- Medication
  - Discontinue/change suspected causative medication
  - Add PRN anti-emetic for nausea
  - Add PRN and/or scheduled pain medication
- IV fluid needs if oral intake is poor, there are signs of dehydration, the patient is NPO or hypotensive

- Imaging (depending on the suspected cause)
  - Head CT scan/MRI
- Labs (depending on the suspected cause)
  - ABG
  - BMP/CMP
  - CBC
  - Digoxin
  - Magnesium
- Safety
  - Fall risk protocol
- Monitoring needs
  - Blood sugars including frequency and parameters to call the provider (if applicable)
  - Continuous O_2 monitoring
  - Vital signs including frequency and parameters to call the provider
- Change diet to
  - Push oral fluids
- Protocols
  - CIWA-Ar if alcohol withdrawal is suspected
- Referrals
  - Neurology
- Ask if the provider wants anything else done
- Read back orders; ask that they enter all orders into the electronic medical record

ISBARR Template	
I **Introduction**	**Introduce Yourself and the Patient** • "Hello, Dr. Hoffman. This is Mike Mitchell. I am the nurse for your patient Becky Russell in Room 201."
S **Situation**	**Sign/Symptom You Are Concerned About** • "Over the past couple of hours, the patient has had a generalized 6/10 throbbing headache. It is better when she is lying flat, and worse when she is upright in bed."

ISBARR Template

	Associated Signs/Symptoms
	• "She is also having mild constant nausea."
B **Background**	**Vitals** • "Her vitals are stable, blood pressure is 137/80, heart rate is 70, respirations are 16, and her temperature is 99.0." **Exam** • "Exam shows no new signs of neurological deficits." **Past Medical History** • "She did have a lumbar puncture earlier today for her MS workup. She doesn't have a history of chronic headaches or headache issues before the lumbar puncture." **Labs and Medications** • "I do not have the results of her CSF testing yet."
A **Assessment**	**Assessment** • "I am concerned about a spinal headache from her lumbar puncture."
R **Recommendations** **R** **Read Back**	**Nurse's Recommendations, Interventions, and Read Back** • "I gave the patient 500mg of PRN Tylenol an hour ago with mild relief of the pain. I have made sure there are dimmed lights in the room and patient has continued to lie flat. Can you order something for her nausea? Did you want anything else done at this time?" • "Thank you, Dr. Hoffman. I will continue Tylenol but will change it to scheduled Tylenol 500mg PO every six hours. I will also start Zofran 4mg PO every eight hours PRN for nausea and call you if her symptoms worsen or persist."

Disclaimer: This dialogue is factitious and any resemblance to actual persons, living or dead, or actual events is purely coincidental.

In order to avoid order discrepancies, it is recommended that all orders be entered by the provider in the electronic medical record.

Select Differential Diagnosis Presentations

Anxiety

Overview: psychiatric disorder that can cause intense fear and worry

Patient may complain of: fatigue, chest pain, palpitations, dyspnea, nausea, vomiting, abdominal pain, constipation/diarrhea, paresthesias, tremors, headache, insomnia, mind racing, dizziness, feelings of impending doom

Objective findings: signs of acute distress, irritability, inability to focus, diaphoresis, tachycardia, hypertension, tachypnea, muscle tension

PMH considerations/risk factors: hx of anxiety, depression, PTSD, insomnia, substance abuse, physical abuse, recent physical or emotional trauma, family hx of psychiatric diseases

Diagnostics: clinical diagnosis; workup to rule out more emergent causes may be indicated

Cerebral Vascular Accident

Overview: partial or complete obstruction of blood flow to the brain due to ischemia or hemorrhage causing brain tissue death

Patient may complain of: vision changes, nausea, vomiting, dysphagia, headache, dizziness, seizures, insomnia, difficulty with memory, speaking, focusing, and understanding; unilateral paralysis of the face, arms, and legs

Objective findings: signs of acute distress, altered mental status, ptosis, dysarthria, hypertension, carotid bruit(s), facial droop, seizures, unilateral weakness and sensation disturbances, immobility, gait disturbances

PMH considerations/risk factors: hx of HTN, CAD, heart failure, hyperlipidemia, arrhythmia, cardiac valve disease, diabetes, obesity, nicotine use, substance abuse, family hx of heart disease

Diagnostics: Head CT/MRI

Dehydration

Overview: abnormal loss of extracellular fluid volume

Patient may complain of: fatigue, thirst, dry mouth, palpitations, constipation, oliguria, muscle cramps, dizziness, headache

Objective findings: fever, altered mental status, lethargy, irritability, decreased skin turgor, generalized skin dryness, dry mucous membranes, (orthostatic) hypotension, tachycardia, oliguria

PMH considerations/risk factors: hx of liver or renal disease/failure, recent vomiting and/or diarrhea, GI bleeding, polyuria, diuretic use, burn injury, or intense physical activity

Diagnostics: BMP/CMP, CBC, urine Na, I/O

Hypermagnesemia

Overview: elevated serum magnesium

Patient may complain of: fatigue, palpitations, nausea, vomiting, muscle spasms, headache; patient is typically asymptomatic unless severe

Objective findings: lethargy, altered mental status, diaphoresis, flushing, hypotension, bradycardia, arrhythmia, prolonged PR interval, wide QRS complex, bradypnea, decreased reflexes; exam is typically unremarkable unless severe

PMH considerations/risk factors: hx of gastroparesis, ileus, intestinal obstruction, CKD, AKI, hypothyroidism, magnesium supplementation

Diagnostics: serum Mg, ECG

Hyponatremia

Overview: low-serum sodium

Patient may complain of: fatigue, thirst, nausea, vomiting, anorexia, muscle cramps and weakness, headache; patient is typically asymptomatic unless severe

Objective findings: altered mental status, lethargy, irritability, tachycardia, weak pulses, bradypnea, decreased reflexes; exam is typically unremarkable unless severe

PMH considerations/risk factors: recent GI loss, hx of CKD, heart failure, diuretic use, SIADH, dehydration

Diagnostics: serum Na

Hypothyroidism

Overview: underactive thyroid gland

Patient may complain of: fatigue, cold intolerance, constipation, weight gain, irregular menstrual cycles, headache, paresthesias

Objective findings: lethargy, skin dryness, facial swelling, goiter, bradycardia, hypotension, hypoactive bowel sounds, decreased reflexes

PMH considerations/risk factors: hx of thyroid dysfunction, autoimmune diseases, radiation therapy of the head and neck, previous thyroidectomy, female gender

Diagnostics: TSH, T3, free T4, TPO; thyroid US may be considered

Increased Intracranial Pressure

Overview: rise in pressure within the cranial cavity

Patient may complain of: vision changes, nausea, vomiting, headache, confusion, seizures

Objective findings: signs of acute distress, altered mental status, GCS changes, sluggish/fixed pupillary response, hypertension, bradycardia, bradypnea

PMH considerations/risk factors: hx of TBI, CVA, CNS infections, hydrocephalus, cancer, seizures, HTN

Diagnostics: ICP monitoring, head CT/MRI

Influenza

Overview: viral respiratory illness

Patient may complain of: chills, fever, fatigue, body aches, sore throat, nasal congestion, nasal drainage, dry coughing, headache

Objective findings: signs of acute distress/illness, lethargy, altered mental status (elderly), fever, tachycardia, pharyngeal erythema, conjunctival erythema, nasal turbinate swelling, rhinorrhea, lymphadenopathy, cough

PMH considerations/risk factors: recent exposure to influenza, pregnancy, hx of immunosuppression, COPD, older/younger age, influenza season, immunization status

Diagnostics: clinical diagnosis; rapid flu test and CBC may be considered

Meningitis

Overview: inflammation and infection of the meninges surrounding the brain and spinal cord

Patient may complain of: chills, fever, fatigue, photophobia, neck pain, anorexia, nausea, vomiting, headache, confusion, dizziness

Objective findings: signs of acute distress/illness, lethargy, fever, irritability, altered mental status, petechial rash, nuchal rigidity (positive Brudzinski, Kernig sign), seizures, signs of increased ICP

PMH considerations/risk factors: hx of TBI, immunosuppression, pregnancy, close quarter living situations, recent travel outside of the United States, alcohol abuse, older/younger age

Diagnostics: CBC, lumbar puncture, head CT

Migraine Headache

Overview: recurrent head pain with or without aura

Patient may complain of: generalized weakness, photophobia, phonophobia, blurred vision, nausea, vomiting, throbbing lateralized headache, paresthesias, dizziness, presence of an aura

Objective findings: irritability, intolerance to light and sound; exam is typically unremarkable

PMH considerations/risk factors: hx of migraines, increased psychological stress, lack of sleep, nicotine use, alcohol abuse/use, family hx of migraines, female gender, younger age (<40 years old)

Diagnostics: clinical diagnosis; head CT/MRI may be considered initially

Otitis Media

Overview: infection or inflammation of the middle ear

Patient may complain of: chills, fever, fatigue, otalgia, hearing changes, tinnitus, nasal congestion, nasal drainage, coughing, anorexia, nausea, headache, dizziness

Objective findings: signs of acute distress/illness, lethargy, fever, irritability, erythematous bulging tympanic membrane with or without effusion, otorrhea (perforation)

PMH considerations/risk factors: hx of otitis media, eustachian tube dysfunction, younger age

Diagnostics: clinical diagnosis

Post-Nasal Drip (Upper Airway Cough Syndrome)

Overview: excessive mucous produced by the nasal mucosa that accumulates in the back of the nose or throat

Patient may complain of: sneezing, nasal congestion, nasal drainage, sore throat, coughing, headache

Objective findings: nasal turbinate swelling, rhinorrhea, halitosis, posterior pharyngeal erythema, cobblestoning and drainage, cough

PMH considerations/risk factors: hx of allergies, asthma, GERD, recent respiratory illness

Diagnostics: clinical diagnosis

Sinusitis

Overview: inflammation of the sinuses, typically due to an infection

Patient may complain of: chills, fever, fatigue, facial pain, nasal congestion, nasal drainage, ear pain, dental pain, sore throat, coughing, sputum production, nausea, headache; acute symptoms last <4 weeks

Objective findings: signs of acute illness, low-grade fever, lethargy, frontal/maxillary tenderness, nasal turbinate swelling, rhinorrhea (purulent can indicate bacterial infection), halitosis, pharyngeal erythema, cough, sputum; signs and symptoms are more severe with a bacterial infection

PMH considerations/risk factors: hx of chronic sinusitis, allergies, asthma, immunosuppression, nicotine use

Diagnostics: clinical diagnosis; workup to rule out more emergent causes may be indicated

Sleep Apnea

Overview: pauses in breathing (varying in number and length of time) while sleeping

Patient may complain of: snoring, daytime fatigue, headaches, inability to concentrate, mood changes, dry mouth, insomnia

Objective findings: elevated BMI, mouth breathing, thick neck, enlarged tonsils/uvula/soft palate, hypertension

PMH considerations/risk factors: hx of obesity, enlarged tonsils, nicotine use, narcotic pain medication use, CVA, family hx of sleep apnea, male gender, older age

Diagnostics: sleep study

Tension Headache

Overview: episodic benign head pain

Patient may complain of: non-throbbing head pain, described as "band like," usually generalized or bilateral

Objective findings: pericranial muscle tenderness; exam is typically unremarkable

PMH considerations/risk factors: hx of headaches, increased psychological stress, lack of sleep, nicotine use, alcohol abuse/use

Diagnostics: clinical diagnosis

Transient Ischemic Attack

Overview: transient obstruction of blood flow to the brain mimicking a CVA

Patient may complain of: vision changes, nausea, vomiting, dysphagia, headache, dizziness, seizures, insomnia, difficulty with memory, speaking, focusing, and understanding; unilateral paralysis of face, arms, and legs; signs and symptoms are transient in nature

Objective findings: signs of acute distress, altered mental status, ptosis, dysarthria, hypertension, carotid bruit(s), facial droop, seizures, unilateral weakness and sensation disturbances, immobility, gait disturbances; may not have abnormal exam findings due to transient nature of the issue

PMH considerations/risk factors: hx of HTN, CAD, heart failure, hyperlipidemia, arrhythmia, cardiac valve disease, diabetes, obesity, nicotine use, substance abuse, family hx of heart disease

Diagnostics: Head CT/MRI

Upper Respiratory Infection

Overview: broad term for infection of the upper respiratory tract, including the nose, throat, and upper airway

Patient may complain of: chills, fever, fatigue, nasal congestion, nasal drainage, sore throat, coughing, sputum production, nausea, vomiting, headache; symptoms have a short duration (<10 days)

Objective findings: signs of acute illness, low-grade fever, lethargy, conjunctival erythema, nasal turbinate swelling, rhinorrhea, halitosis, pharyngeal erythema, cough, sputum; signs and symptoms are typically mild in nature

PMH considerations/risk factors: hx of asthma, COPD, immunosuppression, allergies, nicotine use

Diagnostics: clinical diagnosis; workup to rule out more emergent causes may be indicated

Withdrawal (Alcohol)

Overview: rapid or abrupt decrease in alcohol intake causing physical and psychological disturbances

Patient may complain of: fever, chills, palpitations, anorexia, nausea, vomiting, diarrhea, seizures, headache, alcohol craving, insomnia, anxiety

Objective findings: signs of acute distress, fever, irritability, altered mental status, diaphoresis, tachycardia, hypertension, hepatomegaly, ascites, seizures, tremors, hallucinations/delirium

PMH considerations: hx of alcohol abuse, longer cessation (>48 hrs) since last drink, other substance abuse

Diagnostics: toxicology screen; workup to rule out more emergent causes may be indicated

References

American Academy of Neurology. (2012). *Update: Pharmacologic treatment for episodic migraine prevention in adults.* Retrieved from https://www.aan.com/guidelines/home/getguidelinecontent/545

American Medical Directors Association. (2010). *Know-it-all before you call: Data collection system.* Columbia, MD: Author.

Anderson, D., Larson, D., Ferguson, A., Klaas, J., Kushner, F., Peterson, B., . . . Thomson, R. (2016). Diagnosis and initial treatment of ischemic stroke. *Institute for Clinical Systems Improvement.* Retrieved from https://www.icsi.org/_asset/xql3xv/Stroke.pdf

Bajwa, Z. H, & Wootton, R. J. (2016). Evaluation of headache in adults. In J. F. Dashe (Ed.), *UpToDate.* Retrieved from https://www.uptodate.com/contents/evaluation-of-headache-in-adults

Becker, W. J., Findlay, T., Moga, C., Scott, N. A., Harstall, C., & Taenzer, P. (2015). Guideline for primary care management of headache in adults. *Canadian Family Physician, 61*(8), 670–679.

Beithon, J., Gallenberg, M., Johnson, K., Kildahl, P., Krenik, J., Liebow, M., . . . Swanson, J. (2013). Diagnosis and treatment of headache. *Institute for Clinical Systems Improvement.* Retrieved from https://www.guideline.gov/summaries/summary/43791/diagnosis-and-treatment-of-headache

Bulechek, G. M., Butcher, H. K., Dochterman, J. M., & Wagner, C. (2013). *Nursing intervention classification (NIC).* St. Louis, MO: Elsevier Mosby.

Conti, P. C., Costa, Y. M., Goncalves, D. A., & Svensson, P. (2016). Headaches and myofascial temporomandibular disorders: Overlapping entities, separate managements? *Journal of Oral Rehabilitation, 43,* 702–715.

Cutrer, F. M., & Edlow, J. A. (2018). Evaluation of the adult with non-traumatic headache in the emergency room. In J. Grayzel, & J. F. Dashe (Eds.), *UpToDate.* Retrieved from https://www.uptodate.com/contents/evaluation-of-the-adult-with-nontraumatic-headache-in-the-emergency-department

Desai, S. P. (2009). *Clinician's guide to laboratory medicine* (3rd ed.). Houston, TX: MD2B.

Evans, R. W., & Timm, J. S. (2017). New daily persistent headache caused by a multinodular goiter and headaches associated with thyroid disease. *Headache, 57,* 285–289.

Feleppa, M., Fucci, S., & Bigal, M. E. (2017). Primary headaches in an elderly population seeking medical care for cognitive decline. *Headache, 57,* 209–216.

Garza, I., & Schwedt, T. J. (2016). New daily persistent headache. In J. F. Dashe (Ed.), *UpToDate*. Retrieved from https://www.uptodate.com/contents/new-daily-persistent-headache

Garza, I., & Schwedt, T. J. (2017). Medication overuse headache: Etiology, clinical features, and diagnosis. In J. F. Dashe (Ed.), *UpToDate*. Retrieved from https://www.uptodate.com/contents/medication-overuse-headache-etiology-clinical-features-and-diagnosis

Hainer, B. L, & Matheson, E. M. (2013). Approach to acute headache in adults. *American Family Physician, 87*(10), 682–687.

Hale, A., & Hovey, M. J. (2014). *Fluid, electrolyte and acid-base imbalances.* Philadelphia, PA: F.A. Davis Company.

Jarvis, C. (2015). *Physical examination & health assessment.* St. Louis, MO: Elsevier.

Kelley, K., Latchem, S., Layden, J., Neilson, J., Nunes, V., Riley, S., . . . Westby, M. National Institute for Health and Clinical Excellence. (2012). *Headaches: Diagnosis and management of headaches in young people and adults.* Retrieved from https://www.ncbi.nlm.nih.gov/pubmedhealth/PMH0078140/pdf/PubMedHealth_PMH0078140.pdf

LeBlond, R. F., Brown, D. D., Suneja, M., & Szot, J. F. (2015). *DeGowin's diagnostic examination* (10th ed.). New York, NY: McGraw-Hill.

Lovely, M. P., Stewart-Amidei, C., Arzbaecher, J., Bell, S., Maher, M. E., Maida, M., . . . Nicolaseau, G. (2016). *Care of the adult patient with a brain tumor.* Retrieved from http://aann.org/uploads/Membership/SFG/neurooncology/AANN14_ABT_Module_2016_update.pdf

Management of Concussion-Mild Traumatic Brain Injury Working Group. (2016). *VA/DoD clinical practice guideline for the management of concussion-mild traumatic brain injury.* Retrieved from https://www.healthquality.va.gov/guidelines/Rehab/mtbi/mTBICPGFullCPG50821816.pdf

Marmura, M. J., Silberstein, S. D., & Schwedt, T. J. (2015). The acute treatment of migraine in adults: The American headache society evidence assessment of migraine pharmacotherapies. *Headache, 55,* 3–20.

McCance, K. L., Huether, S. E., Brashers, V. L., & Rote, N. S. (2014). *Pathophysiology: The biologic basis for disease in adults and children* (7th ed.). St. Louis, MO: Elsevier.

National Institute for Health and Care Excellence. (2014). *Head injury: Assessment and early management.* Retrieved from https://www.nice.org.uk/guidance/cg176/resources/head-injury-assessment-and-early-management-pdf-35109755595493

Papadakis, M. A., & McPhee, S. J. (2017). *Current medical diagnosis and treatment* (56th ed.). New York, NY: McGraw-Hill.

Prakash, S., & Rathore, C. (2016). Side-locked headaches: An algorithm-based approach. *Journal of Headache and Pain, 17*(95), 1–14.

Pringsheim, T., Davenport, W., Mackie, G., Worthington, I., Aube, M., Christie, S. N., & Becker W. J. (2012). Canadian headache society prophylactic guidelines development group: Canadian headache society guideline for migraine prophylaxis. *Canadian Journal of Neurological Sciences, 39*(2), 51–59.

Raftery, A. T., Lim, E., & Ostor, A. J. (2014). *Differential diagnosis* (4th ed.). London: Elsevier.

Ramzan, M., & Fisher, M. (2018). Headache, migraine, and stroke. In Dashe, J. F. (Ed.), *UpToDate.* Retrieved from https://www.uptodate.com/contents/headache-migraine-and-stroke

Rosenfeld, R. M., Piccirillo, J. F., Chandrasekhar, S. S., Brook, I., Ashok Kumar, K., Kramper, M., . . . Corrigan, M.D. (2015). Clinical practice guideline: Adult sinusitis. *Otolaryngology Head Neck Surgery, 152*(2), 1–39.

Seller, R. H., & Symons, A. B. (2012). *Differential diagnosis of common complaints* (6th ed.). Philadelphia, PA: Elsevier.

Sun-Edelstein, C., & Lay, C. L. (2018). Post-lumbar puncture headache. In J. F. Dashe, & M. Crowley (Ed.), *UpToDate.* Retrieved from https://www.uptodate.com/contents/post-lumbar-puncture-headache

Taylor, F. R. (2017). Tension-type headache in adults: Acute treatment. In J. F. Dashe (Ed.), *UpToDate.* Retrieved from https://www.uptodate.com/contents/tension-type-headache-in-adults-acute-treatment

Tepper, D. (2016). Thunderclap headaches. *Headache: The Journal of Head and Face Pain, 56*(9), 1563–1564.

Uphold, C. R., & Graham, M. V. (2013). *Clinical guidelines in family practice* (5th ed.). Gainesville, FL: Barmarrae Books.

Working Group of the Clinical Practice Guideline on the Management of Invasive Meningococcal Disease. (2013). *Clinical practice guideline on the management of invasive meningococcal disease.* Retrieved from http://www.guiasalud.es/GPC/GPC_525_EMI_ICS_compl_en.pdf

Yancy, J. R., Sheridan, R., & Koren, K. G. (2014). Chronic daily headache: Diagnosis and management. *American Family Physician, 89*(8), 642–648.

CHAPTER 18

Hematuria

Hematuria is defined as blood in the urine and is separated into two different types: gross and microscopic. Gross hematuria is blood that can be seen with the naked eye, while microscopic hematuria can only be detected through urine dipstick or urinalysis. The etiology of hematuria ranges from benign issues like UTI or urolithiasis, to malignancies of the kidney and bladder. The most common cause of hematuria comes from an unknown etiology. Painless gross hematuria is more suspicious for malignancy, and in this situation the nurse should assess the patient's risk factors for cancer, such as older age, male gender, a history of smoking or pelvic radiation, chronic use of an indwelling catheter, and voiding difficulties. Patients who are taking anticoagulants and antiplatelet drugs are at higher risk for hematuria, but it should not be the assumed cause, and a workup would be done regardless. Hematuria may require evaluation by nephrology or urology, depending on the location of the problem in the GU tract. It is the nurse's priority to quickly detect the hematuria, perform thorough subjective questioning, monitor for other signs of bleeding, collect a clean catch urine sample, and notify the provider.

Differential Diagnosis Considerations

Common: anticoagulant use, BPH, exercise induced, menses, pyelonephritis, trauma, urolithiasis, UTI

Consider: AV malformation, bleeding/clotting disorders, endometriosis, food dye, glomerulonephritis, GU malignancy, hydronephrosis, hypercalciuria, hyperuricosuria, interstitial cystitis, interstitial nephritis, malignant HTN, papillary necrosis, polycystic kidney disease, prostatitis, renal vein thrombus, sarcoidosis, sickle cell anemia, SLE, TB, thrombocytopenia, ureter stricture

Questions to Ask the Patient/Family/Witness/Yourself

- When did you first notice blood in your urine?
- Where do you see the blood? In the toilet? On toilet paper with wiping? Spots in your underwear?
- Do you see blood at the beginning of voiding, mid-void, or at the end of voiding?
- Have there been any blood clots in your urine?
- Do you see blood every time you urinate?
- Is there an odor to your urine?
- What color is your urine (red, pink, cola colored)?
- Do you have any pain when you urinate? Do you have pain in your abdomen, pelvis, flank, or back?
- Have you been urinating more than usual? If so, how often are you going?
- Do you feel like you empty your bladder completely when you urinate?
- How much fluid are you drinking on a daily basis?
- Any recent intake of artificial food coloring, beet root, blackberries, blueberries, rhubarb, or fava beans?
- Do you have a history of blood in your urine? If so, what has been done or used to treat it?
- When was your last menstrual period? (if applicable)
- Have you had any recent: GU infection? GU surgery? trauma to the abdomen, pelvis, back, or flank? radiation therapy? travel outside of the United States? vigorous exercise?
- Have you had any recent invasive interventions such as GU biopsy or a urinary catheter?
- Do you take any anticoagulants?
- Have you taken any new prescribed or over-the-counter medications? Have there been any recent changes to your current medication?

Associated Signs/Symptoms: PAIN: pain anywhere; GENERAL: chills, fatigue, fever, weight changes; CARDIOVASCULAR: chest pain/tightness; RESPIRATORY: dyspnea; GASTROINTESTINAL: nausea, signs of GI bleeding, vomiting; GENITOURINARY:

hesitancy, incontinence, itching, nocturia, penile/vaginal discharge, urgency, retention, vaginal bleeding; PSYCHOLOGICAL: confusion

Recommended Assessments

- Vital signs
- Temperature
- Weight and nutritional status
- I/O
- Pain scale (if applicable)
  - Tolerable pain level
- General
  - Level of consciousness and orientation
  - Inspect: signs of acute distress, acute illness, affect, restlessness
- Skin
  - Inspect: diaphoresis, dryness, ecchymosis, pallor
  - Palpate: temperature, turgor
- Mouth
  - Inspect: mucous membrane moisture level
- Cardiovascular
  - Auscultate: heart sounds, rate, rhythm
- Respiratory
  - Inspect: respiratory effort
  - Auscultate: lung sounds
- Gastrointestinal
  - Inspect: distention
  - Auscultate: bowel sounds
  - Palpate: guarding, masses, (rebound) tenderness
- Rectal (if applicable)
  - Inspect: bleeding, erythema, fissures, hemorrhoids, open lesions, swelling
- Genitourinary
  - Inspect: external drainage, erythema, swelling, lesions
  - Palpate: bladder distention, CVAT
- Extremities
  - Inspect: IV site (if applicable)

Past Medical History Considerations

Puts the patient at risk for differential considerations

- CKD
- Diabetes
- GU/GYN surgery
- Obesity
- Nicotine use
- Radiation therapy to the abdomen/pelvis

Reoccurrence/exacerbation should be considered

- Prostatitis
- Urolithiasis
- UTI

Chronic conditions that can cause hematuria

- Bleeding/clotting disorder
- BPH
- GU malignancy
- Endometriosis
- Interstitial cystitis
- Interstitial nephritis
- Polycystic kidney disease
- Sarcoidosis
- Sickle cell anemia
- SLE
- Ureter stricture

Medication Evaluation

Puts the patient at risk for GU bleeding

- Anticoagulants
- Antiplatelet agents

Can cause hematuria or discoloration of the urine

- Cyclophosphamide
- Isoniazid
- Levodopa
- Methyldopa
- Metronidazole
- Nitrofurantoin
- NSAIDs
- Penicillin
- Phenazopyridine
- Phenytoin
- Quinine
- Rifampin
- Sulfonamides

Lab Evaluation and Trends

- BMP/CMP
- CBC
- PT/INR

Nursing Intervention Considerations

- Verify patent IV if IVF or IV medication treatment is anticipated
  - Flush according to facility protocol; watch for swelling, erythema, pain, and other signs of infiltration
- Bladder scan PVR if urinary retention symptoms are present
- Medications (if ordered or protocol allows)
  - Hold suspected causative medication until discussion with the provider
- Diet
  - Push fluids if there are no contraindications (>2,000mL/day)
  - Avoid bladder irritants such as soda, coffee, tea, chocolate

- Avoid foods that can discolor the urine such as beet root, blackberries, blueberries, rhubarb, fava beans, and foods with artificial coloring
- Positioning
  - Supine or side lying position with knees flexed to chest to take tension off the abdominal wall if the patient has active abdominal pain
  - Reposition every 2–4 hours or establish an individualized turning schedule
- Collect
  - Urine sample
- Monitor
  - Pain levels
  - Vital signs and trends
  - Temperature trends
  - I/O
  - Orientation status changes
  - Agitation levels
  - Skin assessment every 8–24 hours or more frequently if the patient is incontinent
  - Signs of dehydration such as lethargy, decreased skin turgor, dry mucous membranes, tachycardia, and (orthostatic) hypotension
  - Signs and symptoms of GU infection such as fever, chills, dysuria, hematuria, increased urinary frequency and urgency, fatigue, altered mental status, and back/flank pain
  - Signs and symptoms of sepsis such as fever, chills, hypotension, altered mental status, hypoxia, cool clammy skin, dyspnea, oliguria, tachycardia, and tachypnea
  - Signs and symptoms of blood loss such as fatigue, dizziness, dyspnea, melena, hematochezia, hematemesis, hematuria, epistaxis, pallor, ecchymosis, altered mental status, hypotension, tachycardia, tachypnea, and hemoptysis
  - Catheter patency and kinking
  - PVR
  - Urine output color, frequency, and volume

- Safety
  - Perform a fall risk assessment and implement the appropriate strategies
- Supportive care
  - Maintain effective communication between yourself, patient, and family
  - Provide emotional support and reassurance to the patient and family
  - Maintain a calm manner during patient interactions
  - Discuss plan of care with the patient and decide reasonable goals together
  - Notify the patient and family of changes in the plan of care
  - Discuss any religious restrictions that may affect their care (blood transfusion)
  - Promote skin care and integrity
  - **Educational topics (as applicable to the patient):**
    - General information regarding the patient's hematuria and differential diagnosis considerations
    - Procedure and intervention explanation and justification
    - Explanation regarding referrals and specialist who may see them for this issue
    - Medication changes
    - Laboratory monitoring needs
    - Blood transfusion needs
    - Pain scale and pain goals
    - Catheter care
    - Bladder irrigation
    - Bladder scanning and PVR
    - Proper positioning and turning schedule
    - Peri-care and proper hygiene
    - Skin care
    - Safety needs and fall risk
    - Handwashing and infection control measures
    - Increased fluid intake

- Avoidance of bladder irritants
- Avoidance of food/fluid that can discolor the urine
- When to notify the nurse or provider
- Signs and symptoms of GU infection
- Signs and symptoms of abnormal bleeding
- Dehydration prevention
- Pressure injury prevention

ISBARR Recommendation Considerations

- Medication
  - Discontinue/change suspected causative medication
- IV fluid needs if oral intake is poor, there are signs of dehydration, the patient is NPO or hypotensive
- Bladder scanning needs with or without PVR
- Bladder irrigation
- Foley catheter insertion or discontinuation
- Imaging (depending on the suspected cause)
  - Abdominal/pelvic CT scan, KUB, renal/bladder US
- Labs (depending on the suspected cause)
  - BMP/CMP
  - CBC
  - PT/INR
  - Type and cross match
  - Urinalysis
  - Urine culture
- Safety
  - Fall risk protocol
- Monitoring needs
  - Daily weights
  - Strict I/O
  - Vital signs including frequency and parameters to call the provider
- Change diet to
  - Push oral fluids

- Protocols
  - Blood transfusion (if applicable)
- Referrals
  - Nephrology
  - Urology
- Ask if the provider wants anything else done
- Read back orders; ask that they enter all orders into the electronic medical record

ISBARR Template	
I **Introduction**	**Introduce Yourself and the Patient** • "Hello, Dr. Chaudoir, this is Mai Lor. I am the nurse for Mrs. Stephanie Azarian at Golden Living Center in Milwaukee."
S **Situation**	**Sign/Symptom You Are Concerned About** • "I'm calling because a large amount of pink urine was seen in her Depend® this morning." **Associated Signs/Symptoms** • "She is not having any fever, dysuria, or fatigue, but is complaining of mild pelvic cramping and fullness."
B **Background**	**Vitals** • "Vitals are stable. Blood pressure is 130/82, heart rate is 80, respirations are 18, and temperature is 99.4." **Exam** • "She has no abdominal or CVA tenderness. I haven't noticed any orientation changes." **Past Medical History** • "She does have a history of UTIs. Her last one was six months ago." **Labs and Medications** • "She is taking aspirin on a daily basis, but no other anticoagulants. Her creatinine and GFR were done a week ago and were normal."

ISBARR Template	
A **Assessment**	**Assessment** • "I am concerned she is having a recurrent UTI."
R **Recommendations** **R** **Read Back**	**Nurse's Recommendations, Interventions, and Read Back** • "I collected a clean catch urine sample. Did you want me to send it for a urinalysis and culture? Do you want to start antibiotics? Is there anything else you would like me to do?" • "Thank you, Dr. Chaudoir, if I could just read those orders back. You would like the urine to be sent for UA, culture, and sensitivity. Start Macrobid 100mg 1 tab BID for 7 days. I will monitor vital signs, including temperature, every 12 hours and as needed, and will call with any abnormal findings."

Disclaimer: This dialogue is factitious and any resemblance to actual persons, living or dead, or actual events is purely coincidental.

In order to avoid order discrepancies, it is recommended that all orders be entered by the provider in the electronic medical record.

Select Differential Diagnosis Presentations

Benign Prostatic Hyperplasia

Overview: enlargement of the prostate due to hyperplasia

Patient may complain of: urinary hesitancy, diminished stream force, urinary frequency and retention, nocturia, incontinence, hematuria

Objective findings: enlarged prostate with digital rectal exam, bladder distention

PMH considerations/risk factors: hx of BPH, prostatitis, urinary retention, prostate cancer, diabetes, obesity, recent UTI or trauma to pelvis/genitals, older age

Diagnostics: PSA, urinalysis, urine culture, biopsy, PVR

Pyelonephritis

Overview: bacterial infection of the kidney

    Patient may complain of: fever; chills; nausea; vomiting; abdominal/back/flank pain; increased urinary frequency, retention, and urgency; dysuria; hematuria; urine odor; confusion (elderly)

    Objective findings: signs of acute distress/illness, altered mental status (elderly), fever, tachycardia, CVAT, abdominal tenderness, bladder distention

    PMH considerations: hx of frequent UTIs, diabetes, urolithiasis, urinary retention, immunosuppression, pregnancy, poor fluid intake, immobility, recent catheter use or GU surgery, female gender

    Diagnostics: CBC, urinalysis, urine culture, renal US

Urolithiasis

Overview: calculi that form in the urinary tract

    Patient may complain of: severe flank/back pain, may radiate to the abdomen, nausea, vomiting, urinary urgency and frequency, dysuria, hematuria

    Objective findings: signs of acute distress/illness, irritability, fidgeting, CVAT, abdominal tenderness

    PMH considerations/risk factors: hx of urolithiasis, short bowel syndrome, malnutrition, diabetes, gout, obesity, dehydration, bariatric surgery, family hx of urolithiasis, female gender

    Diagnostics: urinalysis, KUB, renal US

Urinary Tract Infection

Overview: broad term for infection of the urinary tract including the urethra, bladder, ureters, and kidneys

    Patient may complain of: fever, chills, abdominal/back/flank/pelvic pain, nausea, vomiting, dysuria, increased urinary frequency, retention and urgency, hematuria, incontinence, urine odor, confusion (elderly)

    Objective findings: fever, altered mental status (elderly), pelvic tenderness, bladder distention; exam is typically unremarkable

PMH considerations/risk factors: hx of frequent UTIs, diabetes, interstitial cystitis, urinary retention, immunosuppression, dehydration, pregnancy, incontinence, recent catheter use, GU surgery or sexual activity, immobility, female gender

Diagnostics: urinalysis/urine dipstick, urine culture

References

American Medical Directors Association. (2010). *Know-it-all before you call: Data collection system.* Columbia, MD: Author.

American Urological Association. (2013). AUA guideline addresses diagnosis, evaluation, and follow-up of asymptomatic microhematuria. *American Family Physician, 87*(9), 652–653.

Bagnall, P. (2014). Haematuria: Classification, causes and investigations. *British Journal of Nursing, 23*(20), 1074–1078.

Bulechek, G. M., Butcher, H. K., Dochterman, J. M., & Wagner, C. (2013). *Nursing intervention classification (NIC).* St. Louis, MO: Elsevier Mosby.

D'Agata, E., Loeb, M. B., & Mitchell, S. L. (2013). Challenges in assessing nursing home residents with advanced dementia for suspected urinary tract infections. *Journal of the American Geriatrics Society, 61*(1), 62–66.

Davis, R., Jones, J. S., Barocas, D. A., Castle, E. P., Lang, E. K., Leveillee, R. J., . . . Weitzel, W. (2012). Diagnosis, evaluation and follow-up of asymptomatic microhematuria (AMH) in adults: AUA guideline. *The Journal of Urology, 188,* 2473–2481.

Desai, S. P. (2009). *Clinician's guide to laboratory medicine* (3rd ed.). Houston, TX: MD2B.

Hale, A., & Hovey, M. J. (2014). *Fluid, electrolyte and acid-base imbalances.* Philadelphia, PA: F.A. Davis Company.

Jarvis, C. (2015). *Physical examination & health assessment.* St. Louis, MO: Elsevier.

Kashtan, C. E. (2015). Thin basement membrane nephropathy (benign familial hematuria). In A. Q. Lam (Ed.), *UpToDate.* Retrieved from https://www.uptodate.com/contents/thin-basement-membrane-nephropathy-benign-familial-hematuria

King, K., & Steggall, M. (2014). Haematuria: From identification to treatment. *British Journal of Nursing, 23*(9), 28–32.

Kurtz, M., Feldman, A. S., & Perazella, M. A. (2017). Etiology and evaluation of hematuria in adults. In A. Q. Lam (Ed.), *UpToDate.* Retrieved from https://www.uptodate.com/contents/etiology-and-evaluation-of-hematuria-in-adults

LeBlond, R. F., Brown, D. D., Suneja, M., & Szot, J. F. (2015). *DeGowin's diagnostic examination* (10th ed.). New York, NY: McGraw-Hill.

Liu, J. J., Jones, S., & Rao, P. K. (2016). Urinalysis in the evaluation of hematuria. *JAMA, 315*(24), 2726–2727.

McCance, K. L., Huether, S. E., Brashers, V. L., & Rote, N. S. (2014). *Pathophysiology: The biologic basis for disease in adults and children* (7th ed.). St. Louis, MO: Elsevier.

Mercieri, A. (2017). Exercise-induced hematuria. In A. Q. Lam (Ed.), *UpToDate.* Retrieved from https://www.uptodate.com/contents/exercise-induced-hematuria

Nielsen, M., & Qaseem, A. (2016). Hematuria as a marker of occult urinary tract cancer: Advice for high-value care from the American college of physicians. *Annals of Internal Medicine, 164*(7), 488–498.

Niemi, M. A., & Cohen, R.A. (2015). Evaluation of microscopic hematuria: A critical review and proposed algorithm. *Advances in Chronic Kidney Disease, 22*(4), 289–296.

Papadakis, M. A., & McPhee, S. J. (2017). *Current medical diagnosis and treatment* (56th ed.). New York, NY: McGraw-Hill.

Raftery, A. T., Lim, E., & Ostor, A. J. (2014). *Differential diagnosis* (4th ed.). London: Elsevier.

Seller, R. H., & Symons, A. B. (2012). *Differential diagnosis of common complaints* (6th ed.). Philadelphia, PA: Elsevier.

Sharp, V. J., Barnes, K. T., & Erickson, B.A. (2013). Assessment of asymptomatic microscopic hematuria in adults. *American Family Physician, 88*(11), 747–754.

Uphold, C. R., & Graham, M. V. (2013). *Clinical guidelines in family practice* (5th ed.). Gainesville, FL: Barmarrae Books.

CHAPTER 19

Hemoptysis

Hemoptysis is defined as coughing up blood that originates from the respiratory tract. It can be a scant trace of blood streaked in the patient's sputum or a large blood volume loss, known as mass hemoptysis. In the current literature, the definition of mass hemoptysis is not universally accepted, and ranges from 500 to 1,000mL within a 24-hour period. It is an emergent situation that can lead to respiratory compromise and is associated with high mortality rates. It is important to assess where the bleeding is coming from and to discern between true hemoptysis and pseudohemoptysis, which is bleeding originating from the nose, pharynx, or GI tract. The nurse's priority is to maintain the patient's airway, provide adequate ventilation, ensure that the patient is hemodynamically stable, and hang urgent blood products if needed. A pulmonology referral may be indicated if a bronchoscopy evaluation is required.

Differential Diagnosis Considerations

Common: anticoagulant use, airway trauma, bronchiectasis, bronchitis, COPD, pneumonia, pseudohemoptysis, pulmonary malignancy, URI

Consider: airway-vascular fistula, anthrax, AV malformation, Behcet disease, bleeding/clotting disorders, bullous emphysema, cocaine use, cystic fibrosis, DIC, Dieulafoy's lesion, endocarditis, foreign body, Goodpasture syndrome, heart failure, Hughes–Stovin syndrome, medication induced, mitral valve stenosis, PE, pulmonary abscess, pulmonary artery rupture, pulmonary HTN, pulmonary pseudoaneurysm, SLE, TB, thrombocytopenia, Wegener's granulomatosis

Questions to Ask the Patient/Family/Witness/Yourself

- When did you first notice you were coughing up blood?
- Was the blood mixed with phlegm/sputum?
- Is the phlegm/sputum clear, white, purulent, red, brown, pink?
- How much blood was there (estimated amount)?
- Were there any blood clots?
- Do you see blood every time you cough up sputum?
- Do you have pain with coughing?
- Do you have a history of coughing up blood? If so, what has been done or used to treat it?
- Have you had any recent: respiratory illness? exposure to chemicals, smoke, or toxins? exposure to respiratory infection or been around anyone who is sick? hospitalization? immobilization such as prolonged time spent in bed or sitting? CV, pulmonary, or thoracic surgery? trauma to the abdomen, chest, face, or throat? travel outside of the United States?
- Have you had any recent invasive interventions such as bronchoscopy, endoscopy, intubation, pulmonary artery catheter (Swan-Ganz), pulmonary biopsy, or thoracic needle aspiration?
- Do you take any anticoagulants?
- Do you use any inhalers? If so, have you been taking them as prescribed?
- Have you taken any new prescribed or over-the-counter medications? Have there been any recent changes to your current medication?
- Do you smoke? How much (ppd)? How long have you been smoking? (if applicable)
- Do you have a history of drug use? What types and how much? Do you use on a daily basis? When was your last use? (if applicable)

Associated Signs/Symptoms: PAIN: pain anywhere; GENERAL: chills, fatigue, fever, weakness, weight changes; EENT: bleeding gums, epistaxis, hoarseness, sore throat; CARDIOVASCULAR: chest pain/tightness, edema, palpitations, PND, orthopnea; RESPIRATORY: cough, painful breathing/coughing, dyspnea, wheezing; GASTROINTESTINAL: heartburn, signs of GI bleeding; GENITOURINARY: hematuria; NEUROLOGICAL: dizziness; SKIN: ecchymosis; ENDOCRINE: night time sweating

Recommended Assessments

- Vital signs
- Temperature
- Weight and nutritional status
- I/O
- Pain scale (if applicable)
  - Tolerable pain level
- General
  - Level of consciousness and orientation
  - Inspect: signs of acute distress, acute illness, affect, restlessness
  - Difficulty speaking due to breathlessness
- Skin
  - Inspect: cyanosis, diaphoresis, dryness, ecchymosis, pallor
  - Palpate: temperature, turgor
- Mouth
  - Inspect: bleeding, dentition, lesions, mucous membrane moisture level
- Nose
  - Inspect: bleeding, turbinate swelling
- Head/face/neck
  - Inspect: signs of trauma
  - Palpate: swelling, tenderness
- Cardiovascular
  - Auscultate: heart sounds, rate, rhythm
- Respiratory
  - Inspect: chest asymmetry, respiratory effort, depth, pattern, use of accessory muscles
  - Auscultate: lung sounds, stridor

- Extremities
  - Inspect: IV site
  - Palpate: capillary refill, edema, pulses

Past Medical History Considerations

- Immunization status: influenza, pertussis, pneumonia

Puts the patient at risk for differential considerations

- AIDS/HIV
- Asthma
- CV/thoracic surgery
- Drug abuse/use
- Epistaxis
- Liver disease
- Immobilization
- Nicotine use
- PUD
- Radiation therapy to the neck/chest

Reoccurrence/exacerbation should be considered

- COPD
- GI bleed
- PE

Chronic conditions that can cause hemoptysis

- Bleeding/clotting disorder
- Cardiac valve disorders
- COPD
- Cystic fibrosis
- Goodpasture syndrome
- Heart failure
- Pulmonary HTN
- Pulmonary malignancy
- SLE

Medication Evaluation

Puts the patient at risk for pulmonary bleeding

- Anticoagulants
- Antiplatelet agents
- Bevacizumab
- NSAIDs

Used to treat common differential considerations

- Antibiotics → various respiratory infections
- Antitussives → acute cough
- Corticosteroids → airway inflammation
- Expectorants → acute cough
- ICS, LABA, LAMA, SABA, SAMA, and combination inhalers → chronic lung disease

Lab Evaluation and Trends

- CBC
- PT/INR

Nursing Intervention Considerations

- Call for help or rapid response/code team if vital signs are unstable or there are signs of urgent distress
- Maintain a patent airway
  - Apply oxygen if hypoxic
  - Encourage cough and deep breathing
  - Encourage slow relaxed deep breathing if hyperventilating
  - Chest splinting with a pillow to promote more effective coughing
  - Suction as needed
  - Provide oral care throughout the day (q2–4hrs)
  - Call respiratory therapy for signs of respiratory distress
- Verify patent IV if IVF or IV medication treatment is anticipated

- Flush according to facility protocol; watch for swelling, erythema, pain, and signs of infiltration
- Large bore IV is preferred if mass hemoptysis is present
- Medications (if ordered or protocol allows)
  - Hold suspected causative medication until discussion with the provider
  - PRN cough suppressant
  - PRN bronchodilator treatment per respiratory therapy if the patient is coughing or short of breath
- Diet
  - NPO if procedure or surgery is anticipated
  - Push fluids if there are no contraindications (>2,000mL/day)
- Activity
  - Encourage activity and ambulation if safety permits
- Positioning
  - HOB raised to comfort for respiratory distress
  - Reposition every 2–4 hours or establish an individualized turning schedule
- Collect
  - Sputum sample
- Monitor
  - Stay with the patient until stable
  - Pain levels
  - Vital signs and trends
  - Oxygen saturation/pulse oximetry
  - Temperature trends
  - Orientation status changes
  - Telemetry/cardiac monitor
  - Agitation levels
  - Peripheral pulses
  - Skin assessment every 8–24 hours
  - Signs of decreased cardiac output such as weak pulses, cool skin, altered mental status, hypotension, oliguria, and mottling

- Signs of respiratory distress such as cyanosis, tachypnea, hypoxia, use of accessory muscles, diaphoresis, and adventitious lung sounds
- Signs and symptoms of blood loss such as fatigue, dizziness, dyspnea, melena, hematochezia, hematemesis, hematuria, epistaxis, pallor, ecchymosis, altered mental status, hypotension, tachycardia, tachypnea, and hemoptysis
- Signs and symptoms of sepsis such as fever, chills, hypotension, altered mental status, hypoxia, cool clammy skin, dyspnea, oliguria, tachycardia, and tachypnea
- Sputum output color, consistency, frequency, and volume
- Safety
  - Perform a fall risk assessment and implement the appropriate strategies
- Environment
  - Provide a calm, quiet environment and reduce stimulation
  - Maintain a well-lit environment
  - Maintain a comfortable room temperature
  - Initiate isolation precautions: droplet, airborne
- Supportive care
  - Maintain effective communication between yourself, patient, and family
  - Provide emotional support and reassurance to the patient and family
  - Maintain a calm manner during patient interactions
  - Discuss plan of care with the patient and decide reasonable goals together
  - Notify the patient and family of changes in the plan of care
  - Identify barriers to care and compliance
  - Discuss any religious restrictions that may affect their care (blood transfusion)
  - Promote skin care and integrity

- **Educational topics (as applicable to the patient):**
  - General information regarding the patient's hemoptysis and differential diagnosis considerations
  - Procedure and intervention explanation and justification
  - Explanation regarding referrals and specialist who may see them for this issue
  - New medication education including reason, side effects, and administration needs
  - Medication changes
  - MDI administration techniques
  - Laboratory monitoring needs
  - Blood transfusion needs
  - Pain scale and pain goals
  - Oxygen therapy and maintenance
  - Relaxation techniques and breathing exercises
  - Cough and deep-breathing techniques
  - Trigger avoidance
  - Telemetry
  - Proper positioning and turning schedule
  - Skin care
  - Safety needs and fall risk
  - Handwashing and infection control measures
  - Isolation precaution needs
  - NPO diet
  - Increased fluid intake
  - Increased physical activity
  - Immunization needs
  - Drug cessation and support
  - Smoking cessation
  - When to notify the nurse or provider
  - Signs and symptoms of respiratory emergencies
  - Signs and symptoms of abnormal bleeding
  - Dehydration prevention
  - Pressure injury prevention

ISBARR Recommendation Considerations

- Ask the provider to come assess the patient STAT if they are unstable or showing signs of mass hemoptysis
- Transfer to the ICU if hemodynamically unstable, advanced medication management is required, or closer monitoring is needed
- Medication
  - Hold oral medications if the patient is unable to tolerate or NPO
  - Discuss changing medication routes with the provider (and pharmacy) if the patient is NPO
  - Discontinue/change suspected causative medication
  - Add corticosteroids for airway inflammation
  - Add PRN and/or scheduled bronchodilator nebulizer treatments per respiratory therapy for coughing, dyspnea, or other signs of respiratory distress
  - Add PRN cough suppressant
  - Add PPI, H2 antagonist or antacid for dyspepsia, heartburn, or other signs/symptoms of GERD
- IV fluid needs if oral intake is poor, there are signs of dehydration, and the patient is NPO or hypotensive
- ECG if cardiac etiology is suspected
- Imaging (depending on the suspected cause)
  - Chest CT scan, chest X-ray
- Labs (depending on the suspected cause)
  - ABG
  - CBC
  - D-dimer
  - PT/INR
  - Sputum culture
  - Type and cross match
- Safety
  - Activity level changes
  - Fall risk protocol
  - Isolation precautions: airborne, droplet

- Monitoring needs
  - Continuous O_2 monitoring
  - Telemetry/continuous cardiac monitoring
  - Daily weights
  - Vital signs including frequency and parameters to call the provider
- Change diet to (depending on the suspected cause)
  - NPO
  - Push oral fluids
- Protocols
  - Blood transfusion (if applicable)
- Referrals
  - Pulmonology
  - Respiratory therapy
- Ask if the provider wants anything else done
- Read back orders; ask that they enter all orders into the electronic medical record

ISBARR Template	
I **Introduction**	**Introduce Yourself and the Patient** • "Hello, Dr. Davis, this is Luciana Fitzgerald. I am the nurse for Ms. Lindy Berry in Room 204. She is your new admission from the ER who is being admitted for a COPD exacerbation."
S **Situation**	**Sign/Symptom You Are Concerned About** • "I am calling to make you aware that Ms. Berry has had three episodes of hemoptysis this morning. Her sputum is frothy and pink with blood streaks. I am estimating 30mL of sputum in the past two to three hours. She says she has had sputum like this on a daily basis for the past month."

ISBARR Template	
	Associated Signs/Symptoms • "She has moderate shortness of breath and wheezing when she is up walking. She is also coughing frequently, but has been denying chest pain."
B **Background**	**Vitals** • "Blood pressure is 138/80, heart rate is 80, respiratory rate is 18, temperature is 99.0, and her O_2 sat is somewhat low at 87% on room air." **Exam** • "Her lungs are course throughout with expiratory wheezing. She does not appear to be in any respiratory distress at rest. I didn't notice any bleeding from her mouth or nose." **Past Medical History** • "She does have a history of severe COPD. She has smoked one to two packs of cigarettes per day for the past 50 years. She also told me she was in India last month on vacation when the hemoptysis started, but wasn't exposed to anything she knows of." **Labs and Medications** • "Her WBC count in the ER was within normal limits. She had no anemia. Her chest X-ray showed hyperinflation, but no masses or infiltrates." • "She is not on any anti-coagulants."
A **Assessment**	**Assessment** • "Her hemoptysis does not seem severe at this time, but I am worried enough about it that I wanted you to be aware. I am suspecting it is from her uncontrolled COPD, but I am also concerned about her risk of lung cancer and her recent travel history."

ISBARR Template	
R Recommendations R Read Back	**Nurse's Recommendations, Interventions, and Read Back** • "I have placed her on 2 liters of oxygen, which has brought O_2 sat up to 92%. I am recommending we put her on droplet precautions. Did you want me to collect a sputum sample? Did you want any other imaging or labs?" • "Thank you, Dr. Davis. I just want to read those orders back to you. You would like me to keep her O_2 level above 90%, and start droplet precautions. I will make sure I have a sputum sample for you to see when you come to see her later today."

Disclaimer: This dialogue is factitious and any resemblance to actual persons, living or dead, or actual events is purely coincidental.

In order to avoid order discrepancies, it is recommended that all orders be entered by the provider in the electronic medical record.

Select Differential Diagnosis Presentations

Bronchitis

Overview: inflammation of the bronchioles typically due to an infection

Patient may complain of: fever, chills, fatigue, sore throat, nasal congestion, chest pain/tightness, coughing, dyspnea, wheezing, sputum production, hemoptysis

Objective findings: signs of acute illness, lethargy, low-grade fever, rhinorrhea, pharyngeal erythema, cough, sputum, adventitious breath sounds, tachypnea

PMH considerations/risk factors: hx of asthma, COPD, allergies, GERD, exposure to lung irritants, nicotine use, older age

Diagnostics: clinical diagnosis; ABG, chest X-ray, spirometry may be considered

Chronic Obstructive Pulmonary Disease Exacerbation

Overview: acute inflammation and swelling of the airway, progressively worsening COPD symptomology

Patient may complain of: worsening fatigue, activity intolerance, sputum production from baseline, chest pain/tightness, coughing, dyspnea, wheezing, hemoptysis, insomnia

Objective findings: signs of acute distress, lethargy, cyanosis, diaphoresis, hypoxia, breathlessness, cough, adventitious breath sounds, sputum, prolonged expirations, use of accessory muscles, barrel chest, digital clubbing

PMH considerations/risk factors: hx of COPD, asthma, allergies, GERD, recent respiratory illness, nicotine use

Diagnostics: clinical diagnosis; chest X-ray, spirometry may be considered

Pneumonia

Overview: infection of the air sacs in one or both lungs causing inflammation and fluid accumulation

Patient may complain of: chills, fever, fatigue, chest pain/tightness, dyspnea, wheezing, coughing, sputum production, hemoptysis, activity intolerance, anorexia, nausea, vomiting, headache

Objective findings: signs of acute distress/illness, lethargy, altered mental status (elderly), fever, tachycardia, tachypnea, use of accessory muscles, cough, sputum, hypoxia, adventitious breath sounds, dullness to percussion over consolidation, pleural friction rub

PMH considerations/risk factors: hx of COPD, asthma, immunosuppression, dysphagia, immunization status, recent/current hospitalization, intubation, nicotine use, alcohol abuse, older/younger age

Diagnostics: CBC, sputum culture, chest X-ray

Pulmonary Embolism

Overview: a blood clot in the pulmonary vasculature

Patient may complain of: chills, fever, chest pain, pain with deep breaths, palpitations, activity intolerance, dyspnea, coughing, hemoptysis, abdominal pain, dizziness

Objective findings: signs of acute distress, fever, pallor, cyanosis, diaphoresis, tachycardia, hypotension, S3/S4 heart sounds, tachypnea, hypoxia, cough, signs of DVT

PMH considerations/risk factors: hx of DVT, PE or CVA, bleeding/clotting disorder, cancer, pregnancy, HRT/birth control use, IV drug use, recent surgery, immobility, nicotine use

Diagnostics: D-dimer, chest CT, V/Q scan, chest X-ray

References

American Medical Directors Association. (2010). *Know-it-all before you call: Data collection system.* Columbia, MD: Author.

Bannister, M., & Ah-See, K. W. (2015). Evidenced-based management of haemoptysis by otolaryngologists. *Journal of Laryngology & Otology, 129*(8), 807–811. doi:10.1017/S0022215115001310

Desai, S. P. (2009). *Clinician's guide to laboratory medicine* (3rd ed.). Houston, TX: MD2B.

Earwood, J. S., & Thompson, T. D. (2015). Hemoptysis: Evaluation and management. *American Family Physician, 91*(4), 243–249.

Gulanick, M., & Myers, J. L. (2017). *Nursing care plans: Diagnosis, interventions, & outcomes* (9th ed.). St. Louis, MO: Elsevier.

Hale, A., & Hovey, M. J. (2014). *Fluid, electrolyte and acid-base imbalances.* Philadelphia, PA: F.A. Davis Company.

Hogrefe, C. (2014). *The initial evaluation and management of hemoptysis.* Retrieved from http://ir.uiowa.edu/cgi/viewcontent.cgi?article=1030&context=fmrc

Ingbar, D. H. (2017). Massive hemoptysis: Initial management. In G. Finlay (Ed.), *UpToDate.* Retrieved from https://www.uptodate.com/contents/massive-hemoptysis-initial-management

Jarvis, C. (2015). *Physical examination & health assessment.* St. Louis, MO: Elsevier.

Larici, A. R., Franchi, P., Occhipinti, M., Contegiacomo, A., del Ciello, A., Calandriello, L., . . . Bonomo, L. (2014). Diagnosis and management of hemoptysis. *Diagnostic and Interventional Radiology, 20,* 299–309.

LeBlond, R. F., Brown, D. D., Suneja, M., & Szot, J. F. (2015). *DeGowin's diagnostic examination* (10th ed.). New York, NY: McGraw-Hill.

Madden, B. P. (2017). Evolutional trends in the management of tracheal and bronchial injuries. *Journal of Thoracic Disease, 9*(1), 67–70.

McCance, K. L., Huether, S. E., Brashers, V. L., & Rote, N. S. (2014) *Pathophysiology: The biologic basis for disease in adults and children* (7th ed.). St. Louis, MO: Elsevier.

Midthun, D. E. (2017). Overview of the risk factors, pathology, and clinical manifestations of lung cancer. In S. R. Vora (Ed.), *UpToDate*. Retrieved from https://www.uptodate.com/contents/overview-of-the-risk-factors-pathology-and-clinical-manifestations-of-lung-cancer

Mucha, S. M., Varghese, L. A., French, R. E., & Shade, D. A. (2014). Separating fact from factitious hemoptysis: A case report. *Critical Care Nurse, 34*(4), 36–42. doi:10.4037/ccn2014212

Ong, Z. Y., Chai, H. Z., How, C. H., & Low, T. B. (2016). A simplified approach to haemoptysis. *Singapore Medical Journal, 57*(8), 415–418.

Papadakis, M.A., & McPhee, S. J. (2017). *Current medical diagnosis and treatment* (56th ed.). New York, NY: McGraw-Hill.

Pinkerman, C., Sander, P., Breeding, J. E., Brink, D., Curtis, R., Hayes, R., . . . Turner A. (2013). Heart failure in adults. *Institute for Clinical Systems Improvement*. Retrieved from https://www.guideline.gov/summaries/summary/47030/heart-failure-in-adults

Raftery, A. T., Lim, E., & Ostor, A. J. (2014). *Differential diagnosis* (4th ed.). London: Elsevier.

Rail, P., Gandhi, V., & Tariq, C. (2016). Massive hemoptysis. *Critical Care Nursing Quarterly, 39*(2), 139–147. doi:10.1097/CNQ.0000000000000107

Seller, R. H., & Symons, A. B. (2012). *Differential diagnosis of common complaints* (6th ed.). Philadelphia, PA: Elsevier.

Simoff, M. J., Lally, B., Slade, M. G., Goldberg, W. G., Lee, P., Michaud, G. C., . . . Chawla, M. (2013). Symptom management in patients with lung cancer: Diagnosis and management of lung cancer, 3rd ed.: American college of chest physicians evidence-based clinical practice guidelines. *Chest, 143*(5), 455–497.

Uphold, C. R., & Graham, M. V. (2013). *Clinical guidelines in family practice* (5th ed.). Gainesville, FL: Barmarrae Books.

Von Gunten, C., & Buckholz, G. (2018). Palliative care: Overview of cough, stridor, and hemoptysis. In D. M. Savarese (Ed.), *UpToDate*. Retrieved from https://www.uptodate.com/contents/palliative-care-overview-of-cough-stridor-and-hemoptysis

Weinberger, S. E. (2017). Etiology and evaluation of hemoptysis in adults. In H. Hollingsworth (Ed.), *UpToDate*. Retrieved from https://www.uptodate.com/contents/etiology-and-evaluation-of-hemoptysis-in-adults

CHAPTER 20

Hyperglycemia

The American Diabetes Association (ADA) defines hyperglycemia as a blood sugar >140mg/dL. Diabetes is the primary cause of hyperglycemia; however, it can also occur during times of severe bodily stress from trauma, infection, or surgery. These secondary glucose elevations are typically transient and self-limiting. Common signs of hyperglycemia include weight loss, polyuria, polyphagia, and polydipsia. Uncontrolled hyperglycemia is associated with increased risk of mortality, delayed healing, longer hospital stays, and infections. The ADA recommends a blood glucose goal of 140–180mg/dL for non-critically ill patients, and 110–140mg/dL for post-operative patients and for those considered critically ill. In order to avoid complications, tight glucose control should be the top priority of the nurse, along with monitoring for hypoglycemia when hyperglycemia is being aggressively treated, and educating the patient about their chronic diabetes management.

Differential Diagnosis Considerations

Common: diabetes mellitus type 1 and 2, DKA, HHS, infectious process, medication induced, medication noncompliance, post-operative state, trauma

Other secondary considerations: alcoholic ketoacidosis, burn injury, Cushing's syndrome, CVA/TIA, dialysis, heat stroke, hypothermia, intestinal obstruction, mesenteric thrombosis, MI, pancreatitis, parental nutrition, PE, renal failure, starvation ketoacidosis, subdural hematoma, substance abuse, thyrotoxicosis

Questions to Ask the Patient/ Family/Witness/Yourself

- When was the last time you ate? What did you eat?
- Have you had any recent: dialysis? dietary changes or noncompliance with diabetic diet? exposure to any infection/illness or been around anyone who is sick? parental nutrition? surgery? trauma? vigorous exercise?
- Have you taken any new prescribed or over-the-counter medications? Have there been any recent changes to your current medication?
- Do you drink alcohol? How many drinks per day/week? What kind and amount of alcohol do you drink? When was your last drink? (if applicable)
- Do you have a history of drug use? What types and how much? Do you use on a daily basis? When was your last use? (if applicable)

If the patient has a history of diabetes:

- Have you been using your diabetes medications as prescribed? If missing doses, how often do you miss doses per day/week?
- Do you check your blood sugar regularly? What is an average blood sugar for you?
- Have you had any episodes of low blood sugar?
- When was your last hemoglobin A1C? What was it?

Associated Signs/Symptoms: PAIN: pain anywhere; GENERAL: chills, fatigue, fever, weakness, weight changes; EENT: dry mouth, vision changes; CARDIOVASCULAR: chest pain/tightness, palpitations; RESPIRATORY: dyspnea; GASTROINTESTINAL: appetite changes, nausea, vomiting; NEUROLOGICAL: dizziness, headache, seizures; ENDOCRINE: polydipsia, polyphagia, polyuria, sweating; PSYCHOLOGICAL: confusion, nervousness

Recommended Assessments

- Vital signs
- Temperature
- Weight and nutritional status
- I/O
- General
  - Level of consciousness and orientation
  - Inspect: signs of acute distress, acute illness, affect, restlessness
- Skin
  - Inspect: diaphoresis, dryness, pallor
  - Palpate: temperature, turgor
- Mouth
  - Inspect: acetone breath, mucous membrane moisture level
- Cardiovascular
  - Auscultate: heart sounds, rate, rhythm
- Respiratory
  - Inspect: respiratory effort, depth, pattern
  - Auscultate: lung sounds
- Gastrointestinal
  - Inspect: distention
  - Auscultate: bowel sounds
  - Palpate: guarding, tenderness
- Extremities
  - Inspect: IV site
  - Palpate: capillary refill, edema, pulses

Past Medical History Considerations
Puts the patient at risk for differential considerations

- Alcohol abuse/use
- Anorexia nervosa
- CKD

- Drug abuse/use
- Surgery

Reoccurrence/exacerbation should be considered

- DKA
- HHS

Chronic conditions that can cause hyperglycemia

- Cushing's syndrome
- Diabetes
- Obesity
- Thyroid disease

Medication Evaluation

Most common causative/exacerbating medication

- Antipsychotics
- Beta blockers
- CCBs
- Cimetidine
- Corticosteroids
- Dextrose
- Lithium
- Phenytoin
- Quinolone antibiotics
- Thiazide diuretics

Used to treat type 1 and 2 diabetes

- DPP-4s
- GLP-1s
- Insulin (long and short acting)
- Metformin
- SGLT2 inhibitors

- Sulfonylureas
- TZDs

Lab Evaluation and Trends

- Bedside capillary glucose trends
- BMP/CMP
- Hemoglobin A1C

Nursing Intervention Considerations

- Call for help or rapid response/code team if vital signs are unstable or there are signs of urgent distress
- Verify patent IV if IVF or IV medication treatment is anticipated
  - Flush according to facility protocol; watch for swelling, erythema, pain, and other signs of infiltration
  - Large bore IV is preferred if DKA or HHS is suspected
- Blood sugar as needed or per DKA protocol (if applicable)
- Medications (if ordered or protocol allows)
  - Hold suspected causative medication until discussion with the provider
  - Scheduled and sliding scale insulin
- Diet
  - Encourage diabetic diet food choices
- Positioning
  - HOB raised to comfort
  - Side lying position if there is a decrease in LOC or the patient is vomiting
  - Reposition every 2–4 hours or establish an individualized turning schedule
- Collect
  - Clean catch urine sample if DKA or HHS is suspected
- Monitor
  - Stay with the patient until stable
  - Vital signs and trends
  - I/O

- Blood sugar trends
- Weight trends
- Orientation status changes
- Agitation levels
- Skin assessment every 8–24 hours
- Wound healing progression (if applicable)
- Signs of dehydration such as lethargy, decreased skin turgor, dry mucous membranes, tachycardia, and (orthostatic) hypotension
- Urine output color, frequency, and volume
- Safety
  - Perform a fall risk assessment and implement the appropriate strategies
- Environment
  - Provide a calm, quiet environment and reduce stimulation
  - Maintain a well-lit environment
  - Maintain a comfortable room temperature
- Supportive care
  - Maintain effective communication between yourself, patient, and family
  - Provide emotional support and reassurance to the patient and family
  - Maintain a calm manner during patient interactions
  - Discuss plan of care with the patient and decide reasonable goals together
  - Notify the patient and family of changes in the plan of care
  - Re-orient the patient as needed
  - Identify barriers to care and compliance
  - Promote skin care and integrity
  - Provide light clothing and bed linen
  - **Educational topics (as applicable to the patient):**
    - General information regarding the patient's hyperglycemia and differential diagnosis considerations

- Procedure and intervention explanation and justification
- Explanation regarding referrals and specialist who may see them for this issue
- New medication education including reason, side effects, and administration needs
- Medication compliance
- Medication changes
- Laboratory monitoring needs
- Telemetry
- Skin care
- Proper positioning and turning schedule
- Safety needs and fall risk
- Handwashing and infection control measures
- Diabetic diet
- Alcohol and/or drug cessation and support
- Blood glucose measurement techniques and frequency
- Diabetic self-care: foot care, vision exams, and blood glucose goals
- Weight loss, physical activity, and exercise needs
- Immunization needs
- When to notify the nurse or provider
- Signs and symptoms of hyper- and hypoglycemia
- Dehydration prevention
- Pressure injury prevention

ISBARR Recommendation Considerations

- Ask the provider to come assess the patient STAT if they are unstable
- Transfer to the ICU if hemodynamically unstable, advanced medication management is required, or closer monitoring is needed
- Medication

- Discontinue/change suspected causative medication
- Add/change scheduled insulin, insulin drip, or oral anti-diabetics
- IV fluid needs if oral intake is poor, there are signs of dehydration, and the patient is NPO or hypotensive
- Labs
  - ABG
  - BMP/CMP
  - Hemoglobin A1C
  - Urinalysis
- Safety
  - Activity-level changes
  - Fall risk protocol
- Monitoring needs
  - Blood sugars including frequency and parameters to call the provider
  - Daily weights
  - Telemetry/continuous cardiac monitoring
  - Strict I/O
  - Vital signs including frequency and parameters to call the provider
- Change diet to
  - Diabetic
- Protocols
  - DKA (if applicable)
- Referrals
  - Dietician
  - Endocrinology
- Ask if the provider wants anything else done
- Read back orders; ask that they enter all orders into the electronic medical record

ISBARR Template	
I **Introduction**	**Introduce Yourself and the Patient** • "Hello, Dr. Klinker, this is Becky Rebro. I am an RN at MKE Assisted Living. I understand you are the provider for Mr. Jeremy Klug on unit 2?"
S **Situation**	**Sign/Symptom You Are Concerned About** • "For the past two days, Mr. Klug has had elevated blood sugars. They have been ranging from 180–440. Today, before lunch, he had a glucose of 250, and at 1730, before dinner, he had a glucose of 440." **Associated Signs/Symptoms** • "He feels a little more fatigued than usual and has had a mild headache for a couple of hours but otherwise denies any polyuria, polyphagia, and polydipsia."
B **Background**	**Vitals** • "I took a set of vitals before calling you. His blood pressure is 140/90, heart rate is 80, and temperature is 98.2." **Exam** • "Overall, he is in no acute distress, his lungs continue to sound course, heart sounds are normal, and skin is pink, warm, and dry." **Past Medical History** • "He does have a history of type 2 diabetes," **Labs and Medications** • "and is currently on 500mg Metformin BID. He took his metformin this morning. Prednisone was prescribed three days ago when he was diagnosed with a COPD exacerbation. He has another two days of the prednisone ordered. His last A1C three months ago was 7.6."

ISBARR Template	
A **Assessment**	**Assessment** • "I am concerned the steroids are causing his sugars to be uncontrolled."
R **Recommendations** **R** **Read Back**	**Nurse's Recommendations, Interventions, and Read Back** • "Did you want to start insulin? Do you want to continue metformin? How often do you want me to check his blood sugars? Do you want any other labs? Do you want anything else done at this time? • "Thank you, Dr. Klinker, I would like to read those orders back to you. Start low dose sliding scale of rapid-acting insulin protocol with each meal. Continue Metformin dose. Check blood sugars before each meal and before bedtime for one week."

Disclaimer: This dialogue is factitious and any resemblance to actual persons, living or dead, or actual events is purely coincidental.

In order to avoid order discrepancies, it is recommended that all orders be entered by the provider in the electronic medical record.

Select Differential Diagnosis Presentations

Diabetes

Overview: a group of disease states as a result of poor (or complete lack of) insulin use or production causing chronic hyperglycemia

Patient may complain of: fatigue, weight changes, vision changes, nausea, vomiting, nocturia, numbness/tingling, polyuria, polyphagia, polydipsia

Objective findings: altered mental status, poor wound healing, decreased skin turgor, dry mucous membranes, acanthosis nigricans, retinal hemorrhages, hypertension, sensation disturbances; exam is typically unremarkable unless severe

PMH considerations/risk factors: hx of metabolic syndrome, obesity, sedentary lifestyle, pregnancy, family hx of diabetes, older/younger age

Diagnostics: A1C, fasting blood glucose

Diabetic Ketoacidosis

Overview: lack of insulin leads to extreme hyperglycemia and the production of ketones, causing the blood to be more acidic

Patient may complain of: fatigue, generalized abdominal pain, nausea, vomiting, dyspnea, polyuria, polyphagia, polydipsia

Objective findings: altered mental status, lethargy, acetone breath, decreased skin turgor, dry mucous membranes, tachycardia, hypotension, tachypnea

PMH considerations/risk factors: hx of type 1 diabetes, medication noncompliance, substance abuse, recent major illness or stress

Diagnostics: anion gap, BMP/CMP, A1C, urine ketones

References

American Diabetes Association. (2015a). Approaches to glycemic treatment. *Diabetes Care, 38*(1), 41–48.

American Diabetes Association. (2015b). Foundations of care: Education, nutrition, physical activity, smoking cessation, psychosocial care, and immunizations. *Diabetes Care, 38*(1), 20–30.

American Diabetes Association. (2017). Standards of medical care in diabetes – 2017. *Diabetes Care, 40*(1). Retrieved from https://professional.diabetes.org/sites/professional.diabetes.org/files/media/dc_40_s1_final.pdf

American Medical Directors Association. (2010). *Know-it-all before you call: Data collection system.* Columbia, MD: Author.

Bajwa, S. S., Baruah, M. P., Kalra, S., & Kapoor, M. C. (2015). Interdisciplinary position statement on management of hyperglycemia in peri-operative and intensive care. *Journal of Anesthesiology Clinical Pharmacology, 31*(2), 155–164.

Bulechek, G. M., Butcher, H. K., Dochterman, J. M., & Wagner, C. (2013). *Nursing intervention classification (NIC).* St. Louis, MO: Elsevier Mosby.

Freeland, B. (2016). Hyperglycemia in the hospital setting. *Medsurg Nursing, 25*(6), 393–396.

Goguen, J., & Gilbert, J. (2013). Hyperglycemic emergencies in adults. *Canadian Journal of Diabetes, 37,* 72–76.

Greco, G., Ferket, B. S., Alessandro, D. A., Shi, W., Horvath, K. A., Rosen, A., … Moskowitz, A. J. (2016). Diabetes and the association of postoperative hyperglycemia with clinical and economic outcomes in cardiac surgery. *Diabetes Care, 39*(3), 408–417.

Gulanick, M., & Myers, J. L. (2017). *Nursing care plans: Diagnosis, interventions, & outcomes* (9th ed.). St. Louis, MO: Elsevier.

Hirsch, I., & Emmett, M. (2016). Diabetic ketoacidosis and hyperosmolar hyperglycemic state in adults: Clinical features, evaluation, and diagnosis. In J. E. Mulder (Ed.), *UpToDate.* Retrieved from https://www.uptodate.com/contents/diabetic-ketoacidosis-and-hyperosmolar-hyperglycemic-state-in-adults-clinical-features-evaluation-and-diagnosis

Inzucchi, S. E., Bergenstal, R. M., Buse, J. B., Diamant, M., Ferrannini, E., Nauck, M., ... Matthews, D. R. (2015). Management of hyperglycemia in type 2 diabetes, 2015: A patient centered approach: Update to a position statement of the American diabetes association and the European association for the study of diabetes. *Diabetes Care, 38*(1), 140–149.

Lee, P. G., & Halter, J. B. (2017). The pathophysiology of hyperglycemia in older adults: Clinical considerations. *Diabetes Care, 40*(4), 444–452.

McCulloch, D. K. (2017). Management of persistent hyperglycemia in type 2 diabetes mellitus. In J. E. Mulder (Ed.), *UpToDate.* Retrieved from https://www.uptodate.com/contents/management-of-persistent-hyperglycemia-in-type-2-diabetes-mellitus

McCulloch, D. K., & Inzucchi, S. E. (2017). Management of diabetes mellitus in hospitalized patients. In J. E. Mulder (Ed.), *UpToDate.* Retrieved from https://www.uptodate.com/contents/management-of-diabetes-mellitus-in-hospitalized-patients

McMahon, M. M., Braunschweig, C., & Compher, C. (2013). A.S.P.E.N. clinical guidelines: Nutrition support of adult patients with hyperglycemia. *Journal of Parenteral and Enteral Nutrition, 37*(1), 23–26.

Umpierrez, G. E., Hellman, R., Korykowski, M. T., Kosiborod, M., Maynard, A. A., Montori, V. M., . . . Van den Berghe, G. (2012). Management of hyperglycemia in hospitalized patients in non-critical care setting: An endocrine society clinical practice guideline. *Journal of Clinical Endocrinology & Metabolism, 97*(1), 16–38.

Umpierrez, G. E., & Pasquel, F. J. (2017). Management of inpatient hyperglycemia and diabetes in older adults. *Diabetes Care, 40*(4), 509–517.

Wolfsdorf, J. I., Allgrove, J., Craig, M. E., Glaser, E. J., Glaser, N., Jain, V., . . . Rosenbloom, A. L. (2014). Diabetic ketoacidosis and hyperglycemic hyperosmolar state. *Pediatric Diabetes, 15*(20), 154–179.

CHAPTER 21

Hypertension

According to the American Heart Association, hypertension is defined as a SBP >140 and/or DBP >90. There are many risk factors for developing hypertension, including age, obesity, a diet high in sodium, smoking, diabetes, CKD, family history, drug use, and alcohol consumption. A patient with persistent hypertension, without treatment, is at risk for MI, heart failure, CVA, kidney disease, and death. Hypertension is usually an asymptomatic disease even when uncontrolled. Hypertensive urgency is when the SBP is >180 and DBP >110, but the patient is asymptomatic and has no signs of end-organ damage. When end-organ damage is evident (intracranial bleeding, MI, pulmonary edema, AKI, heart failure, eclampsia), it is considered a hypertensive emergency. For patients who are younger than 60 years, the Joint National Committee (JNC) has a SBP blood pressure goal of <140 and DBP <90. In patients 60 years and older, the treatment goal is a SBP <150 and DBP <90. The patient's blood pressure should gradually be reduced.

It is important for the nurse to ensure that an accurate blood pressure is obtained with proper technique and cuff size. It is also recommended that trends of the blood pressure are monitored; one elevated pressure does not always warrant immediate treatment. The nurse's priorities are to notify the provider about persistent elevations, monitor for end-organ damage, safely administer scheduled and PRN anti-hypertensives, set blood pressure goals and parameters with the provider, and educate the patient about lifestyle adjustments needed to help control and treat their hypertension.

Differential Diagnosis Considerations

Common: anxiety, fever, hypervolemia, medication induced, medication noncompliance, pain, uncontrolled primary HTN, white coat syndrome

Consider: anemia, aortic dissection, CKD, cocaine use, Cushing's syndrome, CVA/TIA, glomerulonephritis, Guillain-Barré syndrome, heart failure, hypercalcemia, hyperthyroidism, hypoglycemia, increased ICP, MI, pheochromocytoma, preeclampsia, primary aldosteronism, renal artery stenosis, renal failure, Shy-Drager syndrome, sleep apnea, spinal cord injury, stable angina, TBI, unstable angina, withdrawal from alcohol/drugs

Questions to Ask the Patient/ Family/Witness/Yourself

- Do you have daytime sleepiness? History of snoring? Erratic sleep?
- How often do you exercise?
- How much fluid are you drinking on a daily basis?
- Do you have a diet high in salt?
- Do you have a family history of high blood pressure or heart disease?
- Have you had any recent: pregnancy? surgery? trauma?
- Have you taken any new prescribed or over-the-counter medications? Have there been any recent changes to your current medication?
- Do you drink caffeine? How many drinks in a day? When was the last time you had any?
- Do you smoke? How much (ppd)? How long have you been smoking? (if applicable)
- Do you drink alcohol? How many drinks per day/week? What kind and amount of alcohol do you drink? When was your last drink? (if applicable)
- Do you have a history of drug use? What types and how much? Do you use on a daily basis? When was your last use? (if applicable)

If the patient has a history of HTN

- Have you been using your blood pressure medications as prescribed? If missing doses, how often do you miss doses per day/week?

- Do you check your blood pressure at home? What are your average readings?

Associated Signs/Symptoms: PAIN: pain anywhere; GENERAL: chills, fatigue, fever, weakness; EENT: vision changes; CARDIOVASCULAR: chest pain/tightness, edema, palpitations, PND, orthopnea; RESPIRATORY: cough, dyspnea; GASTROINTESTINAL: nausea, vomiting; GENITOURINARY: oliguria; NEUROLOGICAL: dizziness, headache; PSYCHOLOGICAL: confusion, feelings of impending doom

Recommended Assessments

- Vital signs
- Temperature
- Weight
- I/O
- Pain scale (if applicable)
  - Tolerable pain level
- General
  - Level of consciousness and orientation
  - Inspect: signs of acute distress, acute illness, affect, restlessness
- Skin
  - Inspect: cyanosis, diaphoresis, pallor
  - Palpate: temperature, turgor
- Head/face/neck
  - Inspect: JVD, goiter
  - Auscultate: carotid bruits
- Cardiovascular
  - Auscultate: heart sounds, rate, rhythm
  - Palpate: heaves, thrills
- Respiratory
  - Inspect: respiratory effort
  - Auscultate: lung sounds
- Extremities
  - Inspect: IV site
  - Palpate: capillary refill, edema, pulses

Past Medical History Considerations

Puts the patient at risk for differential considerations

- Alcohol abuse/use
- CAD
- Diabetes
- Drug abuse/use
- Nicotine use
- Obesity
- Pregnancy

Reoccurrence/exacerbation should be considered

- MI

Chronic conditions that can cause acute or chronic hypertension

- Anemia
- Angina
- Anxiety
- Cardiac valve disorders
- Chronic pain
- CKD
- Cushing's syndrome
- CVA
- Guillain-Barré syndrome
- Heart failure
- HTN (primary)
- Primary aldosteronism
- Renal artery stenosis
- Sleep apnea
- Spinal cord injury
- TBI
- Thyroid disease

Medication Evaluation
Most common causative/exacerbating medication

- Amphetamines
- Birth control/HRT
- Corticosteroids
- Decongestants
- Erythropoietin
- MAO inhibitors
- NSAIDs
- SSRIs
- Sympathomimetic agents
- Tricyclic antidepressants

Used to treat hypertension

- ACE inhibitors
- Alpha-1 adrenergic antagonist
- Alpha-2 adrenergic agonists
- ARBs
- Beta blockers
- CCBs
- Diuretics
- Nitrates
- Vasodilators

Lab Evaluation and Trends

- BMP/CMP
- CBC

Nursing Intervention Considerations

- Call for help or rapid response/code team if vital signs are unstable or there are signs of urgent distress

- Maintain a patent airway
  - Apply oxygen if hypoxic
  - Call respiratory therapy for signs of respiratory distress
- Verify patent IV if IVF or IV medication treatment is anticipated
  - Flush according to facility protocol; watch for swelling, erythema, pain, and other signs of infiltration
- ECG
- Blood sugar if hypoglycemia is suspected
- Medications (if ordered or protocol allows)
  - Hold suspected causative medication until discussion with the provider
  - PRN anti-hypertensive
- Diet
  - Restrict fluids until discussion with the provider if there are signs of fluid overload
  - Avoid caffeine
  - Encourage heart healthy, low-sodium food choices
- Positioning
  - Sitting upright with legs uncrossed, arm should be supported at heart level. Rest for 5 minutes before taking blood pressure
  - Reposition every 2–4 hours or establish an individualized turning schedule
- Monitor
  - Stay with the patient until stable
  - Vital signs and trends
  - Oxygen saturation/pulse oximetry
  - I/O
  - Blood sugar trends (if applicable)
  - Telemetry/cardiac monitor
  - Weight trends
  - Orientation status changes
  - Agitation levels
  - Peripheral pulses
  - Skin assessment every 8–24 hours

- Signs of decreased cardiac output such as weak pulses, cool skin, altered mental status, oliguria, and mottling
- Signs and symptoms of fluid overload such as cough, adventitious lung sounds, dyspnea, tachypnea, weight gain, edema, JVD, and ascites
- Signs and symptoms of increased ICP such as worsening headache, nausea, vomiting, hypertension, bradypnea, altered mental status, vision changes, fixed or sluggish pupillary response, and GCS changes
- Safety
  - Perform a fall risk assessment and implement the appropriate strategies
- Environment
  - Provide a calm, quiet environment and reduce stimulation
  - Maintain a well-lit environment
  - Maintain a comfortable room temperature
  - Offer aromatherapy and/or music therapy (if appropriate)
  - Utilize a fan (if appropriate)
- Supportive care
  - Maintain effective communication between yourself, patient, and family
  - Provide emotional support and reassurance to the patient and family
  - Maintain a calm manner during patient interactions
  - Discuss plan of care with the patient and decide reasonable goals together
  - Notify the patient and family of changes in the plan of care
  - Identify barriers to care and compliance
  - Re-orient the patient as needed
  - Promote skin care and integrity
  - **Educational topics (as applicable to the patient):**
    - General information regarding the patient's HTN and differential diagnosis considerations

- Explanation regarding referrals and specialist who may see them for this issue
- Procedure and intervention explanation and justification
- New medication education, including reason, side effects, and administration needs
- Medication compliance
- Medication changes
- Oxygen therapy and maintenance
- Relaxation techniques and breathing exercises
- Telemetry
- Skin care
- Proper positioning and turning schedule
- Safety needs and fall risk
- DASH diet, low-tyramine diet if on MAOI
- Caffeine restriction
- Fluid restriction
- Weight loss, physical activity, and exercise needs
- Stress reduction and management
- Smoking cessation
- Alcohol and/or drug cessation and support
- Home blood pressure monitoring
- When to notify the nurse or provider
- Signs and symptoms of cardiac emergencies
- Signs and symptoms of fluid overload
- Signs and symptoms of hypoglycemia
- Pressure injury prevention

ISBARR Recommendation Considerations

- Ask the provider to come assess the patient STAT if they are unstable or showing signs of end-organ damage
- Transfer to the ICU if hemodynamically unstable, advanced medication management is required, or closer monitoring is needed
- Medication

- Discontinue/change suspected causative medication
- Add/change PRN and/or scheduled anti-hypertensive
- Add/change diuretics for signs of fluid overload
- Add PRN and/or scheduled medication for anxiety or irritability
- Add PRN and/or scheduled pain medication
- ECG if not already done or repeat testing is needed
- Labs (depending on the suspected cause)
  - BMP/CMP
  - BNP
  - Cardiac enzymes
  - CBC
  - TSH
- Safety
  - Activity-level changes
  - Fall risk protocol
- Monitoring needs
  - Continuous O_2 monitoring
  - Blood sugars, including frequency and parameters to call the provider (if applicable)
  - Daily weights
  - Telemetry/continuous cardiac monitoring
  - Strict I/O
  - Vital signs, including frequency and parameters to call the provider
- Supportive cares
  - Compression stockings or SCDs
- Change diet to (depending on the suspected cause)
  - Caffeine restriction
  - DASH, low sodium
  - Fluid restriction
  - Low tyramine
- Protocols
  - CIWA-Ar if alcohol withdrawal is suspected
- Referrals
  - Cardiology

- Ask if the provider wants anything else done
- Read back orders; ask that they enter all orders into the electronic medical record

ISBARR Template	
I **Introduction**	**Introduce Yourself and the Patient** • "Hello, Dr. Khan. This is Abby Andris. I am the nurse for your patient Sarah Tilque in Room 609 who was admitted today for severe back pain with an unknown etiology."
S **Situation**	**Sign/Symptom You Are Concerned About** • "She has had significantly high blood pressure readings this morning. Systolically, she has been consistently above 200. Diastolically, above 100. Last blood pressure five minutes ago was 203/100." **Associated Signs/Symptoms** • "She has no complaints of chest pain, headache, or dizziness and is still complaining of 10/10 lower back pain."
B **Background**	**Vitals** • "Heart rate is 98, respirations are 18, and oxygen saturation is 98% on room air." **Exam** • "Her exam was unremarkable; heart sounds are normal, lungs are clear and she has no peripheral edema or signs of respiratory distress." **Past Medical History** • "She does have a history of hypertension and says she was previously noncompliant with her medications before being admitted, only taking her medication two to three times a week." **Labs and Medications** • "Scheduled 10 mg amlodipine and as needed pain medication was given one hour ago with no changes in her pressure. CMP and CBC this morning were both normal."

ISBARR Template	
A **Assessment**	**Assessment** • "I am concerned about her hypertensive urgency."
R **Recommendations** **R** **Read Back**	**Nurse's Recommendations, Interventions, and Read Back** • "I have been taking vital signs every 15 minutes. A 12-lead ECG showed normal sinus rhythm. Did you want to order a PRN IV anti-hypertensive? Did you want to make any other changes to her medication? How often would you like me to check her blood pressure? Did you want her on telemetry? Did you want anything else done at this time?" • "Thank you, Dr. Khan, I would like to read those orders back to you. You would like a blood pressure every 30 minutes until patient has three consecutive systolic blood pressures of <140, we can then switch to every four hours and as needed. Give 20 mg IV labetalol now for one dose. Call back if her blood pressure does not improve after one hour."

Disclaimer: This dialogue is factitious and any resemblance to actual persons, living or dead, or actual events is purely coincidental.

In order to avoid order discrepancies, it is recommended that all orders be entered by the provider in the electronic medical record.

Select Differential Diagnosis Presentations

Angina (Stable)

Overview: chest pain caused by a decrease in myocardial oxygen supply that is improved with rest

Patient may complain of: fatigue, chest pain/tightness/heaviness that is worse with activity, better with rest or NTG, radiation of the pain to the left arm/neck/jaw, palpitations, dyspnea, activity intolerance, nausea, dyspepsia, dizziness, feelings of impending doom, anxiety; symptoms have a short duration

Objective findings: signs of acute distress, lethargy, diaphoresis, hypertension, tachycardia, murmur, weak pulses, sluggish capillary refill, tachypnea

PMH considerations/risk factors: hx of angina, CAD, HTN, heart failure, hyperlipidemia, diabetes, cardiac valve disorders, obesity, increased psychological stress, nicotine use, family hx of heart disease

Diagnostics: cardiac enzymes, ECG, stress test, coronary angiography

Angina (Unstable)

Overview: chest pain caused by a decrease in myocardial oxygen supply that is not improved with rest

Patient may complain of: fatigue, chest pain/tightness/heaviness that is worse with activity, not improved with rest or NTG, radiation of the pain to the left arm/neck/jaw, palpitations, dyspnea, activity intolerance, nausea, dyspepsia, dizziness, feelings of impending doom, anxiety; symptoms have a longer duration than stable angina

Objective findings: signs of acute distress, lethargy, diaphoresis, hypertension, tachycardia, murmur, weak pulses, sluggish capillary refill, tachypnea

PMH considerations/risk factors: hx of angina, CAD, HTN, heart failure, hyperlipidemia, diabetes, cardiac valve disorders, obesity, increased psychological stress, nicotine use, family hx of heart disease

Diagnostics: cardiac enzymes, ECG, stress test, coronary angiography

Anxiety

Overview: psychiatric disorder that can cause intense fear and worry

Patient may complain of: fatigue, chest pain, palpitations, dyspnea, nausea, vomiting, abdominal pain, constipation/diarrhea, paresthesias, tremors, headache, dizziness, insomnia, mind racing, feelings of impending doom

Objective findings: signs of acute distress, irritability, inability to focus, diaphoresis, tachycardia, hypertension, tachypnea, muscle tension

PMH considerations/risk factors: hx of anxiety, depression, PTSD, insomnia, substance abuse, physical abuse, recent physical or emotional trauma, family hx of psychiatric diseases

Diagnostics: clinical diagnosis; workup to rule out more emergent causes may be indicated

Aortic Dissection

Overview: a tear in the intima layer of the aorta

Patient may complain of: severe chest/back pain described as ripping or tearing, abdominal pain, flank pain, dyspnea, nausea, dizziness, (pre)syncope, paresthesias, feelings of impending doom

Objective findings: signs of acute distress, altered mental status, diaphoresis, cool clammy skin, syncope, JVD, murmur, hypotension/hypertension, weak pulses or pulse deficit, sluggish capillary refill, tachypnea

PMH considerations/risk factors: hx of HTN, heart failure, cardiac valve disorders, connective tissue disorders, diabetes, substance abuse, pregnancy, nicotine use, male gender, older age

Diagnostics: ECG, TEE, chest X-ray, chest CT, aortography

Cerebral Vascular Accident

Overview: partial or complete obstruction of blood flow to the brain due to ischemia or hemorrhage causing brain tissue death

Patient may complain of: vision changes, nausea, vomiting, dysphagia, headache, dizziness, seizures, insomnia, difficulty with memory, speaking, focusing, and understanding; unilateral paralysis of the face, arms, and legs

Objective findings: signs of acute distress, altered mental status, ptosis, dysarthria, hypertension, carotid bruit(s), facial droop, seizures, unilateral weakness and sensation disturbances, immobility, gait disturbances

PMH considerations/risk factors: hx of HTN, CAD, heart failure, hyperlipidemia, arrhythmia, cardiac valve disease, diabetes, obesity, nicotine use, substance abuse, family hx of heart disease

Diagnostics: Head CT/MRI

Heart Failure

Overview: broad term to describe pumping malfunction of the heart

Patient may complain of: fatigue, activity intolerance, chest pain, palpitations, dyspnea, orthopnea, PND, coughing, sputum production, weight gain/loss, anorexia, nausea, nocturia, insomnia

Objective findings: signs of acute distress, lethargy, diaphoresis, cyanosis, JVD, bradycardia/tachycardia, hypertension/hypotension, displaced PMI, murmur, gallop, weak pulses, sluggish capillary refill, digital clubbing, edema, breathlessness, tachypnea, cough, adventitious lung sounds, sputum, hepatomegaly, ascites

PMH considerations/risk factors: hx of heart failure, HTN, CAD, cardiac valve disorders, MI, diabetes, arrhythmias, hyper/hypothyroidism, obesity, nicotine use, substance abuse, family hx of heart disease

Diagnostics: BNP, BMP/CMP, TSH, ECG, I/O, chest X-ray, ECHO, cardiac catheterization

Hypercalcemia

Overview: elevated serum calcium

Patient may complain of: fatigue, generalized weakness, anorexia, constipation, nausea, dyspepsia, vomiting, muscle aches; patient is typically asymptomatic unless severe

Objective findings: altered mental status, lethargy, hypertension, bradycardia, shortened QT interval, hypoactive bowel sounds, decreased reflexes; exam is typically unremarkable unless severe

PMH considerations/risk factors: hx of cancer, AIDS/HIV, Addison's disease, hyperparathyroidism

Diagnostics: serum Ca, ECG

Hyperthyroidism

Overview: overactive thyroid gland

Patient may complain of: anxiety, heat intolerance, fatigue, generalized weakness, palpitations, diarrhea, nausea, vomiting, weight loss, muscle cramps, tremors, seizures, insomnia

Objective findings: lethargy, irritability, diaphoresis, hair thinning, exophthalmos, goiter, tachycardia, hypertension, tremors, seizures

PMH considerations/risk factors: hx of Grave's disease, thyroiditis, pregnancy, thyroid cancer, family hx of thyroid dysfunction, female gender, older age

Diagnostics: TSH, T3, T4, thyroid US, radioactive iodine uptake scan

Increased Intracranial Pressure

Overview: rise in pressure within the cranial cavity

Patient may complain of: vision changes, nausea, vomiting, headache, confusion, seizures

Objective findings: signs of acute distress, altered mental status, GCS changes, sluggish/fixed pupillary response, hypertension, bradycardia, bradypnea

PMH considerations/risk factors: hx of TBI, CVA, CNS infections, hydrocephalus, cancer, seizures, HTN

Diagnostics: ICP monitoring, head CT/MRI

Myocardial Infarction

Overview: decreased or no blood flow through the coronary arteries causing cardiac muscle death

Patient may complain of: fatigue, chest pain not improved with rest, radiation of the pain to the left arm/neck/jaw, palpitations, dyspnea, activity intolerance, abdominal pain, nausea, dizziness, anxiety, feelings of impending doom; symptoms have longer duration than stable angina

Objective findings: signs of acute distress, lethargy, irritability, altered mental status, diaphoresis, cool clammy skin, hypertension/

hypotension, tachycardia/bradycardia, arrhythmia, murmur, ST elevations, pathologic Q waves, weak pulses, sluggish capillary refill, tachypnea

PMH considerations/risk factors: hx of MI, CAD, HTN, heart failure, hyperlipidemia, diabetes, cardiac valve disorders, sedentary lifestyle, NSAID use, nicotine use, substance abuse, family hx of heart disease, older age

Diagnostics: cardiac enzymes, ECG, stress test, coronary angiography

Renal Disease/Failure

Overview: broad term to describe damage and malfunction of the kidneys

Patient may complain of: fatigue, itching, dyspnea, anorexia, nausea, vomiting, oliguria, confusion

Objective findings: lethargy, altered mental status, arrhythmia, edema, pericardial rub, hypertension/hypotension, adventitious lung sounds, oliguria or anuria; exam is typically unremarkable unless severe

PMH considerations/risk factors: hx of CKD, diabetes, HTN, CAD, sepsis, BPH, burn injury, heart failure, dehydration, GI/blood loss, NSAID use, ACE inhibitor use, diuretic use, older age

Diagnostics: BMP/CMP, anion gap, urinalysis, renal US

Sleep Apnea

Overview: pauses in breathing (varying in number and length of time) while sleeping

Patient may complain of: snoring, daytime fatigue, headaches, inability to concentrate, mood changes, dry mouth, insomnia

Objective findings: elevated BMI, mouth breathing, thick neck, enlarged tonsils/uvula/soft palate, hypertension

PMH considerations/risk factors: hx of obesity, enlarged tonsils, nicotine use, narcotic pain medication use, CVA, family hx of sleep apnea, male gender, older age

Diagnostics: sleep study

Transient Ischemic Attack

Overview: transient obstruction of blood flow to the brain mimicking a CVA

Patient may complain of: vision changes, nausea, vomiting, dysphagia, headache, dizziness, seizures, insomnia, difficulty with memory, speaking, focusing, and understanding; unilateral paralysis of face, arms, and legs; signs and symptoms are transient in nature

Objective findings: signs of acute distress, altered mental status, ptosis, dysarthria, hypertension, carotid bruit(s), facial droop, seizures, unilateral weakness and sensation disturbances, immobility, gait disturbances; may not have abnormal exam findings due to transient nature of the issue

PMH considerations/risk factors: hx of HTN, CAD, heart failure, hyperlipidemia, arrhythmia, cardiac valve disease, diabetes, obesity, nicotine use, substance abuse, family hx of heart disease

Diagnostics: Head CT/MRI

Withdrawal (Alcohol)

Overview: rapid or abrupt decrease in alcohol intake causing physical and psychological disturbances

Patient may complain of: fever, chills, palpitations, anorexia, nausea, vomiting, diarrhea, seizures, headache, alcohol craving, insomnia, anxiety

Objective findings: signs of acute distress, fever, irritability, altered mental status, diaphoresis, tachycardia, hypertension, hepatomegaly, ascites, seizures, tremors, hallucinations/delirium

PMH considerations: hx of alcohol abuse, longer cessation (>48 hrs) since last drink, other substance abuse

Diagnostics: toxicology screen; workup to rule out more emergent causes may be indicated

Withdrawal (Opioids)

Overview: rapid or abrupt decrease in opioid intake causing physical and psychological disturbances

Patient may complain of: fever, body aches, nasal congestion, nasal drainage, anorexia, abdominal cramping, diarrhea, nausea, vomiting, tremors, opioid craving, anxiety, insomnia

Objective findings: signs of acute distress, fever, irritability, altered mental status, diaphoresis, piloerection, frequent yawning, pupil dilatation, rhinorrhea, hypertension, tachycardia, hyperactive bowel sounds

PMH considerations/risk factors: hx of daily opioid use, chronic pain, other substance abuse

Diagnostics: toxicology screen; workup to rule out more emergent causes may be indicated

References

American Medical Directors Association. (2010). *Know-it-all before you call: Data collection system.* Columbia, MD: Author.

Basile, J., & Bloch, M. J. (2018). Overview of hypertension in adults. In D. J. Sullivan (Ed.), *UpToDate.* Retrieved from https://www.uptodate.com/contents/overview-of-hypertension-in-adults

Cloutier, L., Tobe, S., Lamarre-Cliché, M., Gelfer, M., Bolli, P., Tremblay, G., . . . Leung, A. A. (2016). *Criteria for diagnosis of hypertension and recommendations for follow up.* Retrieved from http://guidelines.hypertension.ca/diagnosis-assessment/diagnosis/

Desai, S. P. (2009). *Clinician's guide to laboratory medicine* (3rd ed.). Houston, TX: MD2B.

Dyal, B., Whyte, M., Blankenship, S. M., & Ford, L. G. (2016). Outcomes of implementing an evidence-based hypertension clinical guideline in an academic nurse managed health center. *Worldviews on Evidence-Based Nursing, 13*(1), 89–93. doi:10.1111/wvn.12135

Elliott, W. J., & Varon, J. (2017). Evaluation and treatment of hypertensive emergencies in adults. In J. P. Forman (Ed.), *UpToDate.* Retrieved from https://www.uptodate.com/contents/evaluation-and-treatment-of-hypertensive-emergencies-in-adults

Feldman-Billard, S., Massin, P., Meas, T., Guillausseau, P., & Héron, E. (2010). Hypoglycemia- induced blood pressure elevation in patients with diabetes. *Archives of Internal Medicine, 170*(9), 829–831. doi:10.1001/archinternmed.2010.98

Franklin, M. M., & McCoy, M. A. (2017). The transition of care from hospital to home for patients with hypertension. *Nurse Practitioner, 42*(2), 12–19. doi:10.1097/01.NPR.0000511701.94615.4f

Frei, S. P., Burmeister, D. B., & Coil, J. F. (2013). Frequency of serious outcomes in patients with hypertension as a chief complaint in the emergency department. *Journal of The American Osteopathic Association, 113*(9), 664–668. doi:10.7556/jaoa.2013.032

Gulanick, M., & Myers, J. L. (2017). *Nursing care plans: Diagnosis, interventions, & outcomes* (9th ed.). St. Louis, MO: Elsevier.

Hale, A., & Hovey, M. J. (2014). *Fluid, electrolyte and acid-base imbalances.* Philadelphia, PA: F.A. Davis Company.

Headley, C. M. (2017). A blood pressure you can believe in. *Nephrology Nursing Journal, 44*(1), 57–72.

James, P. A., Oparil, S., Carter, B. L., Cushman, W. C., Dennison-Himmelfarb, C., Handler, J., . . . Ortiz, E. (2014). 2014 evidence-based guideline for the management of high blood pressure in adults report from the panel members appointed to the eighth joint national committee (JNC 8). *The Journal of the American Medical Association, 311*(5), 507–520.

Jarl, J., Tolentino, J. C., James, K., Clark, M. J., & Ryan, M. (2014). Supporting cardiovascular risk reduction in overweight and obese hypertensive patients through DASH diet and lifestyle education by primary care nurse practitioners. *Journal of The American Association of Nurse Practitioners, 26*(9), 498–503. doi:10.1002/2327-6924.12124

Jarvis, C. (2015). *Physical examination & health assessment.* St. Louis, MO: Elsevier.

Kenning, I., Luehr, D., Margolis, K., O'Connor, P., Pereira, C., Schlichte, A., & Woolley, T. (2014). Hypertension diagnosis and treatment. *Institute for Clinical Systems Improvement.* Retrieved from https://www.icsi.org/_asset/wjqy4g/HTN.pdf

Lagi, A., & Cencetti, S. (2015). Hypertensive emergencies: A new clinical approach. *Clinical Hypertension, 21*(20), 1–7.

Langan, R., & Jones, K. (2015). Common questions about the initial management of hypertension. *American Family Physician, 91*(3), 172–177.

LeBlond, R. F., Brown, D. D., Suneja, M., & Szot, J. F. (2015). *DeGowin's diagnostic examination* (10th ed.). New York, NY: McGraw-Hill.

Leung, A. A., Nerenberg, K., Daskalopoulou, S., McBrien, K., Karnke, K. B., Dasgupta, K., . . . Rabi, D.M. (2016). Hypertension Canada: 2016 Canadian hypertension education program guidelines for blood pressure measurement, diagnosis, assessment of risk, prevention, and treatment of hypertension. *Canadian Journal of Cardiology, 32*, 569–588.

Mann, J. F. (2017). Choice of drug therapy in primary (essential) hypertension. In J. P. Forman (Ed.), *UpToDate*. Retrieved from https://www.uptodate.com/contents/choice-of-drug-therapy-in-primary-essential-hypertension

Mann, J. F., & Hilgers, K. F. (2016). Goal blood pressure in adults with hypertension. In J. P. Forman, D. J. Sullivan (Eds.), *UpToDate*. Retrieved from https://www.uptodate.com/contents/goal-blood-pressure-in-adults-with-hypertension

McCance, K. L., Huether, S. E., Brashers, V. L., & Rote, N. S. (2014). *Pathophysiology: The biologic basis for disease in adults and children* (7th ed.). St. Louis, MO: Elsevier.

National Heart Foundation of Australia. (2016). *Guideline for the diagnosis and management of hypertension in adults.* Retrieved from https://www.heartfoundation.org.au/images/uploads/publications/PRO-167_Hypertension-guideline-2016_WEB.pdf

Oza, R., & Garcellano, M. (2015). Nonpharmacologic management of hypertension: What works? *American Family Physician, 91*(11), 772–776.

Papadakis, M. A., & McPhee, S. J. (2017). *Current medical diagnosis and treatment* (56th ed.). New York, NY: McGraw-Hill.

Qaseem, A., Wilt, T. J., Rich, R., Humphrey, L. L., Frost, J., & Forciea, M. A. (2017). Pharmacologic treatment of hypertension in adults aged 60 years or older to higher versus lower blood pressure targets: A clinical practice guideline from the American college of physicians and American academy of family physicians. *Annals of Internal Medicine, 166*(6), 430–437. Retrieved from http://annals.org/aim/article/2598413/pharmacologic-treatment-hypertension-adults-aged-60-years-older-higher-versus

Raftery, A. T., Lim, E., & Ostor, A. J. (2014). *Differential diagnosis* (4th ed.). London: Elsevier.

Randel, A. (2015). AHA/ACC/ASH release guideline on the treatment of hypertension and CAD. *American Family Physician, 92*(11), 1023–1030.

Rosendorff, C., Lackland, D. T., Allison, M., Aronow, W. S., Black, H. R., & Blumenthal, R. S. (2015). Treatment of hypertension in patients with coronary artery disease: A scientific statement from the American heart association, American college of cardiology, and American society of hypertension. *Journal of the American Society of Hypertension, 9*(6), 453–498.

Scher, H. E., Drew, M. L., & Cottrell, D. B. (2015). Treatment of resistant hypertension in the patient with chronic kidney disease. *Journal for Nurse Practitioners, 11*(6), 597–606. doi:10.1016/j.nurpra.2015.03.018

Sealy, L., & Oliva, A. (2014). Hypertension management guidelines update and research on the importance of blood pressure control. *Home Healthcare Nurse*, 32(10), 603–609. doi:10.1097/NHH.0000000000000163

Seller, R. H., & Symons, A. B. (2012). *Differential diagnosis of common complaints* (6th ed.). Philadelphia, PA: Elsevier.

United States Preventative Services Task Force. (2016). *High blood pressure in adults: Screening*. Retrieved from https://www.uspreventiveservicestaskforce.org/Page/Document/RecommendationStatementFinal/high-blood-pressure-in-adults-screening

Uphold, C. R., & Graham, M. V. (2013). *Clinical guidelines in family practice* (5th ed.). Gainesville, FL: Barmarrae Books.

Varon, J., & Elliott, W. J. (2017). Management of severe asymptomatic hypertension (hypertensive urgencies) in adults. In J. P. Forman (Ed.), *UpToDate*. Retrieved from https://www.uptodate.com/contents/management-of-severe-asymptomatic-hypertension-hypertensive-urgencies-in-adults

Warren, E. (2014). Hypertension: Why we measure it, why we treat it. *Practice Nurse*, 44(12), 14–19.

Weber, M. A., Schiffrin, E. L., White, W. B., Mann, S., Lindholm, L. H., Kenerson, J. G., . . . Harrap, S. B. (2014). Clinical practice guidelines for the management of hypertension in the community: A statement by the American society of hypertension and the international society of hypertension. *The Journal of Clinical Hypertension*, 16(1), 14–26.

CHAPTER 22

Hypoglycemia

The American Diabetes Association defines hypoglycemia as a blood sugar of less than 70mg/dL. It can result from a variety of glucose homeostasis issues, including reduced intake, increased glucose utilization, reduction of glycogen storage, or increased concentration of circulating insulin. Patients with diabetes are more commonly affected by hypoglycemia, particularly when they use medications (such as insulin) that can quickly lower their blood sugar. The elderly population is especially vulnerable to hypoglycemia issues. Each person responds to hypoglycemia differently, and obvious symptoms may not always be present. Common signs and symptoms of hypoglycemia include fatigue, irritability, nausea, lightheadedness, vomiting, confusion, dry mouth, hunger, and headache.

It is possible for patients without diabetes or the use of glucose-lowering medications to develop hypoglycemia, though these disorders are more rare. One hypoglycemia episode does not indicate a hypoglycemic disorder, however, in cases with persistent hypoglycemia, an endocrinology referral will be needed for further workup. No matter the cause, hypoglycemia carries a tremendous risk of mortality and needs to be treated quickly. If glucose testing is not available, and hypoglycemia is suspected, it should be treated as such. It is the nurse's responsibility to recognize signs and symptoms of hypoglycemia, treat them accordingly, and monitor the patient closely.

Differential Diagnosis Considerations

Common: alcohol use, medication induced, physical activity, starvation

Consider: Addison's disease, dialysis, glucagon deficiency, heart failure, insulin autoimmune hypoglycemia, insulinoma, liver failure, nonislet cell tumor, post-prandial syndrome, renal failure, sepsis

Questions to Ask the Patient/ Family/Witness/Yourself

- How is your appetite? Are you able to keep down food and/ or fluids?
- When was the last time you ate? What did you eat?
- How often do you exercise?
- Have you had any recent: dietary changes or have been fasting/ NPO? illness/infection? surgery?
- Have you taken any new prescribed or over-the-counter medications? Have there been any recent changes to your current medication?
- Do you drink alcohol? How many drinks per day/week? What kind and amount of alcohol do you drink? When was your last drink? (if applicable)

If the patient has a history of diabetes:

- Do you have a history of low blood sugars? If so, what have you done or used to treat it?
- Have you been using your diabetes medications as prescribed? Have there been any recent changes with your diabetes medication?
- Do you check your blood sugar regularly? What is an average blood sugar for you?
- When was your last hemoglobin A1C? What was it?

Associated Signs/Symptoms: GENERAL: fatigue, weakness, weight changes; EENT: dry mouth, vision changes; CARDIOVASCULAR: palpitations; RESPIRATORY: dyspnea; GASTROINTESTINAL: nausea, vomiting; NEUROLOGICAL: headache, numbness/tingling, dizziness, seizures, tremors; ENDOCRINE: polydipsia, polyphagia, polyuria, sweating; PSYCHOLOGICAL: confusion, hallucinations, insomnia, nervousness

Recommended Assessments

- Vital signs
- Weight and nutritional status

- I/O
- General
  - Level of consciousness and orientation
  - Inspect: signs of acute distress, acute illness, affect, restlessness
  - Speech changes
- Skin
  - Inspect: diaphoresis, dryness, pallor
- Mouth
  - Inspect: mucous membrane moisture level
  - Palpate: turgor
- Cardiovascular
  - Auscultate: heart sounds, rate, rhythm
- Respiratory
  - Inspect: respiratory effort, depth, pattern
  - Auscultate: lung sounds
- Extremities
  - Inspect: IV site

Past Medical History Considerations
Puts the patient at risk for differential considerations

- Alcohol abuse/use
- CKD
- Diabetes
- Gastric surgery

Chronic conditions that can cause hypoglycemia

- Addison's disease
- Cancer
- CKD
- Eating disorders
- Heart failure
- Liver disease

Medication Evaluation

Most common causative/exacerbating medication

- ACE inhibitors
- Beta blockers
- Haloperidol
- IGF
- Indomethacin
- Insulin
- Lithium
- Meglitinides
- Pentamidine
- Quinine
- Quinolone antibiotics
- Salicylates
- Sulfonylureas

Lab Evaluation and Trends

- Bedside capillary glucose trends
- BMP/CMP
- Hemoglobin A1C

Nursing Intervention Considerations

- Call for help or rapid response/code team if vital signs are unstable or there are signs of urgent distress
- Maintain a patent airway
  - Apply oxygen if hypoxic
- Verify patent IV if IVF or IV medication treatment is anticipated
  - Flush according to facility protocol; watch for swelling, erythema, pain, and other signs of infiltration
- Blood sugar every 15 minutes until hypoglycemia is resolved
- Medications (if ordered or protocol allows)
  - Hold suspected causative medication until discussion with the provider

- If hypoglycemic and has altered mental status or unable to swallow, give 1mg IV/IM/SQ glucagon, and/or 25–50mL IV 50% dextrose, or follow your facility's hypoglycemia protocol (goal is >100)
- Diet
  - Avoid NPO status
  - Encourage diabetic diet food choices
  - If hypoglycemic, alert, and can swallow, give a fast-acting carbohydrate like a glucose tablet, 4oz of fruit juice, 8oz of milk, 4oz of non-diet soda, hard candy, or teaspoon of honey/sugar. Repeat until sugar is normalized (goal is >100)
- Activity
  - Keep the patient in bed until discussion with the provider
- Positioning
  - Side lying position if there is a decrease in LOC or the patient is vomiting
  - Reposition every 2–4 hours or establish an individualized turning schedule
- Monitor
  - Stay with the patient until stable
  - Vital signs and trends
  - I/O
  - Blood sugar trends
  - Orientation status changes
  - Agitation levels
  - Skin assessment every 8–24 hours
- Safety
  - Perform a fall risk assessment and implement the appropriate strategies
- Environment
  - Provide a calm, quiet environment and reduce stimulation
  - Maintain a well-lit environment
  - Maintain a comfortable temperature in the room
  - Utilize a fan (if appropriate)

- Supportive care
  - Maintain effective communication between yourself, patient, and family
  - Provide emotional support and reassurance to the patient and family
  - Maintain a calm manner during patient interactions
  - Discuss plan of care with the patient and decide reasonable goals together
  - Notify the patient and family of changes in the plan of care
  - Re-orient the patient as needed
  - Identify barriers to care and compliance
  - Promote skin care and integrity
  - Provide light clothing and bed linen
- **Educational topics (as applicable to the patient):**
  - General information regarding the patient's hypoglycemia and differential diagnosis considerations
  - Procedure and intervention explanation and justification
  - Explanation regarding referrals and specialist who may see them for this issue
  - Medication changes
  - Medication compliance
  - Laboratory monitoring needs
  - Skin care
  - Proper positioning and turning schedule
  - Safety needs and fall risk
  - Diabetic diet
  - Alcohol and/or drug cessation and support
  - Weight loss, physical activity, and exercise needs
  - Blood glucose measurement techniques and frequency
  - Diabetic self-care: foot care, vision exams, and blood glucose goals
  - Glucagon home kit
  - Immunization needs

- When to notify the nurse or provider
- Signs and symptoms of hyper- and hypoglycemia
- Pressure injury prevention

ISBARR Recommendation Considerations

- Ask the provider to come assess the patient STAT if they are unstable or the hypoglycemia is not resolving
- Transfer to the ICU if hemodynamically unstable, advanced medication management is required, or closer monitoring is needed
- Medication
  - Discontinue/change suspected causative medication
  - Change anti-diabetics (insulin, sulfonylureas)
  - Add PRN 1mg IV/IM/SQ glucagon, and/or 25–50mL IV 50% dextrose
- IV fluid needs (possibly with dextrose) if oral intake is poor, there are signs of dehydration, and the patient is NPO or hypotensive
- Labs
  - BMP/CMP
  - Hemoglobin A1C
- Safety
  - Activity-level changes
  - Fall risk protocol
- Monitoring needs
  - Blood sugars including frequency and parameters to call the provider
  - Daily weights
  - Strict I/O
  - Vital signs including frequency and parameters to call the provider
- Change diet to
  - Diabetic
- Protocols
  - Hypoglycemia (if not already initiated)

- Referrals
  - Dietician
  - Endocrinology
- Ask if the provider wants anything else done
- Read back orders; ask that they enter all orders into the electronic medical record

ISBARR Template	
I Introduction	**Introduce Yourself and the Patient** • "Hello, Dr. Bernier, this is Adam Jost. I am calling about your patient Jessica Navarro in Room 407 at Evergreen Assisted Living."
S Situation	**Sign/Symptom You Are Concerned About** • "I'm calling because Ms. Navarro has been having symptomatic hypoglycemic episodes. Her blood sugar before dinner today was 50. She had a similar episode of hypoglycemia before dinner yesterday. Her blood sugar was 42 at that time and improved after she ate." **Associated Signs/Symptoms** • "During the episode this evening, she was having some mild nausea and lightheadedness."
B Background	**Vitals** • "Blood pressure was 130/80, heart rate 80, respirations 18, and temperature was 98.2." **Exam** • "When I examined her, she was diaphoretic and anxious." **Past Medical History** • "She has a history of insulin-dependent diabetes," **Labs and Medications** • "and is on high-dose pre-meal sliding scale rapid-acting insulin, 20 units of Lantus at night and 5 mg of glipizide once a day. She got her glipizide this morning, 8 units of insulin before lunch, and has 20 units of Lantus due tonight."

ISBARR Template	
A Assessment	**Assessment** • "I am concerned about her hypoglycemia epi-sodes and her risk of hypoglycemia with the use of rapid-acting insulin and glipizide."
R Recommendations **R** Read Back	**Nurse's Recommendations, Interventions, and Read Back** • "I didn't give her any insulin per the sliding scale orders. Her symptoms resolved with a cup of milk after 15 minutes. Her blood sugar is now 102. Do you want any adjustments to her insulin doses or glipizide? Would you like to change how often we check her blood sugar? Do you want anything else done at this time?" • "Thank you, Dr. Bernier. I just want to read those orders back to you. Change rapid-acting insulin to low-dose sliding scale protocol. Continue current dose of Lantus. Check blood sugar every two hours × 3 and as needed with symptomology. I will call you if she has any more episodes of hypoglycemia."

Disclaimer: This dialogue is factitious and any resemblance to actual persons, living or dead, or actual events is purely coincidental.

In order to avoid order discrepancies, it is recommended that all orders be entered by the provider in the electronic medical record.

Select Differential Diagnosis Presentations

Heart Failure

Overview: broad term to describe pumping malfunction of the heart

Patient may complain of: fatigue, activity intolerance, chest pain, palpitations, dyspnea, orthopnea, PND, coughing, sputum production, weight gain/loss, anorexia, nausea, nocturia, insomnia

Objective findings: signs of acute distress, lethargy, diaphoresis, cyanosis, JVD, bradycardia/tachycardia, hypertension/hypotension, displaced PMI, murmur, gallop, weak pulses, sluggish capillary refill, digital clubbing, edema, breathlessness, tachypnea, cough, adventitious lung sounds, sputum, hepatomegaly, ascites

PMH considerations/risk factors: hx of heart failure, HTN, CAD, cardiac valve disorders, MI, diabetes, arrhythmias, hyper/hypothyroidism, obesity, nicotine use, substance abuse, family hx of heart disease

Diagnostics: BNP, BMP/CMP, TSH, ECG, I/O, chest X-ray, ECHO, cardiac catheterization

Liver Disease/Failure

Overview: broad term to describe damage and malfunction of the liver

Patient may complain of: fatigue, itching, anorexia, nausea, vomiting, RUQ abdominal pain, bloating, signs of GI bleeding

Objective findings: altered mental status, lethargy, jaundice, edema, hypertension/hypotension ascites, abdominal distention, hepatomegaly, spider angiomas; exam may be unremarkable

PMH considerations/risk factors: hx of liver disease, hepatitis, diabetes, sepsis, obesity, cancer, Wilson's disease, IV drug use, alcohol abuse

Diagnostics: CMP, hepatitis panel, ammonia, PT/INR, abdominal US/CT, biopsy

Renal Disease/Failure

Overview: broad term to describe damage and malfunction of the kidneys

Patient may complain of: fatigue, itching, dyspnea, anorexia, nausea, vomiting, oliguria, confusion

Objective findings: lethargy, altered mental status, arrhythmia, edema, pericardial rub, hypertension/hypotension, adventitious lung sounds, oliguria or anuria; exam is typically unremarkable unless severe

PMH considerations/risk factors: hx of CKD, diabetes, HTN, CAD, sepsis, BPH, burn injury, heart failure, dehydration, GI/blood loss, NSAID use, ACE inhibitor use, diuretic use, older age

Diagnostics: BMP/CMP, anion gap, urinalysis, renal US

Sepsis

Overview: severe inflammatory response due to an infection causing organ dysfunction

Patient may complain of: chills, fever, fatigue, generalized weakness, palpitations, (pre)syncope, dyspnea, oliguria; symptoms of whatever infection is suspected (i.e., appendicitis, diverticulitis, cholecystitis, pneumonia, cellulitis, meningitis, UTI)

Objective findings: signs of acute distress/illness, lethargy, fever, altered mental status, cyanosis, cool clammy skin or warm to the touch, tachycardia, hypotension, tachypnea, hypoxia, oliguria; signs of whatever infection is suspected

PMH considerations/risk factors: hx of immunosuppression, diabetes, cancer, recent infection or hospitalization, older/younger age

Diagnostics: blood culture, lactate, CBC, BMP/CMP, PT/INR; workup may also relate to whatever infection is suspected

References

American Diabetes Association. (2015). *Hypoglycemia (low blood sugar).* Retrieved from http://www.diabetes.org/living-with-diabetes/treatment-and-care/blood-glucose-control/hypoglycemia-low-blood.html

American Diabetes Association. (2017). Standards of medical care in diabetes – 2017. *Diabetes Care, 40*(1). Retrieved from https://professional.diabetes.org/sites/professional.diabetes.org/files/media/dc_40_s1_final.pdf

American Medical Directors Association. (2010). *Know-it-all before you call: Data collection system.* Columbia, MD: Author.

Andreassen, L. M., Sandberg, S., Kristensen, G. B., Sølvik, U. O், & Kjome, R. S. (2014). Nursing home patients with diabetes: Prevalence, drug treatment and glycemic control. *Diabetes Research & Clinical Practice, 105*(1), 102–109. doi:10.1016/j.diabres.2014.04.012

Cryer, P. E. (2016). Management of hypoglycemia during treatment of diabetes mellitus. In J. E. Mulder (Ed.), *UpToDate.* Retrieved from https://www.uptodate.com/contents/management-of-hypoglycemia-during-treatment-of-diabetes-mellitus

Cryer, P. E., Axelrod, L., Grossman, A. B., Heller, S. R., Montori, V. M., Seaquist, E. R., & Service, F. J. (2009). Evaluation and management of adult hypoglycemic disorders: An endocrine society clinical practice. *The Journal of Clinical Endocrinology & Metabolism, 94*(3), 709–728.

Desai, S. P. (2009). *Clinician's guide to laboratory medicine* (3rd ed.). Houston, TX: MD2B.

Gosmanov, A. R., Gosmanova, E. O., & Kovesdy, C. P. (2016). Evaluation and management of diabetic and non-diabetic hypoglycemia in end-stage renal disease. *Nephrology Dialysis Transplantation, 31*, 8–15.

Gulanick, M., & Myers, J. L. (2017). *Nursing care plans: Diagnosis, interventions, & outcomes* (9th ed.). St. Louis, MO: Elsevier.

Hale, A., & Hovey, M. J. (2014). *Fluid, electrolyte and acid-base imbalances.* Philadelphia, PA: F.A. Davis Company.

Jarvis, C. (2015). *Physical examination & health assessment.* St. Louis, MO: Elsevier.

LeBlond, R. F., Brown, D. D., Suneja, M., & Szot, J. F. (2015). *DeGowin's diagnostic examination* (10th ed.). New York, NY: McGraw-Hill.

Lekarcyk, J. A., Munshi, M., & Himmel, L. (2013). Blood glucose monitoring and underlying question of hypoglycemia are both essential to preventing hypoglycemia in nursing home residents. *Clinical Diabetes, 31*(1), 28–30.

McCance, K. L., Huether, S. E., Brashers, V. L., & Rote, N. S. (2014). *Pathophysiology: The biologic basis for disease in adults and children* (7th ed.). St. Louis, MO: Elsevier.

National Institute of Diabetes and Digestive and Kidney Diseases. (2016). *Low blood sugar (hypoglycemia).* Retrieved from https://www.niddk.nih.gov/health-information/diabetes/overview/preventing-problems/low-blood-glucose-hypoglycemia

Pandey, S. S., & Chauhan, A. (2015). Achieving 100% reporting of hypoglycemia in a tertiary care hospital through a structured action pathway & persistent monitoring tool among nurses. *International Journal of Nursing Education, 7*(2), 111–115. doi:10.5958/0974-9357.2015.00085.9

Papadakis, M. A., & McPhee, S. J. (2017). *Current medical diagnosis and treatment* (56th ed.). New York, NY: McGraw-Hill.

Raftery, A. T., Lim, E., & Ostor, A. J. (2014). *Differential diagnosis* (4th ed.). London: Elsevier.

Sahni, P., Trivedl, N., & Omer, A. (2016). Insulin autoimmune syndrome: A rare cause of postprandial hypoglycemia. *Endocrinology, Diabetes, & Metabolism Case Reports,* 1–4. doi: 10.1530/EDM-16-0064

Seaquist, E. R., Anderson, J., Childs, B., Cryer, P., Dagogo-Jack, S., Fish, L., . . . Vigersky, R. (2013). Hypoglycemia and diabetes: A report of a workgroup of the American diabetes association and the endocrine society. *Diabetes, 36*, 1384–1395.

Seller, R. H., & Symons, A. B. (2012). *Differential diagnosis of common complaints* (6th ed.). Philadelphia, PA: Elsevier.

Service, F. J., Cryer, P. E., & Vella, A. (2017). Hypoglycemia in adults: Clinical manifestations, definition, and causes. In J. E. Mulder (Ed.), *UpToDate*. Retrieved from https://www.uptodate.com/contents /hypoglycemia-in-adults-clinical-manifestations-definition-and-causes

Service, F. J., & Vella, A. (2016). Postprandial (reactive) hypoglycemia. In J. E. Mulder (Ed.), *UpToDate*. Retrieved from https://www.uptodate .com/contents/postprandial-reactive-hypoglycemia

Service, F. J., & Vella, A. (2017). Hypoglycemia in adults without diabetes mellitus: Diagnostic approach. In J. E. Mulder (Ed.), *UpToDate*. Retrieved from https://www.uptodate.com/contents/hypoglycemia -in-adults-without-diabetes-mellitus-diagnostic-approach

Uphold, C. R., & Graham, M. V. (2013). *Clinical guidelines in family practice* (5th ed.). Gainesville, FL: Barmarrae Books.

Wallace, C. R. (2012). Postoperative management of hypoglycemia. *Orthopedic Nursing, 31*(6), 328–335. doi:10.1097/NOR.0b013e31827424df

CHAPTER 23

Hypotension

Hypotension is not a disease in itself, but is a complex clinical sign of an underlying etiology. It is defined as a systolic blood pressure of <90mmHg and/or a diastolic blood pressure of <60mmHg. Orthostatic hypotension is a drop in blood pressure with position change, specifically a systolic reduction of >20mmHg, and/or a diastolic reduction of >10mmHg. Blood pressure can fluctuate quickly and can be affected not only by position change, but also by eating, sleeping, pain, anxiety, and physical activity.

Some patients may have a lower blood pressure without issue, but it can become a problem when the patient develops obvious signs and symptoms of hypotension. The most common signs and symptoms include fatigue, diaphoresis, dizziness, nausea, altered mental status, and vision changes. Regardless of the cause, hypotension is correlated with poor outcomes, morbidity, and mortality. Quick action and emergency treatment may be required. The nurse's priorities are to maintain the patient's airway, breathing and circulation, ensure that an accurate blood pressure is obtained with proper technique and cuff size, assist in identifying the cause, and monitor for shock. In this chapter, nursing intervention considerations and plan of care recommendations should reflect whatever the suspected cause is.

Differential Diagnosis Considerations

Common: arrhythmia, blood loss, dehydration, heart failure, medication induced, MI, neurally mediated syncope, orthostatic hypotension, sepsis, shock (various types)

Consider: AAA rupture, Addison's disease, anaphylaxis, anemia, aortic dissection, BPPV, burn injury, cardiac valve

disorders, CKD, dialysis, DKA, ectopic pregnancy, endur-
ance athleticism, hyperglycemia, hyperkalemia, hypermagnesemia, hypernatremia, hypoglycemia, hypomagnesemia,
hypothyroidism, liver failure, MS, ovarian cyst rupture,
pancreatitis, Parkinson's disease, PE, pericardial tamponade, peripheral neuropathy, pneumothorax, poisoning,
post-prandial effect, pregnancy, prolonged immobility, Shy-
Drager syndrome, spinal cord dysfunction, TBI, transfusion
reaction, vasovagal reflex

Questions to Ask the Patient/ Family/Witness/Yourself

- What makes the hypotension better (certain positions, elevation of legs)?
- What makes the hypotension worse (activity, changing positions, standing)?
- Do you have any dizziness or feel like you will faint when you change positions?
- How is your appetite? Are you able to keep down food and/ or fluids?
- When was the last time you ate? What did you eat?
- How much fluid are you drinking on a daily basis?
- Do you have a diet low in salt?
- How often do you exercise?
- Do you have a history of low blood pressure? If so, what has been done or used to treat it?
- When was your last menstrual period? (if applicable)
- Have you had any recent: illness/infection? dialysis? dietary changes or fasting/NPO status? exposure to any infection/ illness or been around anyone who is sick? immobilization such as prolonged time spent in bed or sitting? immuniza- tions? surgery? trauma?
- Have you had any recent invasive interventions such as a blood transfusion?

- Have you taken any new prescribed or over-the-counter medications? Have there been any recent changes to your current medication?
- What are you allergic to? Have you been exposed to a known allergen?
- Do you drink alcohol? How many drinks per day/week? What kind and amount of alcohol do you drink? When was your last drink? (if applicable)

If the patient has a history of HTN

- Have you been using your blood pressure medications as prescribed? Have you been taking more medication than what is prescribed?
- Do you check your blood pressure at home? What are your average readings?

Associated Signs/Symptoms: PAIN: pain anywhere; GENERAL: fatigue, fever, weakness; EENT: vision changes; CARDIOVASCULAR: chest pain/tightness, palpitations; RESPIRATORY: cough, dyspnea; GASTROINTESTINAL: diarrhea, nausea, signs of GI bleeding, vomiting; GENITOURINARY: dysuria, oliguria, urinary frequency, urinary urgency; MUSCULOSKELETAL: muscle cramps; NEUROLOGICAL: syncope, tremors; SKIN: ecchymosis; ENDOCRINE: polydipsia, polyphagia, polyuria, sweating; PSYCHOLOGICAL: anxiety, confusion

Recommended Assessments

- Vital signs
  - Orthostatic blood pressure
- Temperature
- Weight
- I/O
- Pain scale (if applicable)
  - Tolerable pain level

- General
  - Level of consciousness and orientation
  - Inspect: signs of acute distress, acute illness, affect, restlessness
- Skin
  - Inspect: cyanosis, diaphoresis, dryness, jaundice, mottling, pallor, urticarial rash
  - Palpate: temperature, turgor
- Mouth
  - Inspect: swelling or erythema of the lips, posterior pharynx and/or tongue, mucous membrane moisture level
- Head/face/neck
  - Inspect: JVD, ROM of neck, signs of trauma, tracheal deviation
  - Auscultate: carotid bruits
  - Palpate: swelling, tenderness
- Cardiovascular
  - Auscultate: heart sounds, rate, rhythm
  - Palpate: heaves, thrills
- Respiratory
  - Inspect: chest asymmetry, respiratory effort, depth, pattern, use of accessory muscles
  - Auscultate: lung sounds
- Gastrointestinal
  - Inspect: distention
  - Auscultate: bowel sounds
  - Palpate: guarding, masses, organomegaly, tenderness
- Genitourinary
  - Inspect: external drainage, erythema, swelling, lesions
  - Palpate: bladder distention, CVAT
- Neurological
  - Inspect: tremors
  - Palpate: extremity strength, sensation
- Extremities
  - Inspect: IV site
  - Palpate: capillary refill, edema, pulses

Past Medical History Considerations

- Allergies

Puts the patient at risk for differential considerations

- Alcohol abuse/use
- Bleeding/clotting disorder
- CKD
- Diabetes
- HTN
- Immobilization
- Liver disease

Reoccurrence/exacerbation should be considered

- Anaphylaxis
- Arrhythmias (various)
- GI bleed
- Heart failure
- MI
- PE

Chronic conditions that can cause or mimic signs and symptoms of hypotension

- Addison's disease
- Anemia
- Arrhythmias (various)
- BPPV
- Cardiac valve disorders
- CKD
- Heart failure
- MS
- Parkinson's disease
- Peripheral neuropathy
- Pregnancy
- Spinal cord injury
- TBI
- Thyroid disease

Medication Evaluation

Most common causative/exacerbating medication

- ACE inhibitors
- Alpha-1 adrenergic antagonist
- Alpha-2 adrenergic agonists
- Antipsychotics
- ARBs
- Benzodiazepines
- Beta blockers
- CCBs
- Cholinergic agonists
- Diuretics
- Insulin
- Levodopa
- Neuromuscular blockers
- Nitrates
- Opioids
- Propofol
- Tricyclics antidepressants
- Vasodilators

Lab Evaluation and Trends

- BMP/CMP
- CBC
- PT/INR (if applicable)

Nursing Intervention Considerations

- Call for help or rapid response/code team if vital signs are unstable or there are signs of urgent distress
- Maintain a patent airway
  - Apply oxygen if hypoxic
  - Call respiratory therapy for signs of respiratory distress
- Verify patent IV if IVF or IV medication treatment is anticipated
  - Flush according to facility protocol; watch for swelling, erythema, pain, and other signs of infiltration
  - Large bore IV is preferred

- ECG
- Blood sugar if hypo- or hyperglycemia is suspected
- Medications (if ordered or protocol allows)
  - Hold suspected causative medication until discussion with the provider
  - Rapid or bolus IV fluids per rapid response orders
- Diet
  - Push fluids if there are no contraindications (>2,000mL/day)
- Activity
  - Keep the patient in bed until discussion with the provider
- Positioning
  - Lay supine with feet elevated (preferred)
  - HOB raised to comfort for respiratory distress
  - HOB elevated at least 4 inches if orthostatic hypotension is present
  - Reposition every 2–4 hours or establish an individualized turning schedule
- Monitor
  - Stay with the patient until stable
  - Vital signs and trends
  - Oxygen saturation/pulse oximetry
  - I/O
  - Telemetry/cardiac monitor
  - Blood sugar trends (if applicable)
  - Orientation status changes
  - Agitation levels
  - Peripheral pulses
  - Skin assessment every 8–24 hours
  - Signs of decreased cardiac output such as weak pulses, cool skin, altered mental status, hypotension, oliguria, and mottling
  - Signs of respiratory distress such as cyanosis, tachypnea, hypoxia, use of accessory muscles, diaphoresis, and adventitious lung sounds

- Signs of dehydration such as lethargy, decreased skin turgor, dry mucous membranes, tachycardia, and (orthostatic) hypotension
- Signs and symptoms of blood loss such as fatigue, dizziness, dyspnea, melena, hematochezia, hematemesis, hematuria, epistaxis, pallor, ecchymosis, altered mental status, hypotension, tachycardia, tachypnea, and hemoptysis
- Signs and symptoms of sepsis such as fever, chills, hypotension, altered mental status, hypoxia, cool clammy skin, dyspnea, oliguria, tachycardia, and tachypnea
- Safety
  - Perform a fall risk assessment and implement the appropriate strategies
- Environment
  - Provide a calm, quiet environment and reduce stimulation
  - Maintain a well-lit environment
- Supportive care
  - Maintain effective communication between yourself, patient, and family
  - Provide emotional support and reassurance to the patient and family
  - Maintain a calm manner during patient interactions
  - Discuss plan of care with the patient and decide reasonable goals together
  - Notify the patient and family of changes in the plan of care
  - Re-orient the patient as needed
  - Promote skin care and integrity
  - **Educational topics (as applicable to the patient):**
    - General information regarding the patient's hypotension and differential diagnosis considerations
    - Procedure and intervention explanation and justification
    - Medication changes
    - Laboratory monitoring needs
    - Oxygen therapy and maintenance
    - Relaxation techniques and breathing exercises

- Energy conservation techniques: placing items within reach, sitting to do tasks, taking breaks in between activities, sliding rather than lifting, pushing rather than pulling
- Telemetry
- Avoidance of vagal maneuvers
- Skin care
- Proper positioning and turning schedule
- Safety needs and fall risk
- Handwashing and infection control measures
- Position change techniques and avoidance of standing for long periods of time
- Increased sodium intake (if appropriate)
- Increased fluid intake
- Alcohol and/or drug cessation and support
- Home blood pressure monitoring
- When to notify the nurse or provider
- Signs and symptoms of hyper- and hypoglycemia
- Signs and symptoms of cardiac emergencies
- Signs and symptoms of respiratory emergencies
- Signs and symptoms of abnormal bleeding
- Dehydration prevention
- Pressure injury prevention

ISBARR Recommendation Considerations

- Ask the provider to come assess the patient STAT if they are symptomatic or unstable
- Transfer to the ICU if hemodynamically unstable, advanced medication management is required, or closer monitoring is needed
- Medication
  - Discontinue/change suspected causative medication
  - Change PRN and/or scheduled anti-hypertensive
- IV fluid needs if oral intake is poor, there are signs of dehydration, and the patient is NPO or hypotensive. Rapid infusion or bolus rates should be discussed.

- ECG if not already done or repeat testing is needed
- Labs (depending on the suspected cause)
  - ABG
  - Blood culture
  - BMP/CMP
  - BNP
  - Cardiac enzymes
  - CBC
  - D-dimer
  - Lactate
  - Magnesium
  - PT/INR
  - TSH
- Safety
  - Activity-level changes
  - Fall risk protocol
- Monitoring needs
  - Blood sugars including frequency and parameters to call the provider (if applicable)
  - Continuous O_2 monitoring
  - Daily weights
  - Telemetry/continuous cardiac monitoring
  - Strict I/O
  - Vital signs, including frequency and parameters to call the provider
- Supportive cares
  - Compression stockings or SCDs
- Change diet to
  - Increased sodium intake
  - Push oral fluids
- Referrals
  - Cardiology
- Ask if the provider wants anything else done
- Read back orders; ask that they enter all orders into the electronic medical record

Hypotension

ISBARR Template	
I **Introduction**	**Introduce Yourself and the Patient** • "Hello, Dr. Breen. This is Aaron Rodgers. I am the nurse for your patient Danielle Christel in Room 203. She is your patient who had a positive *C. difficile* stool culture yesterday."
S **Situation**	**Sign/Symptom You Are Concerned About** • "Ms. Christel has been hypotensive for the past hour. This is a new issue for her. Systolically, she has been between 80–90. Diastolically, she has been between 40–60. Last blood pressure, two minutes ago, was 88/50." **Associated Signs/Symptoms** • "She has had seven moderate-sized watery bowel movements in the past three hours but has not had any vomiting or signs of GI bleeding."
B **Background**	**Vitals** • "Other vital signs are stable. Heart rate is 96, respiratory rate is 16, and she is afebrile." **Exam** • "Her oral mucosa is very dry and she has been fatigued. This shift so far, her oral intake is 100cc. It is hard to tell if she has urinated because she is having so much diarrhea. She believes she has urinated along with her bowel movements." **Past Medical History** • "She does not take any medication for hypertension." **Labs and Medications** • "CMP and CBC this morning were both normal. She does have 100cc IV normal saline running and is taking oral metronidazole for the *C. difficile*."

ISBARR Template	
A **Assessment**	**Assessment** • "I am concerned about dehydration causing her hypotension."
R **Recommendations** **R** **Read Back**	**Nurse's Recommendations, Interventions, and Read Back** • "Would you like me to give her a fluid bolus or increase her IV fluid rate? Did you want any other labs? Can I start her on the fall risk protocol because she is fatigued and weak? Would you like anything else done at this time?" • "Thank you, Dr. Breen. I would like to read those orders back to you. You would like a 500cc bolus over 30 minutes STAT, and after it is completed, increase IV infusion rate to 150cc per hour. I will continue to push oral fluids and monitor I/O closely. I will check blood pressure q1hr × 4 and call you if the blood pressure does not improve. I will also implement the fall risk protocol."

Disclaimer: This dialogue is factitious and any resemblance to actual persons, living or dead, or actual events is purely coincidental.

In order to avoid order discrepancies, it is recommended that all orders be entered by the provider in the electronic medical record.

Select Differential Diagnosis Presentations

Abdominal Aortic Aneurysm Rupture

Overview: abnormal dilation of the abdominal aorta leads to vessel rupture

Patient may complain of: severe abdominal/back pain, palpitations, nausea, vomiting, dizziness

Objective findings: signs of acute distress, altered mental status, diaphoresis, tachycardia, hypotension, pulsating abdominal mass, abdominal bruit

PMH considerations/risk factors: hx of CAD, HTN, heart failure, diabetes, connective tissue disorders, trauma to the abdomen, nicotine use, family hx of AAA, male gender, older age

Diagnostics: abdominal US/CT/MRI

Aortic Dissection

Overview: a tear in the intima layer of the aorta

Patient may complain of: severe chest/back pain described as ripping or tearing, abdominal pain, flank pain, dyspnea, nausea, dizziness, (pre)syncope, paresthesias, feelings of impending doom

Objective findings: signs of acute distress, altered mental status, diaphoresis, cool clammy skin, syncope, JVD, murmur, hypotension/hypertension, weak pulses or pulse deficit, sluggish capillary refill, tachypnea

PMH considerations/risk factors: hx of HTN, heart failure, cardiac valve disorders, connective tissue disorders, diabetes, substance abuse, pregnancy, nicotine use, male gender, older age

Diagnostics: ECG, TE, chest X-ray, chest CT, aortography

Arrhythmia

Overview: any irregular heart rhythm

Patient may complain of: fatigue, generalized weakness, (pre) syncope, palpitations, chest pain, dyspnea, dizziness, seizures, anxiety

Objective findings: signs of acute distress, lethargy, irritability, diaphoresis, irregular heart rhythm, bradycardia/tachycardia, murmur, hypertension/hypotension, tachypnea, seizures

PMH considerations/risk factors: hx of arrhythmia, CAD, HTN, heart failure, MI, cardiac valve disorders, diabetes, previous CV surgery, substance abuse, increased psychological stress, nicotine use, family hx of heart disease

Diagnostics: BMP/CMP, CBC, TSH, ECG, ECHO, Holter monitor/loop recorder/event recorder

Benign Paroxysmal Positional Vertigo

Overview: abnormal calcium debris within the inner ear causing obstruction of fluid movement, leading to acute dizziness

Patient may complain of: nausea, vomiting, dizziness with head position changes, balance disturbances; symptoms have a short duration

Objective findings: nystagmus, positive Dix–Hallpike maneuver, gait instability

PMH considerations/risk factors: hx of BPPV, orthostatic hypotension, recent head injury or ear infection, female gender

Diagnostics: clinical diagnosis; workup to rule out more emergent causes may be indicated

Dehydration

Overview: abnormal loss of extracellular fluid volume

Patient may complain of: fatigue, thirst, dry mouth, palpitations, constipation, oliguria, muscle cramps, dizziness, headache

Objective findings: fever, altered mental status, lethargy, irritability, decreased skin turgor, generalized skin dryness, dry mucous membranes, (orthostatic) hypotension, tachycardia, oliguria

PMH considerations/risk factors: hx of liver or renal disease/failure, recent vomiting and/or diarrhea, GI bleeding, polyuria, diuretic use, burn injury, or intense physical activity

Diagnostics: BMP/CMP, CBC, urine Na, I/O

Diabetic Ketoacidosis

Overview: lack of insulin leads to extreme hyperglycemia and the production of ketones, causing the blood to be more acidic

Patient may complain of: fatigue, generalized abdominal pain, nausea, vomiting, dyspnea, polyuria, polyphagia, polydipsia

Objective findings: altered mental status, lethargy, acetone breath, decreased skin turgor, dry mucous membranes, tachycardia, hypotension, tachypnea

PMH considerations/risk factors: hx of type 1 diabetes, medication noncompliance, substance abuse, recent major illness or stress

Diagnostics: anion gap, BMP/CMP, ABG, hemoglobin A1C, urine ketones

Ectopic Pregnancy

Overview: fertilized egg implants outside of the uterus, typically in the fallopian tubes

Patient may complain of: chills, fever, breast tenderness, severe lower abdominal pain, nausea, vomiting, irregular vaginal bleeding, dizziness

Objective findings: signs of acute distress/illness, fever, hypotension, tachycardia, lower abdominal tenderness, vaginal bleeding

PMH considerations/risk factors: hx of infertility, IUD, previous GYN surgeries

Diagnostics: urine or serum Hcg, pelvic US, pelvic exam

Heart Failure

Overview: broad term to describe pumping malfunction of the heart

Patient may complain of: fatigue, activity intolerance, chest pain, palpitations, dyspnea, orthopnea, PND, coughing, sputum production, weight gain/loss, anorexia, nausea, nocturia, insomnia

Objective findings: signs of acute distress, lethargy, diaphoresis, cyanosis, JVD, bradycardia/tachycardia, hypertension/hypotension, displaced PMI, murmur, gallop, weak pulses, sluggish capillary refill, digital clubbing, edema, breathlessness, tachypnea, cough, adventitious lung sounds, sputum, hepatomegaly, ascites

PMH considerations/risk factors: hx of heart failure, HTN, CAD, cardiac valve disorders, MI, diabetes, arrhythmias, hyper/hypothyroidism, obesity, nicotine use, substance abuse, family hx of heart disease

Diagnostics: BNP, BMP/CMP, TSH, ECG, I/O, chest X-ray, ECHO, cardiac catheterization

Hyperkalemia

Overview: elevated serum potassium

Patient may complain of: fatigue, palpitations, diarrhea, nausea, vomiting, dyspepsia, muscle weakness and cramps, paresthesias; patient is typically asymptomatic unless severe

Objective findings: lethargy, hypotension, peaked T waves, arrhythmia, weak pulses, hyperactive bowel sounds; exam is typically unremarkable unless severe

PMH considerations/risk factors: hx of arrhythmia, CKD, AKI, Addison's disease, diabetes, burn injury, recent surgery

Diagnostics: serum K, ECG

Hypermagnesemia

Overview: elevated serum magnesium

Patient may complain of: fatigue, palpitations, nausea, vomiting, muscle spasms, headache; patient is typically asymptomatic unless severe

Objective findings: lethargy, altered mental status, diaphoresis, flushing, hypotension, bradycardia, arrhythmia, prolonged PR interval, wide QRS complex, bradypnea, decreased reflexes; exam is typically unremarkable unless severe

PMH considerations/risk factors: hx of gastroparesis, ileus, intestinal obstruction, CKD, AKI, hypothyroidism, magnesium supplementation

Diagnostics: serum Mg, ECG

Hypernatremia

Overview: elevated serum sodium

Patient may complain of: thirst, muscle spasms and cramps, tremors, seizures, anxiety; patient is typically asymptomatic unless severe

Objective findings: irritability, altered mental status, decreased skin turgor, dry mucous membranes, tachycardia, hypotension, bradypnea, decreased reflexes; exam is typically unremarkable unless severe

PMH considerations: hx of AKI, Cushing's syndrome, GI loss, burn injury, diabetes, diuretic use

Diagnostics: serum Na

Hypomagnesemia

Overview: low serum magnesium

Patient may complain of: fatigue, generalized weakness, nausea, vomiting, constipation, confusion, paresthesias, tremors, seizures; patient is typically asymptomatic unless severe

Objective findings: altered mental status, lethargy, bradycardia, hypotension, wide QRS, peaked T waves, prolonged PR interval, arrhythmia, bradypnea, hypoactive bowel sounds, hyperactive reflexes, tremors; exam is typically unremarkable unless severe

PMH considerations/risk factors: hx of diarrhea, burn injury, alcohol abuse/use, malnutrition, DKA, pancreatitis

Diagnostics: serum Mg, ECG

Hypothyroidism

Overview: underactive thyroid gland

Patient may complain of: fatigue, cold intolerance, constipation, weight gain, irregular menstrual cycles, headache, paresthesias

Objective findings: lethargy, skin dryness, facial swelling, goiter, bradycardia, hypotension, hypoactive bowel sounds, decreased reflexes

PMH considerations/risk factors: hx of thyroid dysfunction, autoimmune diseases, radiation therapy of the head and neck, previous thyroidectomy, female gender

Diagnostics: TSH, T3, free T4, TPO; thyroid US may be considered

Liver Disease/Failure

Overview: broad term to describe damage and malfunction of the liver

Patient may complain of: fatigue, itching, anorexia, nausea, vomiting, RUQ abdominal pain, bloating, signs of GI bleeding

Objective findings: altered mental status, lethargy, jaundice, edema, ascites, abdominal distention, hepatomegaly, spider angiomas, hypertension/hypotension; exam may be unremarkable

PMH considerations/risk factors: hx of liver disease, hepatitis, diabetes, sepsis, obesity, cancer, Wilson's disease, IV drug use, alcohol abuse

Diagnostics: CMP, hepatitis panel, ammonia, PT/INR, abdominal US/CT, biopsy

Myocardial Infarction

Overview: decreased or no blood flow through the coronary arteries causing cardiac muscle death

Patient may complain of: fatigue, chest pain not improved with rest, radiation of the pain to the left arm/neck/jaw, palpitations, dyspnea, activity intolerance, abdominal pain, nausea, dizziness, anxiety, feelings of impending doom; symptoms have longer duration than stable angina

Objective findings: signs of acute distress, lethargy, irritability, altered mental status, diaphoresis, cool clammy skin, hypertension/hypotension, tachycardia/bradycardia, arrhythmia, murmur, ST elevations, pathologic Q waves, weak pulses, sluggish capillary refill, tachypnea

PMH considerations/risk factors: hx of MI, CAD, HTN, heart failure, hyperlipidemia, diabetes, cardiac valve disorders, sedentary lifestyle, NSAID use, nicotine use, substance abuse, family hx of heart disease, older age

Diagnostics: cardiac enzymes, ECG, stress test, coronary angiography

Ovarian Cyst Rupture

Overview: rupture of a fluid-filled sac on the ovary

Patient may complain of: generalized weakness, nausea, vomiting, sudden onset of unilateral pelvic pain typically after sexual intercourse, vaginal bleeding

Objective findings: signs of acute distress, irritability, unilateral abdominal/pelvic tenderness; tachycardia, hypotension, positive Cullen's sign (abdominal ecchymosis) if there is intraabdominal bleeding

PMH considerations/risk factors: hx of ovarian cysts or polycystic ovarian syndrome (PCOS), fertility treatments, nicotine use, family hx of ovarian cancer, younger age (<40 years)

Diagnostics: clinical diagnosis; pelvic US, pelvic exam may be considered

Pancreatitis

Overview: inflammation of the pancreas

Patient may complain of: fatigue, chills, fever, epigastric/upper abdominal pain, radiation of the pain to the back, worse with movement, nausea, vomiting, dyspepsia, diarrhea

Objective findings: signs of acute distress/illness, lethargy, fever, diaphoresis, pallor, jaundice, tachycardia, hypotension, upper abdominal/epigastric tenderness, abdominal distention, positive Cullen's sign or Grey Turner sign (abdominal ecchymosis)

PMH considerations/risk factors: hx of chronic pancreatitis, hypertriglyceridemia, cholelithiasis, GI cancer, recent GI surgery or trauma to the abdomen, nicotine use, alcohol abuse/use

Diagnostics: amylase, lipase, abdominal CT/US

Pneumothorax

Overview: abnormal air or fluid in the pleural cavity causing lung collapse

Patient may complain of: sudden onset of chest pain, palpitations, dyspnea, coughing, anxiety, feelings of impending doom

Objective findings: signs of acute distress, tachycardia, hypotension, tachypnea, diminished/absent unilateral breath sounds, uneven chest excursion, tracheal deviation, hypoxia, cough

PMH considerations/risk factors: hx of Marfan syndrome, COPD, cystic fibrosis, asthma, TB, trauma to the chest/back, thin body habitus, recent thoracentesis or pulmonary biopsy, family hx of pneumothorax, nicotine use, male gender

Diagnostics: chest X-ray

Pulmonary Embolism

Overview: a blood clot in the pulmonary vasculature

Patient may complain of: chills, fever, chest pain, pain with deep breaths, palpitations, activity intolerance, dyspnea, coughing, hemoptysis, abdominal pain, dizziness

Objective findings: signs of acute distress, fever, pallor, cyanosis, diaphoresis, tachycardia, S3/S4 heart sounds, hypotension, tachypnea, hypoxia, cough, signs of DVT

PMH considerations/risk factors: hx of DVT, PE or CVA, bleeding/clotting disorder, cancer, pregnancy, HRT/birth control use, IV drug use, recent surgery, immobility, nicotine use

Diagnostics: D-dimer, chest CT, V/Q scan, chest X-ray

Renal Disease/Failure

Overview: broad term to describe damage and malfunction of the kidneys

Patient may complain of: fatigue, itching, dyspnea, anorexia, nausea, vomiting, oliguria, confusion

Objective findings: lethargy, altered mental status, arrhythmia, edema, pericardial rub, hypertension/hypotension, adventitious lung sounds, oliguria or anuria; exam is typically unremarkable unless severe

PMH considerations/risk factors: hx of CKD, diabetes, HTN, CAD, sepsis, BPH, burn injury, heart failure, dehydration, GI/blood loss, NSAID use, ACE inhibitor use, diuretic use, older age

Diagnostics: BMP/CMP, anion gap, urinalysis, renal US

Sepsis

Overview: severe inflammatory response due to an infection causing organ dysfunction

Patient may complain of: chills, fever, fatigue, generalized weakness, palpitations, (pre)syncope, dyspnea, oliguria; symptoms of whatever infection is suspected (i.e., appendicitis, diverticulitis, cholecystitis, pneumonia, cellulitis, meningitis, UTI)

Objective findings: signs of acute distress/illness, lethargy, fever, altered mental status, cyanosis, cool clammy skin or warm to the touch, tachycardia, hypotension, tachypnea, hypoxia, oliguria; signs of whatever infection is suspected

PMH considerations/risk factors: hx of immunosuppression, diabetes, cancer, recent infection or hospitalization, older/younger age

Diagnostics: blood culture, lactate, CBC, BMP/CMP, PT/INR; workup may also relate to whatever infection is suspected

References

Alagiakrishnan, K. (2015). Current pharmacological management of hypotensive syndromes in the elderly. *Drugs Aging, 32*, 337–348.

American Heart Association. (2017). *Low blood pressure-when blood pressure is too low*. Retrieved from http://www.heart.org/HEARTORG/Conditions/HighBloodPressure/GettheFactsAboutHighBloodPressure/Low-Blood-Pressure---When-Blood-Pressure-Is-Too-Low_UCM_301785_Article.jsp#.Wt0uB8aZO3U

American Medical Directors Association. (2010). *Know-it-all before you call: Data collection system*. Columbia, MD: Author.

Barnason, S., Williams, J., Patrick, V. C., Storer, A., Brim, C., Halpren, J., . . . Bradford, J. Y. (2012). *Clinical practice guideline: Non-invasive blood pressure measurement with automated devices*. Retrieved from https://www.ena.org/docs/default-source/resource-library/practice-resources/cpg/nibpmcpg.pdf?sfvrsn=8fe4af94_12

Cheung, W. K., Chau, L. S., Mak, I. I., Wong, M. Y., Wong, S. L., & Tiwari, A. F. (2015). Clinical management for patients admitted to a critical care unit with severe sepsis or septic shock. *Intensive and Critical Care Nursing, 31*, 359–365.

Colwell, C. (2018). Initial evaluation of shock in the adult trauma patient and management of non-hemorrhagic shock. In J. Grayzel (Ed.), *UpToDate*. Retrieved from https://www.uptodate.com/contents/initial-evaluation-of-shock-in-the-adult-trauma-patient-and-management-of-non-hemorrhagic-shock

Dennis, C. J., Chung, K. K., Holland, S. R., Yoon, B. S., Milligan, D. J., Nitzschke, S. L., . . . Renz, E. M. (2012). Risk factors for hypotension in urgently intubated burn patients. *Burns, 38,* 1181–1185.

Desai, S. P. (2009). *Clinician's guide to laboratory medicine* (3rd ed.). Houston, TX: MD2B.

Diroll, D. (2014). Oxygen as an adjunct to treat intradialytic hypotension during hemodialysis. *Nephrology Nursing Journal, 41*(4), 420–423.

Gaieski, D. F., & Mikkelsen, M. E. (2018). Evaluation of and initial approach to the adult patient with undifferentiated hypotension and shock. In G. Finlay (Ed.), *UpToDate.* Retrieved from https://www.uptodate .com/contents/evaluation-of-and-initial-approach-to-the-adult-patient -with-undifferentiated-hypotension-and-shock

Gulanick, M., & Myers, J. L. (2017). *Nursing care plans: Diagnosis, interventions, & outcomes* (9th ed.). St. Louis, MO: Elsevier.

Hale, A., & Hovey, M. J. (2014). *Fluid, electrolyte and acid-base imbalances.* Philadelphia, PA: F.A. Davis Company.

Jarvis, C. (2015). *Physical examination & health assessment.* St. Louis, MO: Elsevier.

Kaufman, H., & Kaplan, N. M. (2015a). Mechanism, causes, and evaluation of orthostatic hypotension. In J. L. Wilterdink (Ed.), *UpToDate.* Retrieved from https://www.uptodate.com/contents/mechanisms -causes-and-evaluation-of-orthostatic-hypotension

Kaufman, H., & Kaplan, N. M. (2015b). Treatment of orthostatic and postprandial hypotension. In J. L. Wilterdink (Ed.), *UpToDate.* Retrieved from https://www.uptodate.com/contents/treatment -of-orthostatic-and-postprandial-hypotension

Kolarik, M., & Roberts, E. (2017). Permissive hypotension and trauma: Can fluid restriction reduce the incidence of ARDS? *Journal of Trauma Nursing, 24*(1), 19–E2. doi:10.1097/JTN.0000000000000257

Kotanko, P., & Henrich, W. L. (2018). Intradialytic hypotension in an otherwise stable patient. In M. Sheridan (Ed.), *UpToDate.* Retrieved from https:// www.uptodate.com/contents/intradialytic-hypotension-in-an-otherwise -stable-patient

LeBlond, R. F., Brown, D. D., Suneja, M., & Szot, J. F. (2015). *DeGowin's diagnostic examination* (10th ed.). New York, NY: McGraw-Hill.

Magner, D. R. (2012). Orthostatic hypotension pathophysiology, problems and prevention. *Home Healthcare Nurse, 30*(9), 525–530.

McCance, K. L., Huether, S. E., Brashers, V. L., & Rote, N. S. (2014). *Pathophysiology: The biologic basis for disease in adults and children* (7th ed.). St. Louis, MO: Elsevier.

Metzler, M., Duerr, S., Granata, R., Krismer, F., Robertson, D., & Wenning, G. K. (2013). Neurogenic orthostatic hypotension: Pathophysiology, evaluation, and management. *Journal of Neurology, 260,* 2212–2219.

National Heart, Lung, and Blood Institute. (2010). *Explore hypotension.* Retrieved from https://www.nhlbi.nih.gov/health/health-topics/topics/hyp

Papadakis, M. A., & McPhee, S. J. (2017). *Current medical diagnosis and treatment* (56th ed.). New York, NY: McGraw-Hill.

Seifert, P. C., & Wadlund, D. L. (2015). Crisis management of hypotension in the OR. *AORN Journal, 102*(1), 64–73.

Seller, R. H., & Symons, A. B. (2012). *Differential diagnosis of common complaints* (6th ed.). Philadelphia, PA: Elsevier.

Shibao, C., Lipsitz, L. A., & Biahhioni, I. (2013). ASH position paper: Evaluation and treatment of orthostatic hypotension. *The Journal of Clinical Hypertension, 15*(3), 147–153.

Uphold, C. R., & Graham, M. V. (2013). *Clinical guidelines in family practice* (5th ed.). Gainesville, FL: Barmarrae Books.

Vrtis, M. C. (2013). Preventing and responding to acute kidney injury. *American Journal of Nursing, 113*(4), 38–49. doi:10.1097/01.NAJ.0000428745.71298.16

CHAPTER 24

Insomnia

Insomnia is a common complaint that can cause patients significant suffering. Chronic insomnia can also predispose the patient to diabetes, obesity, and metabolic syndrome. The diagnosis of insomnia includes three components: daytime dysfunction, persistent difficulty falling asleep and/or staying asleep, and waking up too early despite adequate sleep opportunities. Acute insomnia is defined as meeting these criteria for less than 1 month, and chronic insomnia is defined as meeting these criteria for more than 1 month. There are two types of insomnia: primary and secondary. Primary insomnia is often related to stress, substance abuse, medication, trauma, and pain. Once the primary concern has resolved, the insomnia should typically resolve as well. Secondary insomnia can be caused by comorbidities such as COPD, CVA, heart failure, diabetes, Alzheimer's disease, and Parkinson's disease.

Although cognitive behavioral therapy is considered the best and safest strategy for insomnia treatment, it is not always available, especially in the acute care setting. It is important for the nurse to properly assess the patient's insomnia history, create an environment conducive for sleeping, educate the patient on sleep hygiene, and offer short-term medication therapy as appropriate.

Differential Diagnosis Considerations

Common (primary): caffeine intake, environment change/stressors, medication induced, pain, psychological stress/trauma, withdrawal from alcohol/drugs

Other secondary considerations: Alzheimer's disease/dementia, anxiety, asthma, chronic fatigue syndrome, circadian rhythm disorders, COPD, CVA, depression, diabetes, fibromyalgia, GERD, headache, heart failure, hyperthyroidism, menopause, neuropathy, nocturia, nocturnal hypoglycemia, Parkinson's disease, pregnancy, pruritus, PTSD, restless leg syndrome, sleep apnea, TBI

Questions to Ask the Patient/ Family/Witness/Yourself

- When did you start having problems with sleeping?
- Is it happening every night? If not, how many nights a week are you having issues?
- Why do you think you are having problems sleeping?
- Is it harder to fall asleep, stay asleep, or both?
- How many hours of sleep (on average) do you get in a night?
- Do you have a specific routine before you go to sleep?
- What time do you normally go to bed and try to go to sleep?
- How long does it take you to fall asleep?
- How many times do you wake up in the night? How long are you awake each time?
- What time do you usually wake up and not fall back asleep?
- Do you nap during the day?
- Do you have daytime sleepiness or a history of snoring?
- What do you think will help you sleep better?
- Do you have a past history of sleeping issues? If so, what have you done or used to treat it?
- Have you had any recent: hospitalization/change in environment? physical or psychological trauma/stress? pregnancy?
- Have you taken any new prescribed or over-the-counter medications? Have there been any recent changes to your current medication?
- Do you drink caffeine? How many drinks in a day? When was the last time you had any?
- Do you drink alcohol? How many drinks per day/week? What kind and amount of alcohol to do you drink? When was your last drink? (if applicable)
- Do you have a history of drug use? What types and how much? Do you use on a daily basis? When was your last use? (if applicable)

Associated Signs/Symptoms: PAIN: pain anywhere; CARDIOVASCULAR: chest pain/tightness, PND, orthopnea; RESPIRATORY: cough, sputum production, dyspnea, wheezing;

GASTROINTESTINAL: heartburn, nausea, vomiting; GENITO-
URINARY: nocturia; NEUROLOGICAL: headache; SKIN: itching,
rash; PSYCHOLOGICAL: anxiety, depression, mood changes

Recommended Assessments

- Vital signs
- Temperature
- Pain scale (if applicable)
  - Tolerable pain level
- General
  - Level of consciousness and orientation
  - Inspect: signs of acute distress, acute illness, affect,
    restlessness

Note: Other examinations may be necessary if there is a secondary cause

Past Medical History Considerations

Puts the patient at risk for differential considerations

- Alcohol use/abuse
- BPH
- Diabetes
- Drug use/abuse
- Nicotine use

Chronic conditions that can cause insomnia

- Alzheimer's disease/dementia
- Anxiety
- Asthma
- Chronic pain
- Chronic fatigue syndrome
- COPD
- CVA
- Depression
- Diabetes
- Fibromyalgia

- GERD
- Heart failure
- HTN
- Menopause
- Migraines
- Neuropathy
- Parkinson's disease
- Pregnancy
- PTSD
- Restless leg syndrome
- Sleep apnea
- TBI
- Thyroid disease

Medication Evaluation

Most common causative/exacerbating medication

- Antidepressants
- Beta blockers
- Bronchodilators
- CCBs
- CNS stimulants
- Corticosteroids
- Decongestants
- Diuretics
- Levothyroxine
- Opioids
- Theophylline

Used to treat insomnia

- Antihistamines
- Benzodiazepines
- Doxepin
- Melatonin
- Non-benzodiazepine hypnotics
- Suvorexant

Lab Evaluation and Trends

- Bedside capillary glucose trends

Nursing Intervention Considerations

- Blood sugar if hypoglycemia is suspected
- Medications (if ordered or protocol allows)
  - Hold suspected causative medication until discussion with the provider
  - PRN sleep medication
  - If hypoglycemic and has altered mental status or unable to swallow, give 1mg IV/IM/SQ glucagon, and/or 25–50mL IV 50% dextrose, or follow your facility's hypoglycemia protocol (goal is >100)
- Diet
  - Avoid caffeine
  - Avoid bladder irritants such as soda, coffee, tea, chocolate
  - Avoid fluid intake 2–3 hours before sleep
  - If hypoglycemic, alert, and can swallow, give a fast-acting carbohydrate like a glucose tablet, 4oz of fruit juice, 8oz of milk, 4oz of non-diet soda, hard candy, or teaspoon of honey/sugar. Repeat until sugar is normalized (goal is >100)
- Positioning
  - To the patient's comfort
- Monitor
  - Pain levels
  - I/O
  - Orientation status changes
  - Blood sugar trends (if applicable)
  - Agitation levels
- Safety
  - Perform a fall risk assessment and implement the appropriate strategies

- Environment
  - Provide a calm, quiet environment and reduce stimulation
  - Maintain a dimly lit environment
  - Decrease stimulation and interruptions at night
  - Remove distractions
  - Put "Do Not Disturb" notice on the patient's door if safety permits
  - Avoid bothersome odors in the room
  - Maintain a comfortable room temperature
  - Offer aromatherapy and/or music therapy (if appropriate)
  - Utilize a fan (if appropriate)
  - Avoid the use of electronics
- Supportive care
  - Maintain effective communication between yourself, patient, and family
  - Provide emotional support and reassurance to the patient and family
  - Maintain a calm manner during patient interactions
  - Discuss plan of care with the patient and decide reasonable goals together
  - Notify the patient and family of changes in the plan of care
  - Identify barriers to care and compliance
  - Offer back rubs, warmed blankets, warm drinks, and new bed linens
  - Allow the patient to wear their own nighttime clothes
  - Encourage the patient to void immediately before trying to sleep
  - **Educational topics (as applicable to the patient):**
    - General information regarding the patient's insomnia and differential diagnosis considerations
    - Explanation regarding referrals and specialist who may see them for this issue
    - New medication education, including reason, side effects, and administration needs

- Medication changes
- Pain scale and pain goals
- Relaxation techniques and breathing exercises
- Safety needs and fall risk
- Caffeine restriction
- Avoidance of bladder irritants
- Alcohol and/or drug cessation and support
- Sleep hygiene
- Stress reduction and management
- Stimulus control
- Signs and symptoms of hypoglycemia

ISBARR Recommendation Considerations

- Medication
  - Discontinue/change suspected causative medication
  - Add PRN and/or scheduled sleeping medication
  - Add PRN and/or scheduled pain medication
- Safety
  - Fall risk protocol
- Monitoring needs
  - Blood sugars including frequency and parameters to call the provider (if applicable)
- Change diet
  - Add a bedtime snack
  - Caffeine restriction
- Protocols
  - CIWA-Ar if alcohol withdrawal is suspected
- Referrals
  - Psychiatry
  - Sleep medicine
- Ask if the provider wants anything else done
- Read back orders; ask that they enter all orders into the electronic medical record

ISBARR Template	
I **Introduction**	**Introduce Yourself and the Patient** • "Hello, Dr. Woda. This is Aimee Penitmalli. I am the nurse for your patient Kelli Jones at Shady Acres Assisted Living."
S **Situation**	**Sign/Symptom You Are Concerned About** • "Ms. Jones told me today that she has had a lot of issues sleeping for the last week. It is hard for her to fall asleep and stay asleep. She has been waking up around four in the morning every day and estimates she only gets three to four hours of sleep a night because she wakes up so often." **Associated Signs/Symptoms** • "She also told me she has been having more anxiety and stress for the past week since finding out she has cancer."
B **Background**	**Vitals** • "Her last set of vitals were taken a week ago and were unremarkable." **Exam** • "She appears fatigued but her physical exam is otherwise unchanged from her baseline." **Past Medical History** • "She does have a history of insomnia and depression" **Labs and Medications** • "and is taking 50mg of Zoloft daily but is not on anything for sleep specifically."
A **Assessment**	**Assessment** • "I believe her worsening insomnia is related to her increased stress about her cancer diagnosis."

ISBARR Template	
R **Recommendations** **R** **Read Back**	**Nurse's Recommendations, Interventions, and Read Back** • "I have been working with her on sleep hygiene and avoiding naps during the day. We also discussed limiting her caffeine. Are we able to start something to help her sleep for the short term? Is there anything else you would like done at this time?" • "Thank you, Dr. Woda. I would just like to read that order back to you. Start 0.5mg one tab PO lorazepam qhs PRN. Is that correct?"

Disclaimer: This dialogue is factitious and any resemblance to actual persons, living or dead, or actual events is purely coincidental.

In order to avoid order discrepancies, it is recommended that all orders be entered by the provider in the electronic medical record.

Select Differential Diagnosis Presentations

Anxiety

Overview: psychiatric disorder that can cause intense fear and worry

Patient may complain of: fatigue, chest pain, palpitations, dyspnea, nausea, vomiting, abdominal pain, constipation/diarrhea, paresthesias, tremors, headache, dizziness, insomnia, mind racing, feelings of impending doom

Objective findings: signs of acute distress, irritability, inability to focus, diaphoresis, tachycardia, hypertension, tachypnea, muscle tension

PMH considerations/risk factors: hx of anxiety, depression, PTSD, insomnia, substance abuse, physical abuse, recent physical or emotional trauma, family hx of psychiatric diseases

Diagnostics: clinical diagnosis; workup to rule out more emergent causes may be indicated

Diabetes

Overview: a group of disease states as a result of poor (or complete lack of) insulin use or production causing chronic hyperglycemia

Patient may complain of: fatigue, weight changes, vision changes, nausea, vomiting, nocturia, numbness/tingling, polyuria, polyphagia, polydipsia

Objective findings: altered mental status, poor wound healing, decreased skin turgor, dry mucous membranes, acanthosis nigricans, retinal hemorrhages, hypertension, sensation disturbances; exam is typically unremarkable unless severe

PMH considerations/risk factors: hx of metabolic syndrome, obesity, sedentary lifestyle, pregnancy, family hx of diabetes, older/younger age

Diagnostics: hemoglobin A1C, fasting blood glucose

Gastroesophageal Reflux Disease

Overview: abnormal reflux of acid from the stomach back into the esophagus

Patient may complain of: sore throat, sour taste in mouth, dysphagia, chest pain or heartburn that may be worse lying flat or after meals, nausea, dyspepsia, epigastric pain, chronic coughing, insomnia

Objective findings: epigastric tenderness; exam is typically unremarkable

PMH considerations/risk factors: hx of GERD, hiatal hernia, obesity, diabetes, pregnancy, nicotine use, alcohol abuse/use

Diagnostics: clinical diagnosis

Heart Failure

Overview: broad term to describe pumping malfunction of the heart

Patient may complain of: fatigue, activity intolerance, chest pain, palpitations, dyspnea, orthopnea, PND, coughing, sputum production, weight gain/loss, anorexia, nausea, nocturia, insomnia

Objective findings: signs of acute distress, lethargy, diaphoresis, cyanosis, JVD, bradycardia/tachycardia, hypertension/hypotension, displaced PMI, murmur, gallop, weak pulses, sluggish capillary refill, digital clubbing, edema, breathlessness, tachypnea, cough, adventitious lung sounds, sputum, hepatomegaly, ascites

PMH considerations/risk factors: hx of heart failure, HTN, CAD, cardiac valve disorders, MI, diabetes, arrhythmias, hyper/hypothyroidism, obesity, nicotine use, substance abuse, family hx of heart disease

Diagnostics: BNP, BMP/CMP, TSH, ECG, I/O, chest X-ray, ECHO, cardiac catheterization

Hyperthyroidism

Overview: overactive thyroid gland

Patient may complain of: anxiety, heat intolerance, fatigue, generalized weakness, palpitations, diarrhea, nausea, vomiting, weight loss, muscle cramps, tremors, seizures, insomnia

Objective findings: lethargy, irritability, diaphoresis, hair thinning, exophthalmos, goiter, tachycardia, hypertension, tremors, seizures, insomnia

PMH considerations/risk factors: hx of Grave's disease, thyroiditis, pregnancy, thyroid cancer, family hx of thyroid dysfunction, female gender, older age

Diagnostics: TSH, T3, T4, thyroid US, radioactive iodine uptake scan

Parkinson's Disease

Overview: progressive movement disorder of the central nervous system

Patient may complain of: fatigue, generalized weakness, vision changes, dysphagia, constipation, urinary retention, gait instability, joint rigidity, tremors, confusion, hallucinations, insomnia; symptoms are progressive in nature

Objective findings: altered mental status, lethargy, flat affect, dysarthria, (orthostatic) hypotension, bradykinesia, generalized muscle and joint rigidity, postural instability, resting tremor, psychosis

PMH considerations/risk factors: hx of Parkinson's disease, trauma to the head, family hx of Parkinson's, male gender, older age

Diagnostics: clinical diagnosis; head MRI may be ordered initially

Sleep Apnea

Overview: pauses in breathing (varying in number and length of time) while sleeping

Patient may complain of: snoring, daytime fatigue, headaches, inability to concentrate, mood changes, dry mouth, insomnia

Objective findings: elevated BMI, mouth breathing, thick neck, enlarged tonsils/uvula/soft palate, hypertension

PMH considerations/risk factors: hx of obesity, enlarged tonsils, nicotine use, narcotic pain medication use, CVA, family hx of sleep apnea, male gender, older age

Diagnostics: sleep study

Withdrawal (Alcohol)

Overview: rapid or abrupt decrease in alcohol intake causing physical and psychological disturbances

Patient may complain of: fever, chills, palpitations, anorexia, nausea, vomiting, diarrhea, seizures, headache, alcohol craving, insomnia, anxiety

Objective findings: signs of acute distress, fever, irritability, altered mental status, diaphoresis, tachycardia, hypertension, hepatomegaly, ascites, seizures, tremors, hallucinations/delirium

PMH considerations: hx of alcohol abuse, longer cessation (>48hrs) since last drink, other substance abuse

Diagnostics: toxicology screen; workup to rule out more emergent causes may be indicated

Withdrawal (Opioids)

Overview: rapid or abrupt decrease in opioid intake causing physical and psychological disturbances

Patient may complain of: fever, body aches, nasal congestion, nasal drainage, anorexia, abdominal cramping, diarrhea, nausea, vomiting, tremors, opioid craving, anxiety, insomnia

Objective findings: signs of acute distress, fever, irritability, altered mental status, diaphoresis, piloerection, frequent yawning, pupil dilatation, rhinorrhea, hypertension, tachycardia, hyperactive bowel sounds

PMH considerations/risk factors: hx of daily opioid use, chronic pain, other substance abuse

Diagnostics: toxicology screen; workup to rule out more emergent causes may be indicated

References

Agency for Healthcare Research and Quality. (2015). *Management of insomnia disorder: Executive summary.* Rockville, MD: Author

American Sleep Association. (2017a). *About insomnia.* Retrieved from https://www.sleepassociation.org/patients-general-public/insomnia/insomnia/

American Sleep Association. (2017b). *Sleep hygiene tips.* Retrieved from https://www.sleepassociation.org/patients-general-public/insomnia/sleep-hygiene-tips/

Anderson, S. L., & Vande Griend, J. P. (2014). Quetiapine for insomnia: A review of the literature. *American Journal of Health-System Pharmacy, 71*(5), 394–402. doi:10.2146/ajhp130221

Arnedt, J. T. (2017). Insomnia in patients with a substance use disorder. In A. F. Eichler (Ed.), *UpToDate.* Retrieved from https://www.uptodate.com/contents/insomnia-in-patients-with-a-substance-use-disorder

Asnis, G. M., Thomas, M., & Henderson, M. A. (2016). Pharmacotherapy treatment options for insomnia: A primer for clinicians. *International Journal of Molecular Sciences, 17*(1), 1–11. doi:10.3390/ijms17010050

Australian Sleep Association. (n.d.). *Insomnia.* Retrieved from www.sleep.org.au

Bonnet, M. H., & Arand, D. L. (2017). Overview of insomnia in adults. In A. F. Eichler (Ed.), *UpToDate.* Retrieved from https://www.uptodate.com/contents/overview-of-insomnia-in-adults

Bonnet, M. H., & Arand, D. L. (2018). Clinical features and diagnosis of insomnia in adults. In A. F. Eichler (Ed.), *UpToDate*. Retrieved from https://www.uptodate.com/contents/clinical-features-and-diagnosis-of-insomnia-in-adults?search=insomnia&source=search_result&selectedTitle=3~150&usage_type=default&display_rank=3

Bonnet, M. H., & Arand, D. L. (2018). Treatment of insomnia in adults. In A. F. Eichler (Ed.), *UpToDate*. Retrieved from https://www.uptodate.com/contents/treatment-of-insomnia-in-adults

Brasure, M., MacDonald, R., Fuchs, E., Olson, C. M., Carlyle, M., Diem, S., ... Wilt, T. J. (2015). Management of insomnia disorder: Comparative effectiveness review. AHRQ Publication No.15(16)-EHC027-EF. Rockville, MD: Author

Canadian Agency for Drugs and Technologies in Health. (2016). *Treatment of older adults with insomnia, agitation, or delirium with benzodiazepines: A review of the clinical effectiveness and guidelines.* Retrieved from https://www.ncbi.nlm.nih.gov/pubmedhealth/PMH0084861

De Crescenzo, F., Foti, F. Ciabattini, M., Del Giovane, C. Watanabe, N., Sane Schepsi, M., ... Amato, L. (2016). Comparative efficacy and acceptability of pharmacological treatments for insomnia in adults: A systematic review and network meta-analysis. *Cochrane Database of Systematic Reviews,* (9), 1–20. doi:10.1002/14651858.CD012364.

Desai, S. P. (2009). *Clinician's guide to laboratory medicine* (3rd ed.). Houston, TX: MD2B.

Gilsenan, I. (2012). Nursing interventions to alleviate insomnia. *Nursing Older People*, 24(4), 14–18.

Gilsenan, I. (2016). How to promote patients' sleep in the hospital. *Nursing Standard, 31*(28), 42–44.

Hale, A., & Hovey, M. J. (2014). *Fluid, electrolyte and acid-base imbalances.* Philadelphia, PA: F.A. Davis Company.

Jarvis, C. (2015). *Physical examination & health assessment.* St. Louis, MO: Elsevier.

LeBlond, R. F., Brown, D. D., Suneja, M., & Szot, J. F. (2015). *DeGowin's diagnostic examination* (10th ed.). New York, NY: McGraw-Hill.

Lie, J. D., Tu, K. N., Shen, D. D., & Wong, B. M. (2015). Pharmacological treatment of insomnia. *P&T, 40*(11), 759–771.

Loh, K. P., Burhenn, P., Hurria, A., Zachariah, F., & Mohile, S. G. (2016). How do I best manage insomnia and other sleep disorders in older adults with cancer? *Journal of Geriatric Oncology, 7*, 413–421.

McCance, K. L., Huether, S. E., Brashers, V. L., & Rote, N. S. (2014). *Pathophysiology: The biologic basis for disease in adults and children* (7th ed.). St. Louis, MO: Elsevier.

McCulloch, D. K., Wang, B., Cohen, A., Allen, S., Arenz, B., Arnold, B., … Thayer, C. (2015). *Sleep disorder guideline.* Retrieved from https://www.ghc.org/static/pdf/public/guidelines/sleep.pdf

Papadakis, M. A., & McPhee, S. J. (2017). *Current medical diagnosis and treatment* (56th ed.). New York, NY: McGraw-Hill.

Phelps, A. J., Varker, T., Metcalf, O., & Dell, L. (2017). What are effective psychological interventions for veterans with sleep disturbances? A rapid evidence assessment. *Military Medicine, 182*(1), 1541–1550. doi:10.7205/MILMED-D-16-00010

Qaseem, A., Kansagara, D., Forciea, M. A., Cooke, M., & Denberg, T. D. Clinical Guidelines Committee of the American College of Physicians. (2016). Management of chronic insomnia disorder in adults: A clinical practice guideline from the American college of physicians. *Annals of Internal Medicine, 19*(165), 125–133.

Raftery, A. T., Lim, E., & Ostor, A. J. (2014). *Differential diagnosis* (4th ed.). London: Elsevier.

Ramar, K., & Olson, E. J. (2013). Management of common sleep disorders. *American Family Physician, 88*(4), 231–238.

Sateia, M. J., Buysse, D. J., Krystal, A. D., Neubauer, D. N., & Heald, J. L. (2017). Clinical practice guideline for the pharmacologic treatment of chronic insomnia in adults: An American academy of sleep medicine clinical practice guideline. *Journal of Clinical Sleep Medicine, 13*(2), 307–349.

Seller, R. H., & Symons, A. B. (2012). *Differential diagnosis of common complaints* (6th ed.). Philadelphia, PA: Elsevier.

Sharma, M. P., & Andrade, C. (2012). *Behavioral interventions for insomnia: Theory and practice.* Retrieved from https://www.ncbi.nlm.nih.gov/pmc/articles/PMC3554970/

Toward Optimized Practice Insomnia Group. (2015). *Assessment to management of adult insomnia: Clinical practice guideline.* Retrieved from http://www.topalbertadoctors.org/download/439/insomnia_management_guideline.pdf

Trauer, J. M., Qian, M. Y., Doyle, J. S., Rajaratnam, S. W., & Cunnington, D. (2015). Cognitive behavioral therapy for chronic insomnia: A systematic review and meta-analysis. *Annals of Internal Medicine, 163*(3), 191–204. doi:10.7326/M14-2841

Uphold, C. R., & Graham, M. V. (2013). *Clinical guidelines in family practice* (5th ed.). Gainesville, FL: Barmarrae Books.

CHAPTER 25

Nausea and Vomiting

Nausea and vomiting can be very stressful and uncomfortable symptoms. Nausea can occur alone or in conjunction with vomiting and other GI distress. Major complications of frequent nausea and vomiting include dehydration, electrolyte disturbances, poor oral intake, aspiration pneumonia, suture tension, wound dehiscence, increased intracranial pressure, and esophageal trauma. It can also diminish the patient's quality of life and inhibit them from performing ADLs. Priorities for the nurse are to recognize complications of the nausea and vomiting, maintain an open airway, prevent aspiration, promote oral intake as tolerated, and help identify the cause. Acute nausea and vomiting issues are usually self-limiting and improves with pharmacologic and nonpharmacologic treatment. Chronic nausea and vomiting issues are less common and not seen as often in the acute care setting.

Differential Diagnosis Considerations

Common: anxiety, cholecystitis, constipation, dysmenorrhea, food/lactose intolerance, gastritis, gastroenteritis, GERD, *Helicobacter pylori* infection, IBS, intestinal obstruction, medication induced, migraine headache, motion sickness, orthostatic hypotension, pain, post-operative state, pregnancy, PUD, urolithiasis, UTI, withdrawal from alcohol/drugs

Consider: acoustic neuroma, anorexia nervosa, appendicitis, BPPV, bulimia nervosa, cyclic vomiting syndrome, depression, digoxin toxicity, diverticulitis, DKA, ectopic pregnancy, esophagitis, functional GI disorders, gastroparesis, GI malignancy, glaucoma, heart failure, hepatitis, hypercalcemia, hyperglycemia, hyperkalemia, hypermagnesemia, hyperthyroidism, hypoglycemia, hypokalemia, hypomagnesemia, hyponatremia, IBD, increased ICP, labyrinthitis, liver disease/failure, Ménière's disease, meningitis, mesenteric ischemia, MI, otitis media, ovarian cyst rupture, pancreatitis, parathyroid disorders, peritonitis, pyelonephritis, pyloric stenosis, radiation therapy, renal failure, seizure disorder, stable angina, thyroid disorders, unstable angina, uremia

Questions to Ask the Patient/ Family/Witness/Yourself

- When did the nausea/vomiting start? Did it start gradually or suddenly?
- Is the nausea/vomiting constant or does it come and go? If intermittent, how long does it last? How often is it happening per hour/day?
- What makes the nausea/vomiting better (certain positions, eating, medication, rest)?
- What triggers the nausea/vomiting or makes it worse (activity, eating, certain positions, light/sound, medication, smells, psychological stress)?
- How severe is your nausea/vomiting (mild/moderate/severe)?
- When is the last time you vomited? Was there blood within the vomit? (if applicable)
- When was your last bowel movement? What did it look like (consistency, amount, color)?
- How is your appetite? Are you able to keep down food and/or fluids?
- When was the last time you ate? What did you eat?
- How much fluid are you drinking on a daily basis?
- When was your last menstrual period? (if applicable)
- In the past 2 days, have you ingested any fried rice, raw milk, uncooked shellfish, undercooked beef, pork, or poultry?
- Do you have a history of lactose intolerance? If so, have you recently ingested any milk, cheese, yogurt, ice cream, or other dairy products?
- Do you have a history of nausea/vomiting? If so, what have you done or used to treat it?

- Have you had any recent: dietary changes? exposure to GI infection, contaminated drinking water, or been around anyone who is sick? pregnancy? radiation therapy? surgery?
- Have you taken any new prescribed or over-the-counter medications? Have there been any recent changes to your current medication?
- Do you drink alcohol? How many drinks per day/week? What kind and amount of alcohol do you drink? When was your last drink? (if applicable)
- Do you have a history of drug use? What types and how much? Do you use on a daily basis? When was your last use? (if applicable)

Associated Signs/Symptoms: PAIN: pain anywhere; GENERAL: chills, fever, weight changes; EENT: ear pain, tinnitus, hearing changes, eye pain, vision changes; CARDIOVASCULAR: chest pain/tightness; RESPIRATORY: cough, dyspnea; GASTROINTESTINAL: appetite changes, bloating, constipation, diarrhea, heartburn, signs of GI bleeding, swallowing difficulties; GENITOURINARY: dysuria, hematuria, penile/vaginal discharge, urinary frequency, urgency, or retention, vaginal bleeding; NEUROLOGICAL: dizziness, headache; PSYCHOLOGICAL: anxiety, confusion, depression

Recommended Assessments

- Vital signs
  - Orthostatic blood pressure (if applicable)
- Temperature
- Weight and nutritional status
- I/O
- Pain scale (if applicable)
  - Tolerable pain level
- General
  - Level of consciousness and orientation
  - Inspect: signs of acute distress, acute illness, affect, restlessness

- Skin
  - Inspect: diaphoresis, dryness, jaundice, pallor
  - Palpate: temperature, turgor
- Eyes
  - Inspect: conjunctival erythema, nystagmus, pupillary response
- Mouth
  - Inspect: bleeding, dentition, halitosis, swelling and erythema of posterior pharynx, mucous membrane moisture level
- Ears
  - Inspect: erythema, external drainage
  - Palpate: external tenderness
- Cardiovascular
  - Auscultate: heart sounds, rate, rhythm
- Respiratory
  - Inspect: respiratory effort
  - Auscultate: lung sounds
- Gastrointestinal
  - Inspect: distention, scarring
  - Auscultate: bowel sounds
  - Palpate: guarding, masses, organomegaly, (rebound) tenderness
- Genitourinary
  - Palpate: bladder distention, CVAT
- Extremities
  - Inspect: IV site (if applicable)

Past Medical History Considerations

- Allergies

Puts the patient at risk for differential considerations

- Abdominal surgery
- Alcohol abuse/use
- Brain malignancy
- Cholelithiasis

- CKD
- CVA/TIA
- Diabetes
- Diverticulosis
- Drug abuse/use
- Immobilization
- Nicotine use
- Ovarian cysts
- Radiation therapy to the abdomen/pelvis
- TBI

Reoccurrence/exacerbation should be considered

- Diverticulitis
- *H. pylori* infection
- Intestinal obstruction
- MI
- Otitis media
- Ovarian cyst rupture
- Urolithiasis
- UTI

Chronic conditions that can cause nausea and vomiting

- Anxiety
- BPPV
- Chronic pain
- Constipation
- Depression
- Dysmenorrhea
- Dyspepsia
- Eating disorders
- Epilepsy
- GERD
- GI malignancy
- Glaucoma
- Heart failure
- Hepatitis

- IBD
- IBS
- Lactose intolerance
- Liver disease
- Ménière's disease
- Migraines
- Pancreatitis
- Parathyroid disorders
- Pregnancy
- PUD
- Thyroid disease

Medication Evaluation

Most common causative/exacerbating medication

- Antiarrhythmics
- Antibiotics
- Anticonvulsants
- Antidiabetics
- Ascorbic acid
- Beta blockers
- Bisphosphonates
- Birth control/HRT
- CCBs
- Chemotherapy
- Digoxin
- Diuretics
- Iron supplements
- NSAIDs
- Opioids
- Potassium supplements

Used to treat nausea/vomiting

- Benzodiazepines
- Cyclizine
- Dexamethasone

- Diphenhydramine
- Dolasetron
- Doxylamine
- Droperidol
- Erythromycin
- Ginger
- Meclizine
- Metoclopramide
- Olanzapine
- Ondansetron
- Prochlorperazine
- Promethazine
- Pyridoxine
- Scopolamine
- Tropisetron

Lab Evaluation and Trends
- Bedside capillary glucose trends
- BMP/CMP

Nursing Intervention Considerations
- Call for help or rapid response/code team if vital signs are unstable or there are signs of urgent distress
- Maintain a patent airway
  - Apply oxygen if hypoxic
  - Encourage slow relaxed deep breathing if hyperventilating
  - Suction as needed
  - Provide oral care throughout the day (q2–4hrs)
- Verify patent IV if IVF or IV medication treatment is anticipated
  - Flush according to facility protocol; watch for swelling, erythema, pain, and other signs of infiltration
- Blood sugar if hypo- or hyperglycemia is suspected

- Medications (if ordered or protocol allows)
  - Hold suspected causative medication until discussion with the provider
  - PRN anti-emetic for nausea, IV/IM if vomiting
  - PRN stool softener, laxative, enema, suppository if constipated
- Diet
  - NPO if intestinal obstruction is suspected
  - NPO if procedure or surgery is anticipated
  - Push fluids if there are no contraindications (>2,000mL/day)
  - Offer bland, simple foods that the patient can tolerate
  - Avoid foods that trigger symptoms
  - Avoid eating food and drinking fluid together
- Positioning
  - Supine or side lying position with knees flexed to chest to take tension off the abdominal wall if the patient has active abdominal pain
  - Side lying position if there is a decrease in LOC or the patient is vomiting
  - HOB raised for 2–3 hours after meals or at night
  - Reposition every 2–4 hours or establish an individualized turning schedule
- Monitor
  - Pain levels
  - Vital signs and trends
  - Temperature trends
  - I/O
  - Blood sugar trends (if applicable)
  - Bowel sounds
  - Weight trends
  - Orientation status changes
  - Agitation levels
  - Skin assessment every 8–24 hours
  - Signs of dehydration such as lethargy, decreased skin turgor, dry mucous membranes, tachycardia, and (orthostatic) hypotension

- Signs and symptoms of increased ICP such as worsening headache, nausea, vomiting, hypertension, bradypnea, altered mental status, vision changes, fixed or sluggish pupillary response, and GCS changes
- Emesis output color, consistency, frequency, and volume
- Stool output color, consistency, frequency, and volume
- Urine output color, frequency, and volume
- Safety
  - Perform a fall risk assessment and implement the appropriate strategies
- Environment
  - Provide a calm, quiet environment and reduce stimulation
  - Provide distractions
  - Avoid bothersome odors in the room
  - Maintain a comfortable room temperature
  - Offer aromatherapy (isopropyl alcohol preferred) and/or music therapy (if appropriate)
  - Utilize a fan (if appropriate)
- Supportive care
  - Maintain effective communication between yourself, patient, and family
  - Provide emotional support and reassurance to the patient and family
  - Maintain a calm manner during patient interactions
  - Discuss plan of care with the patient and decide reasonable goals together
  - Notify the patient and family of changes in the plan of care
  - Promote skin care and integrity
  - Provide light clothing and bed linen
  - **Educational topics (as applicable to the patient):**
    - General information regarding the patient's nausea/vomiting and differential diagnosis considerations
    - New medication education including reason, side effects, and administration needs

- Medication changes
- Pain scale and pain goals
- Relaxation techniques and breathing exercises
- Trigger avoidance
- Skin care
- Proper positioning and turning schedule
- Safety needs and fall risk
- BRAT diet, NPO diet, clear liquid diet
- Avoidance of food/fluid that trigger symptoms
- Increased fluid intake
- Smoking cessation
- Alcohol and/or drug cessation and support
- Stress reduction and management
- When to notify the nurse or provider
- Signs and symptoms of hyper- and hypoglycemia
- Signs and symptoms of GI/GU infection
- Dehydration prevention
- Constipation prevention
- Pressure injury prevention

ISBARR Recommendation Considerations

- Medication (depending on the suspected cause)
  - Hold oral medications if the patient is unable to tolerate or NPO
  - Discuss changing medication routes with the provider (and pharmacy) if the patient is NPO
  - Discontinue/change suspected causative medication
  - Add PPI, H2 antagonist or antacid for dyspepsia, heartburn, or other signs/symptoms of GERD
  - Add PRN anti-emetic for nausea
  - Add PRN and/or scheduled enema, fiber supplement, stool softener, or laxative for constipation

- IV fluid needs if oral intake is poor, there are signs of dehydration, and the patient is NPO or hypotensive
- Imaging (depending on the suspected cause)
  - KUB, abdominal CT scan or US, HIDA scan
- Labs (depending on the suspected cause)
  - Amylase, lipase
  - BMP/CMP
  - Digoxin
  - Hcg (urine or serum)
  - *H. pylori* breath/stool/serum
  - Toxicology screening
  - Urinalysis
  - Urine culture
- Safety
  - Fall risk protocol
- Monitoring needs
  - Blood sugars including frequency and parameters to call the provider (if applicable)
  - Daily weights
  - Strict I/O
  - Vital signs including frequency and parameters to call the provider
- Change diet to (depending on the suspected cause)
  - NPO
  - BRAT or bland
  - Clear liquid diet
  - Push oral fluids
- Protocols
  - CIWA-Ar if alcohol withdrawal is suspected
- Referrals
  - Dietician
- Ask if the provider wants anything else done
- Read back orders; ask that they enter all orders into the electronic medical record

ISBARR Template	
I **Introduction**	**Introduce Yourself and the Patient** • "Hello, Dr. Creighton. This is Beth Ann Turner. I am the nurse for your patient Julie Jansen in Room 302. Ms. Jansen is here for 24-hour observation after her appendectomy earlier today."
S **Situation**	**Sign/Symptom You Are Concerned About** • "I'm calling because she has been having constant nausea for the past hour and had one episode of vomiting with a small emesis." **Associated Signs/Symptoms** • "She is having 3/10 abdominal pain surrounding her sutures. She says her last bowel movement was yesterday."
B **Background**	**Vitals** • "Vitals are stable. Blood pressure is 120/83, heart rate is 80, respiratory rate is 16. She is afebrile with a temperature of 98.2." **Exam** • "Her exam reveals mild tenderness over entire abdomen but it is soft. Bowel sounds are heard throughout. Her steri-strips are clean, dry, and intact. She appears nauseated but her mucous membranes are moist and I see no other signs of dehydration." **Past Medical History** • "She has no history of GI issues." **Labs and Medications** • "I gave her a dose of 2 mg IV morphine about 90 minutes ago. She has normal saline running at 100cc/hour."
A **Assessment**	**Assessment** • "I am suspecting her nausea is related to the morphine."

ISBARR Template	
R Recommendations R Read Back	**Nurse's Recommendations, Interventions, and Read Back** • "I have put a fan in her room which she says has helped. She has been sipping water but has not had any food since the surgery. Can I have an order for a PRN anti-emetic? Did you want to use something else for pain? Did you want anything else done at this time?" • "Thank you, Dr. Creighton. I would like to repeat those orders back to you. Start 4 mg IV ondansetron every eight hours PRN for nausea. Continue diet as tolerated by the patient. Is that correct?"

Disclaimer: This dialogue is factitious and any resemblance to actual persons, living or dead, or actual events is purely coincidental.
In order to avoid order discrepancies, it is recommended that all orders be entered by the provider in the electronic medical record.

Select Differential Diagnosis Presentations

Appendicitis

Overview: inflammation of the appendix

Patient may complain of: chills, fever, fatigue, umbilical abdominal pain (initially), RLQ abdominal pain, anorexia, nausea, vomiting, diarrhea

Objective findings: signs of acute distress/illness, lethargy, low-grade fever, RLQ tenderness with guarding, positive McBurney's point tenderness, positive psoas and obturator sign

PMH considerations/risk factors: hx of IBD, previous GI surgery, younger age (<30 years)

Diagnostics: CBC, abdominal CT

Benign Paroxysmal Positional Vertigo

Overview: abnormal calcium debris within the inner ear causing obstruction of fluid movement, leading to acute dizziness

Patient may complain of: nausea, vomiting, dizziness with head position changes, balance disturbances; symptoms have a short duration

Objective findings: nystagmus, positive Dix–Hallpike maneuver, gait instability

PMH considerations/risk factors: hx of BPPV, orthostatic hypotension, recent head injury or ear infection, female gender

Diagnostics: clinical diagnosis; workup to rule out more emergent causes may be indicated

Cholecystitis

Overview: inflammation of the gallbladder

Patient may complain of: fever, chills, fatigue, RUQ/epigastric pain, right shoulder pain, nausea, vomiting, anorexia, dyspepsia

Objective findings: signs of acute distress/illness, lethargy, fever, diaphoresis, jaundice, tachycardia, RUQ/epigastric tenderness with guarding, positive Murphy's sign, palpable gallbladder

PMH considerations/risk factors: hx of cholelithiasis, obesity, female gender

Diagnostics: CBC, CMP, abdominal CT/US, HIDA scan

Diabetic Ketoacidosis

Overview: lack of insulin leads to extreme hyperglycemia and the production of ketones, causing the blood to be more acidic

Patient may complain of: fatigue, generalized abdominal pain, nausea, vomiting, dyspnea, polyuria, polyphagia, polydipsia

Objective findings: altered mental status, lethargy, acetone breath, decreased skin turgor, dry mucous membranes, tachycardia, hypotension, tachypnea

PMH considerations/risk factors: hx of type 1 diabetes, medication noncompliance, substance abuse, recent major illness or stress

Diagnostics: anion gap, BMP/CMP, ABG, hemoglobin A1C, urine ketones

Diverticulitis

Overview: inflammation of diverticulum

Patient may complain of: fever, chills, LLQ abdominal pain (typically), constipation/diarrhea, nausea, vomiting

Objective findings: signs of acute distress/illness, fever, palpable abdominal mass, LLQ tenderness with guarding

PMH considerations/risk factors: hx of IBD, IBS, diverticulosis, GI cancer, obesity, nicotine use, older age

Diagnostics: CBC, occult stool, abdomen CT/US

Ectopic Pregnancy

Overview: fertilized egg implants outside of the uterus, typically in the fallopian tubes

Patient may complain of: chills, fever, breast tenderness, severe lower abdominal pain, nausea, vomiting, irregular vaginal bleeding, dizziness

Objective findings: signs of acute distress/illness, fever, hypotension, tachycardia, lower abdominal tenderness, vaginal bleeding

PMH considerations/risk factors: hx of infertility, IUD, previous GYN surgeries

Diagnostics: urine or serum Hcg, pelvic US, pelvic exam

Esophagitis (Various Types)

Overview: inflammation of the esophagus

Patient may complain of: painful swallowing, dysphagia, chest pain, heartburn, upper abdominal/epigastric pain, dyspepsia, nausea, vomiting, signs of GI bleeding, dry coughing

Objective findings: oral herpes or thrush (depending on etiology), poor dentition, cough; exam is typically unremarkable

PMH considerations/risk factors: hx of esophagitis, GERD, hiatal hernia, cancer, immunosuppression, allergic diseases (food allergies, asthma, eczema), obesity, radiation therapy of the head, neck, and chest, alcohol abuse/use, nicotine use, NSAID use

Diagnostics: endoscopy with biopsy

Gastritis

Overview: inflammation of the stomach

Patient may complain of: anorexia, nausea, vomiting, dyspepsia, epigastric pain, signs of GI bleeding

Objective findings: nonspecific epigastric tenderness; exam is typically unremarkable

PMH considerations/risk factors: hx of PUD, *H. pylori* infection, NSAID use, alcohol abuse/use, recent travel outside of the United States, older age

Diagnostics: *H. pylori* serum/breath/stool testing, endoscopy with biopsy

Gastroenteritis

Overview: broad term for infection (typically viral) of the stomach and intestines

Patient may complain of: chills, fever, fatigue, anorexia, nausea, vomiting, diarrhea, generalized abdominal pain, dyspepsia

Objective findings: fever, lethargy, decreased skin turgor, dry mucous membranes, generalized abdominal tenderness without guarding

PMH considerations/risk factors: recent ingestion of undercooked food/contaminated water, hx of immunosuppression, recent antibiotic use, older age

Diagnostics: clinical diagnosis; stool cultures may be considered if symptoms are severe or prolonged

Gastroesophageal Reflux Disease

Overview: abnormal reflux of acid from the stomach back into the esophagus

Patient may complain of: sore throat, sour taste in mouth, dysphagia, chest pain or heartburn that may be worse lying flat or after meals, nausea, dyspepsia, epigastric pain, chronic coughing, insomnia

Objective findings: epigastric tenderness; exam is typically unremarkable

PMH considerations/risk factors: hx of GERD, hiatal hernia, obesity, diabetes, pregnancy, nicotine use, alcohol abuse/use

Diagnostics: clinical diagnosis

Helicobacter pylori Infection

Overview: gram-negative bacterial infection in the stomach that disrupts the gastric mucosal lining making it vulnerable to peptic damage

Patient may complain of: abdominal pain, bloating, nausea, anorexia, dyspepsia, signs of GI bleeding

Objective findings: nonspecific epigastric tenderness; exam is typically unremarkable

PMH considerations/risk factors: hx of PUD, immunosuppression, recent travel outside of the United States, low socioeconomic status, ingestion of contaminated drinking water, NSAID use

Diagnostics: H. pylori serum/breath/stool testing, endoscopy with biopsy

Hypercalcemia

Overview: elevated serum calcium

Patient may complain of: fatigue, generalized weakness, anorexia, constipation, nausea, dyspepsia, vomiting, muscle aches; patient is typically asymptomatic unless severe

Objective findings: altered mental status, lethargy, hypertension, bradycardia, shortened QT interval, hypoactive bowel sounds, decreased reflexes; exam is typically unremarkable unless severe

PMH considerations/risk factors: hx of cancer, AIDS/HIV, Addison's disease, hyperparathyroidism

Diagnostics: serum Ca, ECG

Hyperkalemia

Overview: elevated serum potassium

Patient may complain of: fatigue, palpitations, diarrhea, nausea, vomiting, dyspepsia, muscle weakness and cramps, paresthesias; patient is typically asymptomatic unless severe

Objective findings: lethargy, hypotension, peaked T waves, arrhythmia, weak pulses, hyperactive bowel sounds; exam is typically unremarkable unless severe

PMH considerations/risk factors: hx of arrhythmia, CKD, AKI, Addison's disease, diabetes, burn injury, recent surgery

Diagnostics: serum K, ECG

Hypermagnesemia

Overview: elevated serum magnesium

Patient may complain of: fatigue, palpitations, nausea, vomiting, muscle spasms, headache; patient is typically asymptomatic unless severe

Objective findings: lethargy, altered mental status, diaphoresis, flushing, hypotension, bradycardia, arrhythmia, prolonged PR interval, wide QRS complex, bradypnea, decreased reflexes; exam is typically unremarkable unless severe

PMH considerations/risk factors: hx of gastroparesis, ileus, intestinal obstruction, CKD, AKI, hypothyroidism, magnesium supplementation

Diagnostics: serum Mg, ECG

Hypokalemia

Overview: low serum potassium

Patient may complain of: fatigue, palpitations, nausea, vomiting, constipation, muscle weakness and cramping, seizures, anxiety; patient is typically asymptomatic unless severe

Objective findings: lethargy, irritability, altered mental status, wide QRS, arrhythmia, bradypnea, hypoactive bowel sounds, decreased reflexes; exam is typically unremarkable unless severe

PMH considerations/risk factors: hx of CKD, diabetes, diarrhea, alcohol abuse/use, eating disorders, NPO status, diuretic use

Diagnostics: serum K, ECG

Hypomagnesemia

Overview: low serum magnesium

Patient may complain of: fatigue, generalized weakness, nausea, vomiting, constipation, confusion, paresthesias, tremors, seizures; patient is typically asymptomatic unless severe

Objective findings: altered mental status, lethargy, bradycardia, hypotension, wide QRS, peaked T waves, prolonged PR interval, arrhythmia, bradypnea, hypoactive bowel sounds, hyperactive reflexes, tremors; exam is typically unremarkable unless severe

PMH considerations/risk factors: hx of diarrhea, burn injury, alcohol abuse/use, malnutrition, DKA, pancreatitis

Diagnostics: serum Mg, ECG

Hyponatremia

Overview: low serum sodium

Patient may complain of: fatigue, thirst, nausea, vomiting, anorexia, muscle cramps and weakness, headache; patient is typically asymptomatic unless severe

Objective findings: altered mental status, lethargy, irritability, tachycardia, weak pulses, bradypnea, decreased reflexes; exam is typically unremarkable unless severe

PMH considerations/risk factors: hx of gastrointestinal loss, hx of CKD, heart failure, diuretic use, SIADH, dehydration

Diagnostics: serum Na

Increased Intracranial Pressure

Overview: rise in pressure within the cranial cavity

Patient may complain of: vision changes, nausea, vomiting, headache, confusion, seizures

Objective findings: signs of acute distress, altered mental status, GCS changes, sluggish/fixed pupillary response, hypertension, bradycardia, bradypnea

PMH considerations/risk factors: hx of TBI, CVA, CNS infections, hydrocephalus, cancer, seizures, HTN

Diagnostics: ICP monitoring, head CT/MRI

461

Inflammatory Bowel Disease

Overview: chronic inflammation of all or different parts of the gastrointestinal tract

Patient may complain of: chills, fever, fatigue, weight loss, anorexia, abdominal pain/cramping, nausea, vomiting, dyspepsia, constipation/diarrhea, change in bowel habits, signs of GI bleeding

Objective findings: signs of acute distress/illness, lethargy, fever, signs of malnourishment, diaphoresis, pallor, tachycardia, abdominal tenderness, hematochezia

PMH considerations/risk factors: hx of Crohn's disease or ulcerative colitis, food intolerance/allergies, bleeding/clotting disorders, NSAID use, recent travel outside of the United States, nicotine use, family hx of IBS, younger age

Diagnostics: occult stool, CRP, CBC, endoscopy with biopsy

Intestinal Obstruction

Overview: inability of digestive material to move through the GI tract normally

Patient may complain of: abdominal pain, anorexia, nausea, vomiting, inability to pass gas, constipation/diarrhea

Objective findings: signs of acute distress/illness, decreased skin turgor, dry mucous membranes, tachycardia, abdominal distention and tenderness, hypoactive or absent bowel sounds, fecal impaction (rectal exam)

PMH considerations/risk factors: hx of hernia, GI cancer, IBD, previous GI surgery, radiation therapy to the abdomen, opioid use

Diagnostics: KUB, abdominal CT

Irritable Bowel Syndrome

Overview: recurrent benign intestinal pain syndrome with associated bowel habit changes

Patient may complain of: abdominal pain and cramping, constipation/diarrhea, bloating, dyspepsia, heartburn, nausea, sensation of incomplete bowel movements

Objective findings: irritable, mild abdominal bloating and generalized tenderness; exam is typically unremarkable

PMH considerations/risk factors: hx of IBS, IBD, depression, anxiety, family hx of IBS, female gender, younger age

Diagnostics: may not require any diagnostic testing; colonoscopy with biopsy, stool cultures, and CRP may be considered

Liver Disease/Failure

Overview: broad term to describe damage and malfunction of the liver

Patient may complain of: fatigue, itching, anorexia, nausea, vomiting, RUQ abdominal pain, bloating, signs of GI bleeding

Objective findings: altered mental status, lethargy, jaundice, edema, ascites, abdominal distention, hepatomegaly, spider angiomas, hypertension/hypotension; exam may be unremarkable

PMH considerations/risk factors: hx of liver disease, hepatitis, diabetes, sepsis, obesity, cancer, Wilson's disease, IV drug use, alcohol abuse

Diagnostics: CMP, hepatitis panel, ammonia, PT/INR, abdominal US/CT, biopsy

Ménière's Disease

Overview: inner ear disease thought to be caused by a buildup of fluid in the labyrinth

Patient may complain of: hearing changes, tinnitus, ear fullness, nausea, vomiting, dizziness

Objective findings if symptomatic: signs of acute distress/illness, nystagmus, hearing difficulty, Romberg positive

PMH considerations/risk factors: hx of Ménière's disease, allergies, TBI, migraines, CVA/TIA, MS, BPPV, younger age

Diagnostics: audiometry, MRI

Migraine Headache

Overview: recurrent head pain with or without aura

Patient may complain of: generalized weakness, photophobia, phonophobia, blurred vision, nausea, vomiting, throbbing lateralized headache, paresthesias, dizziness, presence of an aura

Objective findings: irritability, intolerance to light and sound; exam is typically unremarkable

PMH considerations/risk factors: hx of migraines, increased psychological stress, lack of sleep, nicotine use, alcohol abuse/use, family hx of migraines, female gender, younger age (<40 years)

Diagnostics: clinical diagnosis; head CT/MRI may be considered initially

Myocardial Infarction

Overview: decreased or no blood flow through the coronary arteries causing cardiac muscle death

Patient may complain of: fatigue, chest pain not improved with rest, radiation of the pain to the left arm/neck/jaw, palpitations, dyspnea, activity intolerance, abdominal pain, nausea, dizziness, anxiety, feelings of impending doom; symptoms have longer duration than stable angina

Objective findings: signs of acute distress, lethargy, irritability, altered mental status, diaphoresis, cool clammy skin, hypertension/hypotension, tachycardia/bradycardia, arrhythmia, murmur, ST elevations, pathologic Q waves, weak pulses, sluggish capillary refill, tachypnea

PMH considerations/risk factors: hx of MI, CAD, HTN, heart failure, hyperlipidemia, diabetes, cardiac valve disorders, sedentary lifestyle, NSAID use, nicotine use, substance abuse, family hx of heart disease, older age

Diagnostics: cardiac enzymes, ECG, stress test, coronary angiography

Pancreatitis

Overview: inflammation of the pancreas

Patient may complain of: fatigue, chills, fever, epigastric/upper abdominal pain, radiation of the pain to the back, worse with movement, nausea, vomiting, dyspepsia, diarrhea

Objective findings: signs of acute distress/illness, lethargy, fever, diaphoresis, pallor, jaundice, tachycardia, hypotension, upper abdominal/epigastric tenderness, abdominal distention, positive Cullen's sign or Grey Turner sign (abdominal ecchymosis)

PMH considerations/risk factors: hx of chronic pancreatitis, hypertriglyceridemia, cholelithiasis, GI cancer, recent GI surgery or trauma to the abdomen, nicotine use, alcohol abuse/use

Diagnostics: amylase, lipase, abdominal CT/US

Peptic Ulcer Disease

Overview: ulcers that develop in the lining of a stomach and/or duodenum

Patient may complain of: chest pain, dyspepsia, epigastric pain, heartburn, pain relief with food or antacids, nausea, signs of GI bleeding

Objective findings: nonspecific epigastric tenderness; exam is typically unremarkable

PMH considerations/risk factors: hx of PUD, *H. pylori* infection, NSAID use, recent travel outside of the United States, nicotine use, alcohol abuse/use

Diagnostics: CBC, *H. pylori* serum/breath/stool testing, occult stool, endoscopy with biopsy

Pyelonephritis

Overview: bacterial infection of the kidney

Patient may complain of: fever; chills; nausea; vomiting; abdominal/back/flank pain; increased urinary frequency, retention, and urgency; dysuria; hematuria; urine odor; confusion (elderly)

Objective findings: signs of acute distress/illness, altered mental status (elderly), fever, tachycardia, CVAT, abdominal tenderness, bladder distention

PMH considerations: hx of frequent UTIs, diabetes, urolithiasis, urinary retention, immunosuppression, pregnancy, poor fluid intake, immobility, recent catheter use or GU surgery, female gender

Diagnostics: CBC, urinalysis, urine culture, renal US

Renal Disease/Failure

Overview: broad term to describe damage and malfunction of the kidneys

Patient may complain of: fatigue, itching, dyspnea, anorexia, nausea, vomiting, oliguria, confusion

Objective findings: lethargy, altered mental status, arrhythmia, edema, pericardial rub, hypertension/hypotension, adventitious lung sounds, oliguria or anuria; exam is typically unremarkable unless severe

PMH considerations/risk factors: hx of CKD, diabetes, HTN, CAD, sepsis, BPH, burn injury, heart failure, dehydration, GI/blood loss, NSAID use, ACE inhibitor use, diuretic use, older age

Diagnostics: BMP/CMP, anion gap, urinalysis, renal US

Urolithiasis

Overview: calculi that form in the urinary tract

Patient may complain of: severe flank/back pain, may radiate to the abdomen; nausea; vomiting; urinary urgency, retention and frequency; dysuria; hematuria

Objective findings: signs of acute distress/illness, irritability, fidgeting, CVAT, abdominal tenderness

PMH considerations/risk factors: hx of urolithiasis, short bowel syndrome, malnutrition, diabetes, gout, obesity, dehydration, bariatric surgery, family hx of urolithiasis, female gender

Diagnostics: urinalysis, KUB, renal US

Urinary Tract Infection

Overview: broad term for infection of the urinary tract including the urethra, bladder, ureters, and kidneys

Patient may complain of: fever; chills; abdominal/back/flank/ pelvic pai; nausea; vomiting; dysuria; increased urinary frequency, retention and urgency; hematuria; incontinence; urine odor; confusion (elderly)

Objective findings: fever, altered mental status (elderly), pelvic tenderness, bladder distention; exam is typically unremarkable

PMH considerations/risk factors: hx of frequent UTIs, diabetes, interstitial cystitis, urinary retention, immunosuppression, dehydration, pregnancy, incontinence, recent catheter use, GU surgery or sexual activity, immobility, female gender

Diagnostics: urinalysis/urine dipstick, urine culture

Withdrawal (Alcohol)

Overview: rapid or abrupt decrease in alcohol intake causing physical and psychological disturbances

Patient may complain of: fever, chills, palpitations, anorexia, nausea, vomiting, diarrhea, seizures, headache, alcohol craving, insomnia, anxiety

Objective findings: signs of acute distress, fever, irritability, altered mental status, diaphoresis, tachycardia, hypertension, hepatomegaly, ascites, seizures, tremors, hallucinations/ delirium

PMH considerations: hx of alcohol abuse, longer cessation (>48 hrs) since last drink, other substance abuse

Diagnostics: toxicology screen; workup to rule out more emergent causes may be indicated

Withdrawal (Opioids)

Overview: rapid or abrupt decrease in opioid intake causing physical and psychological disturbances

Patient may complain of: fever, body aches, nasal congestion, nasal drainage, anorexia, abdominal cramping, diarrhea, nausea, vomiting, tremors, opioid craving, anxiety, insomnia

Objective findings: signs of acute distress, fever, irritability, altered mental status, diaphoresis, piloerection, frequent

yawning, pupil dilatation, rhinorrhea, hypertension, tachycardia, hyperactive bowel sounds

PMH considerations/risk factors: hx of daily opioid use, chronic
pain, other substance abuse

Diagnostics: toxicology screen; workup to rule out more emergent causes may be indicated

References

Aapro, M., Grall, R. J., Herrstedt, J., Molassiotis, A., & Roila, F. (2016).
MASCC/ESMO antiemetic guideline 2016. Retrieved from http://www
.mascc.org/antiemetic-guidelines

American Medical Directors Association. (2010). *Know-it-all before you
call: Data collection system.* Columbia, MD: Author.

Camilleri, M., Parkman, H. P., Shafi, M. A., Abell, T. L., & Gerson, L.
(2013). Clinical guideline: Management of gastroparesis. *American
Journal of Gastroenterology, 108*(1), 18–37.

Collins, A. S. (2011). Postoperative nausea and vomiting in adults: Impli-
cations for critical care. *Critical Care Nurse, 31*(6), 36–45.

Collins, E. (2015). Nausea and vomiting in palliative care. *BMJ, 351,* 1–11.

Desai, S. P. (2009). *Clinician's guide to laboratory medicine* (3rd ed.).
Houston, TX: MD2B.

Egerton-Warburton, D., Meek, R., Mee, M. J. & Braitberg, G. (2014).
Antiemetic use for nausea and vomiting in adult emergency department
patients: Randomized controlled trial comparing ondansetron, metoclopramide, and placebo. *Annals of Emergency Medicine, 64*(5), 526–532.

Fantasia, H. C. (2014). A new pharmacologic treatment for nausea and
vomiting of pregnancy. *Nursing for Women's Health, 18*(1), 73–77.

Feinleib, J., Kwan, L. H., & Yamani, A. (2017). Postoperative nausea and
vomiting. In M. Crowley (Ed.), *UpToDate.* Retrieved from https://www
.uptodate.com/contents/postoperative-nausea-and-vomiting

Furyk, J., Meek, R., & McKenzie, S. (2014). Drug treatment of adults
with nausea and vomiting in primary care. *BMJ, 349,* 1–6.

Furyk, J. S., Meek, R. A., & Egerton-Warburton, S. (2015). Drugs for
the treatment of nausea and vomiting in adults in the emergency department setting. *Cochrane Database of Systematic Reviews, 9,* 1–53.

Gan, T. J., Diemunsch, P., Habib, A. S., Kovac, A., Kranke, P., Meyer, T. A., . . .
Tramer, M. R. (2014). Consensus guidelines for the management of
postoperative nausea and vomiting. *Society for Ambulatory Anesthesiology,
118*(1), 85–113.

Gulanick, M., & Myers, J. L. (2017). *Nursing care plans: Diagnosis, interventions, & outcomes* (9th ed.). St. Louis, MO: Elsevier.

Hale, A., & Hovey, M. J. (2014). *Fluid, electrolyte and acid-base imbalances.* Philadelphia, PA: F.A. Davis Company.

Hesketh, P. J. (2018). Prevention and treatment of chemotherapy-induced nausea and vomiting in adults. In D. M. Savarese (Ed.), *UpToDate.* Retrieved from https://www.uptodate.com/contents/prevention-and -treatment-of-chemotherapy-induced-nausea-and-vomiting-in-adults

Hines, S., Steels, E., Chang, A., & Gibbons, K. (2012). Aromatherapy for treatment of postoperative nausea and vomiting. *Cochrane Database of Systematic Reviews, 4,* 1–55.

Hooper, V. D. (2015). SAMBA consensus guidelines for the management of postoperative nausea and vomiting: An executive summary for perianesthesia nurses. *Journal of Perianesthesia Nursing, 30*(5), 377–382.

Jarvis, C. (2015). *Physical examination & health assessment.* St. Louis, MO: Elsevier.

Kelly, B., & Ward, K. (2013). Nausea and vomiting in palliative care. *Nursing Times, 109*(39), 16–19.

LeBlond, R. F., Brown, D. D., Suneja, M., & Szot, J. F. (2015). *DeGowin's diagnostic examination* (10th ed.). New York, NY: McGraw-Hill.

Longstreth, G. F. (2016). Approach to the adult with nausea and vomiting. In S. Grover (Ed.), *UpToDate.* Retrieved from https:// www.uptodate.com/contents/approach-to-the-adult-with-nausea-and -vomiting

Mayhall, E. A., Gray, R., Lopes, V., & Matterson, K. A. (2015). Comparison of antiemetics for nausea and vomiting of pregnancy in an emergency department setting. *American Journal of Emergency Medicine,* 33, 882–886.

McCance, K. L., Huether, S. E., Brashers, V. L., & Rote, N. S. (2014). *Pathophysiology: The biologic basis for disease in adults and children* (7th ed.). St. Louis, MO: Elsevier.

Odom-Forren, J., Hooper, V., Moser, D. K., Hall, L. A., Lennie, T. A., Holtman, J., . . . Apfel, C. C. (2014). Post discharge nausea and vomiting: Management strategies and outcomes over 7 days. *Journal of PeriAnesthesia Nursing, 29*(4), 275–284.

Papadakis, M. A., & McPhee, S. J. (2017). *Current medical diagnosis and treatment* (56th ed.). New York, NY: McGraw-Hill.

PDQ Supportive and Palliative Care Editorial Board. (2017). *Treatment-related nausea and vomiting.* Retrieved from https://www.ncbi.nlm.nih.gov /books/NBK66056/

5

Raftery, A. T., Lim, E., & Ostor, A. J. (2014). *Differential diagnosis* (4th ed.). London: Elsevier.

Seller, R. H., & Symons, A. B. (2012). *Differential diagnosis of common complaints* (6th ed.). Philadelphia, PA: Elsevier.

Smith, J. A., Refuerzo, J. S., & Fox, K. A. (2018). Treatment and outcome of nausea and vomiting in pregnancy. In V. A. Barss (Ed.), *UpToDate*. Retrieved from https://www.uptodate.com/contents/treatment-and-outcome-of-nausea-and-vomiting-of-pregnancy

Uphold, C. R., & Graham, M. V. (2013). *Clinical guidelines in family practice* (5th ed.). Gainesville, FL: Barmarrae Books.

CHAPTER 26

Palpitations

Palpitations are defined as a subjective sensation and awareness of a rapid, irregular, fluttering, or bounding heartbeat. Etiology can be benign in nature but cardiac arrhythmias need to be ruled out. A patient with known cardiac disease has a higher likelihood of an arrhythmia compared to a younger patient with minimal risk factors. An ECG will be needed for the diagnostic workup. If possible, it should be done while the patient is symptomatic. It is the nurse's priority to maintain and monitor the patient's hemodynamic stability, perform an ECG, collect a thorough description of the patient's symptoms, and help the provider determine the cause. A referral to cardiology or electrophysiology may be needed if a cause is not found and the patient remains symptomatic.

Differential Diagnosis Considerations

Common: anxiety, arrhythmia, beta blocker withdrawal, caffeine intake, cardiac valve disorders, cardiomyopathy, dehydration, exercise, fever, heart failure, hypoglycemia, medication induced, MI, orthostatic hypotension, pacemaker syndrome, psychological stress, PVCs, stable angina, unstable angina, withdrawal from alcohol/drugs

Consider: AAA rupture, amphetamine use, anemia, atrial myxoma, AV fistula, cocaine use, depression, digoxin toxicity, hyperkalemia, hypermagnesemia, hyperthyroidism, hypokalemia, mastocytosis, myocarditis, Paget's disease, PE, pericarditis, pheochromocytoma, pneumothorax, POTS, pregnancy, sepsis

Questions to Ask the Patient/ Family/Witness/Yourself

- When did the palpitations start? Did it start gradually or suddenly?
- What were you doing before/when the symptoms started?
- Are the palpitations constant or do they come and go? If intermittent, how long do they last? How often is it happening per hour/day?
- Can you describe the palpitations (flip-flopping, fluttering, bounding, or throbbing)?
- Can you tap the rhythm of your heart with your finger on the table?
- What makes the palpitations better (bearing down, certain positions, eating, medication, rest)?
- What triggers the palpitations or makes them worse (activity, anxiety, caffeine, changing positions)?
- Do you have dizziness or feel like you are going to faint?
- How is your appetite? Are you able to keep down food and/or fluids?
- How much fluid are you drinking on a daily basis?
- Do you have a history of palpitations? If so, what has been done or used to treat it?
- Have you had any recent: CV surgery? pregnancy? psychological stress/trauma? sleep habit changes? vigorous exercise?
- Have you taken any new prescribed or over-the-counter medications? Have there been any recent changes to your current medication?
- Any family history of palpitations or other heart conditions?
- Do you drink caffeine? How many drinks in a day? When was the last time you had any?
- Do you smoke? How much (ppd)? How long have you been smoking? (if applicable)
- Do you drink alcohol? How many drinks per day/week? What kind and amount of alcohol do you drink? When was your last drink? (if applicable)

- Do you have a history of drug use? What types and how much? Do you use on a daily basis? When was your last use? (if applicable)

Associated Signs/Symptoms: PAIN: pain anywhere; GENERAL: fatigue, fever, weakness, weight changes; CARDIOVASCULAR: chest pain/tightness, edema, PND, orthopnea; RESPIRATORY: dyspnea, cough, painful breathing/coughing; GASTROINTESTINAL: diarrhea, signs of GI bleeding nausea, vomiting; NEUROLOGICAL: dizziness, headache, (pre)syncope; PSYCHOLOGICAL: anxiety, confusion, feelings of impending doom

Recommended Assessments

- Vital signs
  - Orthostatic blood pressure (if applicable)
- Temperature
- Weight
- I/O
- Pain scale (if applicable)
  - Tolerable pain level
- General
  - Level of consciousness and orientation
  - Inspect: signs of acute distress, acute illness, affect, restlessness
  - Difficulty speaking due to breathlessness
- Skin
  - Inspect: cyanosis, diaphoresis, dryness, pallor
  - Palpate: temperature, turgor
- Head/face/neck
  - Inspect: JVD, tracheal deviation
  - Auscultate: carotid bruits
- Mouth
  - Inspect: mucous membrane moisture level
- Cardiovascular
  - Auscultate: heart sounds, rate, rhythm
  - Palpate: heaves, thrills

- Respiratory
  - Inspect: chest asymmetry, respiratory effort, depth, pattern, use of accessory muscles
  - Auscultate: lung sounds
- Extremities
  - Inspect: IV site
  - Palpate: capillary refill, edema, pulses

Past Medical History Considerations
Puts the patient at risk for differential considerations

- Alcohol abuse/use
- CAD
- CKD
- Diabetes
- Drug abuse/use
- HTN
- Nicotine use
- Pacemaker/ICD

Reoccurrence/exacerbation should be considered

- Arrhythmias (various)
- MI
- PE

Chronic conditions that can cause palpitations

- Anemia
- Angina
- Anxiety
- Arrhythmias (various)
- Cardiac valve disorders
- Depression
- Heart failure
- POTS
- Pregnancy
- Thyroid disease

Medication Evaluation

Most common causative/exacerbating medication

- Albuterol
- Antiarrhythmics
- Anticholinergics
- Antihistamines
- Beta blocker withdrawal
- Decongestants
- Digoxin
- Phentermine
- Sympathomimetic agents
- Tricyclic antidepressants
- Vasodilators

Lab Evaluation and Trends

- Bedside capillary glucose trends
- BMP/CMP
- CBC

Nursing Intervention Considerations

- Call for help or rapid response/code team if vital signs are unstable or there are signs of urgent distress
- Maintain a patent airway
  - Apply oxygen if hypoxic
  - Encourage slow relaxed deep breathing if hyperventilating
  - Call respiratory therapy for signs of respiratory distress
- Verify patent IV if IVF or IV medication treatment is anticipated
  - Flush according to facility protocol; watch for swelling, erythema, pain, and other signs of infiltration
  - Large bore IV is preferred
- ECG STAT
- Blood sugar if hypoglycemia is suspected

- Medications (if ordered or protocol allows)
  - Hold suspected causative medication until discussion with the provider
  - If hypoglycemic and has altered mental status or unable to swallow, give 1mg IV/IM/SQ glucagon, and/or 25–50mL IV 50% dextrose, or follow your facility's hypoglycemia protocol (goal is >100)
- Diet
  - NPO if procedure or surgery is anticipated
  - Push fluids if there are no contraindications (>2,000mL/day)
  - Avoid caffeine
  - Avoid foods that trigger symptoms
  - If hypoglycemic, alert, and can swallow, give a fast-acting carbohydrate like a glucose tablet, 4oz of fruit juice, 8oz of milk, 4oz of non-diet soda, hard candy, or teaspoon of honey/sugar. Repeat until sugar is normalized (goal is >100)
- Activity
  - Keep the patient in bed until discussion with the provider
- Positioning
  - HOB raised to comfort for respiratory distress
  - Lay supine with feet elevated if the patient has hypotension
  - Reposition every 2–4 hours or establish an individualized turning schedule
- Monitor
  - Stay with the patient until stable
  - Pain levels
  - Vital signs and trends
  - Oxygen saturation/pulse oximetry
  - Temperature trends
  - I/O
  - Telemetry/cardiac monitor
  - Blood sugar trends (if applicable)

- Weight trends
- Orientation status changes
- Agitation levels
- Peripheral pulses
- Skin assessment every 8–24 hours
- Signs of decreased cardiac output such as weak pulses, cool skin, altered mental status, hypotension, oliguria, and mottling
- Signs of respiratory distress such as cyanosis, tachypnea, hypoxia, use of accessory muscles, diaphoresis, and adventitious lung sounds
- Signs of dehydration such as lethargy, decreased skin turgor, dry mucous membranes, tachycardia, and (orthostatic) hypotension
- Safety
  - Perform a fall risk assessment and implement the appropriate strategies
- Environment
  - Provide a calm, quiet environment and reduce stimulation
  - Provide distractions
  - Avoid bothersome odors in the room
  - Maintain a comfortable room temperature
  - Offer aromatherapy and/or music therapy (if appropriate)
  - Utilize a fan (if appropriate)
- Supportive care
  - Maintain effective communication between yourself, patient, and family
  - Provide emotional support and reassurance to the patient and family
  - Maintain a calm manner during patient interactions
  - Discuss plan of care with the patient and decide reasonable goals together
  - Notify the patient and family of changes in the plan of care
  - Reorient the patient as needed

- Promote skin care and integrity
- Provide light clothing and bed linen
- Encourage vagal maneuvers (if appropriate)
- Offer back rubs, warmed blankets, warm drinks, and new bed linens
- **Educational topics (as applicable to the patient):**
  - General information regarding the patient's palpitations and differential diagnosis considerations
  - Procedure and intervention explanation and justification
  - Explanation regarding referrals and specialist who may see them for this issue
  - New medication education including reason, side effects, and administration needs
  - Medication changes
  - Medication compliance
  - Pain scale and pain goals
  - Relaxation techniques and breathing exercises
  - Oxygen therapy and maintenance
  - Trigger avoidance
  - Telemetry
  - Energy conservation techniques: placing items within reach, sitting to do tasks, taking breaks in between activities, sliding rather than lifting, pushing rather than pulling
  - Vagal maneuvers
  - Skin care
  - Proper positioning and turning schedule
  - Safety needs and fall risk
  - Avoidance of food/fluid that trigger symptoms
  - NPO diet
  - Increased fluid intake
  - Caffeine restriction
  - Smoking cessation

- Alcohol and/or drug cessation and support
- Stress reduction and management
- When to notify the nurse or provider
- Signs and symptoms of hypoglycemia
- Signs and symptoms of cardiac emergencies
- Signs and symptoms of respiratory emergencies
- Dehydration prevention
- Pressure injury prevention

ISBARR Recommendation Considerations

- Ask the provider to come assess the patient STAT if they are symptomatic or unstable
- Transfer to the ICU if hemodynamically unstable, advanced medication management is required, or closer monitoring is needed
- Medication
  - Hold oral medications if the patient is unable to tolerate or NPO
  - Discuss changing medication routes with the provider (and pharmacy) if the patient is NPO
  - Discontinue/change suspected causative medication
  - Add PRN and/or scheduled medication for anxiety or irritability
- IV fluid needs if oral intake is poor, there are signs of dehydration, and the patient is NPO or hypotensive
- ECG if repeat testing is needed
- Imaging (depending on the suspected cause)
  - Chest X-ray
- Labs (depending on the suspected cause)
  - ABG
  - BMP/CMP

- BNP
- Cardiac enzymes
- CBC
- D-dimer
- Digoxin
- Magnesium
- Toxicology screening
- TSH
- Safety
  - Activity-level changes
  - Fall risk protocol
- Monitoring needs
  - Blood sugars including frequency and parameters to call the provider (if applicable)
  - Continuous O_2 monitoring
  - Telemetry/continuous cardiac monitoring
  - Strict I/O
  - Daily weights
  - Vital signs including frequency and parameters to call the provider
- Supportive cares
  - Compression stockings or SCDs
- Change diet to (depending on the suspected cause)
  - NPO
  - Caffeine restriction
  - Push oral fluids
- Protocols:
  - CIWA-Ar if alcohol withdrawal is suspected
- Referrals
  - Cardiology or electrophysiology
- Ask if the provider wants anything else done
- Read back orders; ask that they enter all orders into the electronic medical record

Palpitations

ISBARR Template	
I **Introduction**	**Introduce Yourself and the Patient** • "Hello, Dr. Handler. This is Emily Hegeman. I am the nurse for your patient Alex Raskin in Room 302."
S **Situation**	**Sign/Symptom You Are Concerned About** • "He started complaining of palpitations 30 minutes ago, saying they come and go and last for 1–2 minutes at a time. He is having an episode every few minutes and describes it as his heart racing with no known trigger." **Associated Signs/Symptoms** • "He is saying he feels anxious, but denied being dizzy, having chest pain, or shortness of breath."
B **Background**	**Vitals** • "Vitals show mild tachycardia. Heart rate has been between 90–115, blood pressure is 142/88, respirations are 18, and his temperature is 98.9." **Exam** • "He appears mildly diaphoretic and anxious but otherwise has no other signs of acute distress. Heart rhythm sounds regular and lungs are clear." **Past Medical History** • "His only cardiac history is hypertension that is usually controlled with lisinopril. He also has a history of diabetes, hypothyroidism, and anxiety. Says he has had similar palpitations when he feels anxious." **Labs and Medications** • "CMP this morning was normal. I took a blood sugar which was 96. He took his last dose of lorazepam (0.5mg) as needed eight hours ago."

ISBARR Template	
A **Assessment**	**Assessment** • "I am suspecting his palpitations are related to anxiety."
R **Recommendations** **R** **Read Back**	**Nurse's Recommendations, Interventions, and Read Back** • "Did you want an ECG or any labs? Do you want the patient placed on telemetry? Do you want anything else done at this time?" • "Thank you, Dr. Handler. I would like to read those orders back to you. You would like an ECG with the next palpitation episode, call you with the results, place the patient on telemetry protocol, and order a CBC, CMP, and TSH for his morning labs. Also change PRN lorazepam to every six hours as needed and give another dose now. Is that correct?"

Disclaimer: This dialogue is factitious and any resemblance to actual persons, living or dead, or actual events is purely coincidental.

In order to avoid order discrepancies, it is recommended that all orders be entered by the provider in the electronic medical record.

Select Differential Diagnosis Presentations

Abdominal Aortic Aneurysm Rupture

Overview: abnormal dilation of the abdominal aorta leads to vessel rupture

Patient may complain of: severe abdominal/back pain, palpitations, nausea, vomiting, dizziness

Objective findings: signs of acute distress, altered mental status, diaphoresis, tachycardia, hypotension, pulsating abdominal mass, abdominal bruit

PMH considerations/risk factors: hx of CAD, HTN, heart failure, diabetes, connective tissue disorders, trauma to the abdomen, nicotine use, family hx of AAA, male gender, older age

Diagnostics: abdominal US/CT/MRI

Angina (Stable)

Overview: chest pain caused by a decrease in myocardial oxygen supply that is improved with rest

Patient may complain of: fatigue, chest pain/tightness/heaviness that is worse with activity, better with rest or NTG, radiation of the pain to the left arm/neck/jaw, palpitations, dyspnea, activity intolerance, nausea, dyspepsia, dizziness, feelings of impending doom, anxiety; symptoms have a short duration

Objective findings: signs of acute distress, lethargy, diaphoresis, hypertension, tachycardia, murmur, weak pulses, sluggish capillary refill, tachypnea

PMH considerations/risk factors: hx of angina, CAD, HTN, heart failure, hyperlipidemia, diabetes, cardiac valve disorders, obesity, increased psychological stress, nicotine use, family hx of heart disease

Diagnostics: cardiac enzymes, ECG, stress test, coronary angiography

Angina (Unstable)

Overview: chest pain caused by a decrease in myocardial oxygen supply that is not improved with rest

Patient may complain of: fatigue, chest pain/tightness/heaviness that is worse with activity, not improved with rest or NTG, radiation of the pain to the left arm/neck/jaw, palpitations, dyspnea, activity intolerance, nausea, dyspepsia, dizziness, feelings of impending doom, anxiety; symptoms have a longer duration than stable angina

Objective findings: signs of acute distress, lethargy, diaphoresis, hypertension, tachycardia, murmur, weak pulses, sluggish capillary refill, tachypnea

PMH considerations/risk factors: hx of angina, CAD, HTN, heart failure, hyperlipidemia, diabetes, cardiac valve disorders, obesity, increased psychological stress, nicotine use, family hx of heart disease

Diagnostics: cardiac enzymes, ECG, stress test, coronary angiography

Anxiety

Overview: psychiatric disorder that can cause intense fear and worry

Patient may complain of: fatigue, chest pain, palpitations, dyspnea, nausea, vomiting, abdominal pain, constipation/diarrhea, paresthesias, tremors, dizziness, headache, insomnia, mind racing, feelings of impending doom

Objective findings: signs of acute distress, irritability, inability to focus, diaphoresis, tachycardia, hypertension, tachypnea, muscle tension

PMH considerations/risk factors: hx of anxiety, depression, PTSD, insomnia, substance abuse, physical abuse, recent physical or emotional trauma, family hx of psychiatric diseases

Diagnostics: clinical diagnosis; workup to rule out more emergent causes may be indicated

Arrhythmia

Overview: any irregular heart rhythm

Patient may complain of: fatigue, generalized weakness, (pre)syncope, palpitations, chest pain, dyspnea, dizziness, anxiety

Objective findings: signs of acute distress, lethargy, irritability, diaphoresis, irregular heart rhythm, bradycardia/tachycardia, murmur, hypertension/hypotension, tachypnea

PMH considerations/risk factors: hx of arrhythmia, CAD, HTN, heart failure, MI, cardiac valve disorders, diabetes, previous CV surgery, substance abuse, increased psychological stress, nicotine use, family hx of heart disease

Diagnostics: BMP/CMP, CBC, TSH, ECG, ECHO, Holter monitor/loop recorder/event recorder

Dehydration

Overview: abnormal loss of extracellular fluid volume

Patient may complain of: fatigue, thirst, dry mouth, palpitations, constipation, oliguria, muscle cramps, dizziness, headache

Objective findings: fever, altered mental status, lethargy, irritability, decreased skin turgor, generalized skin dryness, dry mucous membranes, (orthostatic) hypotension, tachycardia, oliguria

PMH considerations/risk factors: hx of liver or renal disease/failure, recent vomiting and/or diarrhea, GI bleeding, polyuria, diuretic use, burn injury, or intense physical activity

Diagnostics: BMP/CMP, CBC, urine Na, I/O

Heart Failure

Overview: broad term to describe pumping malfunction of the heart

Patient may complain of: fatigue, activity intolerance, chest pain, palpitations, dyspnea, orthopnea, PND, coughing, sputum production, weight gain/loss, anorexia, nausea, nocturia, insomnia

Objective findings: signs of acute distress, lethargy, diaphoresis, cyanosis, JVD, bradycardia/tachycardia, hypertension/hypotension, displaced PMI, murmur, gallop, weak pulses, sluggish capillary refill, digital clubbing, edema, breathlessness, tachypnea, cough, adventitious lung sounds, sputum, hepatomegaly, ascites

PMH considerations/risk factors: hx of heart failure, HTN, CAD, cardiac valve disorders, MI, diabetes, arrhythmias, hyper/hypothyroidism, obesity, nicotine use, substance abuse, family hx of heart disease

Diagnostics: BNP, BMP/CMP, TSH, ECG, I/O, chest X-ray, ECHO, cardiac catheterization

Hyperkalemia

Overview: elevated serum potassium

Patient may complain of: fatigue, palpitations, diarrhea, nausea, vomiting, dyspepsia, muscle weakness and cramps, paresthesias; patient is typically asymptomatic unless severe

Objective findings: lethargy, hypotension, peaked T waves, arrhythmia, weak pulses, hyperactive bowel sounds; exam is typically unremarkable unless severe

PMH considerations/risk factors: hx of arrhythmia, CKD, AKI, Addison's disease, diabetes, burn injury, recent surgery

Diagnostics: serum K, ECG

Hypermagnesemia

Overview: elevated serum magnesium

Patient may complain of: fatigue, palpitations, nausea, vomiting, muscle spasms, headache; patient is typically asymptomatic unless severe

Objective findings: lethargy, altered mental status, diaphoresis, flushing, hypotension, bradycardia, arrhythmia, prolonged PR interval, wide QRS complex, bradypnea, decreased reflexes; exam is typically unremarkable unless severe

PMH considerations/risk factors: hx of gastroparesis, ileus, intestinal obstruction, CKD, AKI, hypothyroidism, magnesium supplementation

Diagnostics: serum Mg, ECG

Hyperthyroidism

Overview: overactive thyroid gland

Patient may complain of: anxiety, heat intolerance, fatigue, generalized weakness, palpitations, diarrhea, nausea, vomiting, weight loss, muscle cramps, seizures, tremors, insomnia

Objective findings: lethargy, irritability, diaphoresis, hair thinning, exophthalmos, goiter, tachycardia, hypertension, tremors, seizures

PMH considerations/risk factors: hx of Grave's disease, thyroiditis, pregnancy, thyroid cancer, family hx of thyroid dysfunction, female gender, older age

Diagnostics: TSH, T3, T4, thyroid US, radioactive iodine uptake scan

Hypokalemia

Overview: low serum potassium

Patient may complain of: fatigue, palpitations, nausea, vomiting, constipation, muscle weakness and cramping, seizures, anxiety; patient is typically asymptomatic unless severe

Objective findings: lethargy, irritability, altered mental status, wide QRS, arrhythmia, bradypnea, hypoactive bowel sounds, decreased reflexes; exam is typically unremarkable unless severe

PMH considerations/risk factors: hx of CKD, diabetes, diarrhea, alcohol abuse/use, eating disorders, NPO status, diuretic use

Diagnostics: serum K, ECG

Myocardial Infarction

Overview: decreased or no blood flow through the coronary arteries causing cardiac muscle death

Patient may complain of: fatigue, chest pain not improved with rest, radiation of the pain to the left arm/neck/jaw, palpitations, dyspnea, activity intolerance, abdominal pain, nausea, dizziness, anxiety, feelings of impending doom; symptoms have longer duration than stable angina

Objective findings: signs of acute distress, lethargy, irritability, altered mental status, diaphoresis, cool clammy skin, hypertension/hypotension, tachycardia/bradycardia, arrhythmia, murmur, ST elevations, pathologic Q waves, weak pulses, sluggish capillary refill, tachypnea

PMH considerations/risk factors: hx of MI, CAD, HTN, heart failure, hyperlipidemia, diabetes, cardiac valve disorders, sedentary lifestyle, NSAID use, nicotine use, substance abuse, family hx of heart disease, older age

Diagnostics: cardiac enzymes, ECG, stress test, coronary angiography

Pneumothorax

Overview: abnormal air or fluid in the pleural cavity causing lung collapse

Patient may complain of: sudden onset of chest pain, palpitations, dyspnea, coughing, anxiety, feelings of impending doom

Objective findings: signs of acute distress, tachycardia, hypotension, tachypnea, diminished/absent unilateral breath sounds, uneven chest excursion, tracheal deviation, hypoxia, cough

PMH considerations/risk factors: hx of Marfan syndrome, COPD, cystic fibrosis, asthma, TB, trauma to the chest/back, thin body habitus, recent thoracentesis or pulmonary biopsy, family hx of pneumothorax, nicotine use, male gender

Diagnostics: chest X-ray

Pulmonary Embolism

Overview: a blood clot in the pulmonary vasculature

Patient may complain of: chills, fever, chest pain, pain with deep breaths, palpitations, activity intolerance, dyspnea, coughing, hemoptysis, abdominal pain, dizziness

Objective findings: signs of acute distress, fever, pallor, cyanosis, diaphoresis, tachycardia, S3/S4 heart sounds, hypotension, tachypnea, hypoxia, cough, signs of DVT

PMH considerations/risk factors: hx of DVT, PE or CVA, bleeding/clotting disorder, cancer, pregnancy, HRT/birth control use, IV drug use, recent surgery, immobility, nicotine use

Diagnostics: D-dimer, chest CT, V/Q scan, chest X-ray

Withdrawal (Alcohol)

Overview: rapid or abrupt decrease in alcohol intake causing physical and psychological disturbances

Patient may complain of: fever, chills, palpitations, anorexia, nausea, vomiting, diarrhea, seizures, headache, alcohol craving, insomnia, anxiety

Objective findings: signs of acute distress, fever, irritability, altered mental status, diaphoresis, tachycardia, hypertension, hepatomegaly, ascites, seizures, tremors, hallucinations/delirium

PMH considerations: hx of alcohol abuse, longer cessation (>48 hrs) since last drink, other substance abuse

Diagnostics: toxicology screen; workup to rule out more emergent causes may be indicated

References

Barkoudah, E., & Collins, J. P. (2012). Management of palpitations in urgent care. *The Journal of Urgent Care Medicine, 7*–12. Retrieved from https://scholar.harvard.edu/files/barkoudah/files/management_of_palpitations.pdf

Cowan, C., Campbell, J., Cheong, V. L., Chung, G., Fay, M., Fitzmaurice, D., . . . Schiff, R. (2014). *Atrial fibrillation: The management of atrial fibrillation. Clinical guidelines: Methods, evidence and recommendations.* Retrieved from https://www.ncbi.nlm.nih.gov/pubmedhealth/PMH0068959/pdf/PubMedHealth_PMH0068959.pdf

Desai, S. P. (2009). *Clinician's guide to laboratory medicine* (3rd ed.). Houston, TX: MD2B.

Everett, R. J., Sheppard, M. N., & Lefroy, D. C. (2013). Chest pain and palpitations: Take a closer look. *Circulation, 128,* 271–277.

Gulanick, M., & Myers, J. L. (2017). *Nursing care plans: Diagnosis, interventions, & outcomes* (9th ed.). St. Louis, MO: Elsevier.

Hale, A., & Hovey, M. J. (2014). *Fluid, electrolyte and acid-base imbalances.* Philadelphia, PA: F.A. Davis Company.

Heart Rhythm Society. (n.d.). *Symptoms & diagnosis.* Retrieved from http://www.hrsonline.org/Patient-Resources/Symptoms-Diagnosis

Helton, M. R. (2015). Diagnosis and management of common types of supraventricular tachycardia. *American Family Physician, 92*(9), 793–802.

Jarvis, C. (2015). *Physical examination & health assessment.* St. Louis, MO: Elsevier.

LeBlond, R. F., Brown, D. D., Suneja, M., & Szot, J. F. (2015). *DeGowin's diagnostic examination* (10th ed.). New York, NY: McGraw-Hill.

Lee, G., & Campbell-Cole, C. (2014). Recognizing and managing atrial fibrillation in the community. *British Journal of Community Nursing, 19*(9), 422–426.

Levy, S., & Olshansky, B. (2017). Arrhythmia management for the primary care clinician. In B. C. Downey (Ed.), *UpToDate.* Retrieved from https://www.uptodate.com/contents/arrhythmia-management-for-the-primary-care-clinician

Manolis, A. S. (2017). Ventricular premature beats. In B. C. Downey (Ed.), *UpToDate.* Retrieved from https://www.uptodate.com/contents/ventricular-premature-beats

McCance, K. L., Huether, S. E., Brashers, V. L., & Rote, N. S. (2014). *Pathophysiology: The biologic basis for disease in adults and children* (7th ed.). St. Louis, MO: Elsevier.

Page, R. L., Joglar, J. A., Caldwell, M. A., Calkins, H., Conti, J. B., Deal, B. J., . . . Tracy, C. M. (2016). 2015 ACC/AHA/HRS guideline for the management of adult patients with supraventricular tachycardia. *Heart Rhythm, 13*(4), 136–221.

Papadakis, M. A., & McPhee, S. J. (2017). *Current medical diagnosis and treatment* (56th ed.). New York, NY: McGraw-Hill.

Probst, M. A., Kanzaria, H. K., Hoffman, J. R., Mower, W. R., Moheimani, R. S., Sun, B. C., & Quigley, D. D. (2015). Emergency physicians' perceptions and decision-making processes regarding patients presenting with palpitations. *Journal of Emergency Medicine, 49*(2), 236–243.

Probst, M. A., Mower, W. R., Kanzaria, H. K., Hoffman, J. R., Buch, E. F., & Sun, B. C. (2014). Analysis of emergency department visits for palpitations (from the national hospital ambulatory medical care survey). *The American Journal of Cardiology, 113*, 1685–1690.

Raftery, A. T., Lim, E., & Ostor, A. J. (2014). *Differential diagnosis* (4th ed.). London: Elsevier.

Raviele, A., Giada, F., Bergfeldt, L., Blanc, J. J., Blomstrom-Lundqvist, C., Mont, L., . . . Viskin, S. (2011). Management of patient with palpitations: A position paper from the European heart rhythm association. *Europace, 13*, 920–934.

Reagan, B. W., Huang, R. L., & Clair, W. K. (2012). Palpitations: An annoyance that may require clairvoyance. *Circulation, 125*, 958–965.

Rohde, J., Hartley, S. E., Hanigan, S., Lin, J., Morganstern, L. B., Seagull, F. J., . . . Crawford, T. C. (2014). *Management of acute atrial fibrillation and atrial flutter in non-pregnant hospitalized adults.* Retrieved from www.med.umich.edu/1info/IHP/practiveguides/Afib/afibfinal.pdf

Seller, R. H., & Symons, A. B. (2012). *Differential diagnosis of common complaints* (6th ed.). Philadelphia, PA: Elsevier.

Steinberg, J. S., Varma, N., Cygankiewicz, I., Aziz, P., Balsam, P., Baranchuk, A., . . . Piotrowicz, R. (2017). 2017 ISHNE-HRS expert consensus statement on ambulatory ECG and external cardiac monitoring/telemetry. *Heart Rhythm, 22*(3), 1–40.

Uphold, C. R., & Graham, M. V. (2013). *Clinical guidelines in family practice* (5th ed.). Gainesville, FL: Barmarrae Books.

Zimetbaum, P. (2016). Overview of palpitations in adults. In H. Libman (Ed.), *UpToDate.* Retrieved from https://www.uptodate.com/contents/overview-of-palpitations-in-adults

CHAPTER 27

Pressure Injury

Formally known as pressure ulcers, pressure injuries are localized areas over bony prominences that are damaged as a result of pressure, shearing, and impaired blood flow. In 2016, the National Pressure Ulcer Advisory Panel changed the terminology to include skin damage not associated with ulceration such as suspected deep tissue injury and unstageable wounds. Pressure injuries can cause pain and infection, diminish quality of life, and prolong hospital stays. Common sites for pressure injuries include the occipital bone, helix, nose, scapula, elbow, iliac crest, sacrum, coccyx, calcaneus, and the lateral/medial malleolus. Patients at the highest risk for developing pressure injuries are those who have impaired mobility, an inability to reposition themselves in bed, impaired perfusion, sensory loss, are malnourished, have cognitive impairment, incontinence, are obese, have had recent surgery, use multiple medical devices, have a history of spinal cord injury, and are of older age. A validated risk assessment tool (i.e., Braden, Norton, and Waterlow scales) should be used in conjunction with clinical judgment to determine the patient's risk for these injuries.

Once a pressure injury is recognized, it is imperative for the nurse to initiate treatment strategies immediately in order to prevent the injury from progressing. Key treatment strategies include early identification and monitoring of the injury with frequent skin assessments, utilizing pressure redistribution devices, pain management, repositioning, nutritional support, infection prevention, and patient and family education. Referrals to a surgeon, wound care nurse, and dietician may also be needed.

Differential Diagnosis Considerations

Consider: arterial ulcer, burn injury, cellulitis, diabetic ulcer, incontinence dermatitis, intertrigo, skin malignancy, skin tears, venous ulcer

Questions to Ask the Patient/ Family/Witness/Yourself

- Are you having any pain in the area? If so, can you describe the pain (pressure, sharp, dull, achy, ripping, burning)?
- What makes the pain better (certain positions, medication, rest)?
- What makes the pain worse (certain positions, movement, touching)?
- How severe is your pain? Can you rate it on a scale from 0 to 10?
- How is your appetite? Are you able to keep down food and/or fluids?
- Have you ever had a pressure injury like this in the past?
- Have you had any recent: difficulty moving in bed? immobilization such as prolonged time spent in bed or sitting? surgery? trauma to the area?

Associated Signs/Symptoms: PAIN: pain anywhere else; GENERAL: chills, fever, weight changes; GENITOURINARY: incontinence; MUSCULOSKELETAL: joint stiffness, swelling; SKIN: itching; NEUROLOGICAL: numbness/tingling

Recommended Assessments

- Vital signs
- Temperature
- Weight and nutritional status
- I/O
- Pain scale (if applicable)
  - Tolerable pain level
- General
  - Level of consciousness and orientation
  - Inspect: signs of acute distress, acute illness, affect, restlessness
- Skin
  - Assess all bony prominences
  - Stage the injury according to the National Pressure Ulcer Advisory Panel:

- Stage 1: intact skin with non-blanchable redness lasting >1 hour after relief of pressure
- Stage 2: partial thickness tissue loss with exposed dermis (with or without infection); blistering may be present
- Stage 3: full thickness tissue loss with destruction extending to the subcutaneous fat (with or without infection); undermining and tunneling may be present
- Stage 4: full thickness tissue loss with bone, tendon, or joint exposure (with or without infection); undermining and tunneling are often present
- Unstageable: full thickness tissue loss in which the wound bed is covered by slough and/or eschar
- Suspected deep tissue injury: localized area of non-blanchable purple or maroon discoloration; could also present as a blood-filled blister
- Measure: wound width, length, and depth. Use of transparency tracing or photograph is preferred
- Inspect: wound bed/margins/surrounding skin for erythema, cyanosis, necrosis, slough, eschar, drainage, undermining, tunneling, odor, moisture level
- Palpate: turgor, response to blanching, warmth, edema, induration, tenderness
- Neurological
  - Palpate: sensation surrounding the injured area
- Extremities
  - Palpate: capillary refill, edema, pulses, temperature

Past Medical History Considerations
Puts the patient at risk for pressure injuries and differential considerations

- Alzheimer's disease/dementia
- ALS
- CKD

- CVA/TIA
- Diabetes
- Guillain-Barré syndrome
- Heart failure
- Immobilization
- Incontinence
- MS
- Neuropathy
- Obesity
- PVD
- Skin malignancy
- Spinal cord injury

Medication Evaluation
May slow or negatively affect wound healing

- Anticoagulants
- Antiplatelet agents
- Biologic/immunosuppressive agents
- Chemotherapy
- Corticosteroids
- NSAIDs

Lab Evaluation and Trends

- Albumin
- Bedside capillary glucose trends

Nursing Intervention Considerations

- Medications (if ordered or protocol allows)
  - PRN pain medication
- Diet
  - Push fluids if there are no contraindications (>2,000mL/day)
  - High-protein diet, target 1.5g/kg/day, specific recommendations from the dietician should be discussed

- Activity
  - Encourage activity and ambulation if safety permits
- Positioning
  - Side lying position (30–40 degrees) preferred if the patient tolerates it
  - HOB should be at the lowest degree tolerated to avoid sliding and sheering (<30 degrees preferred)
  - Float the patient's heels
  - Avoid positioning directly onto medical devices, such as tubes, drainage systems, or other foreign objects
  - Utilize elbow and heel pads, chair cushions, specialty air/foam mattress if available
  - Reposition every 2–4 hours or establish an individualized turning schedule
- Collect
  - Wound drainage sample (if applicable)
- Monitor
  - Pain levels
  - Temperature trends
  - I/O
  - Weight trends
  - Blood sugar trends (if applicable)
  - Agitation levels
  - Peripheral pulses
  - Skin assessment every 8 hours or more frequently if the patient is incontinent
  - Wound healing progression
  - Signs and symptoms of skin infection such as fever, erythema, swelling, heat, pain, wounds, and purulent drainage
  - Signs and symptoms of sepsis such as fever, chills, hypotension, altered mental status, hypoxia, cool clammy skin, dyspnea, oliguria, tachycardia, and tachypnea
- Safety
  - Perform a fall risk assessment and implement the appropriate strategies

- Environment
  - Avoid elevated room temperature to prevent diaphoresis and excessive moisture
- Supportive care
  - Maintain effective communication between yourself, patient, and family
  - Provide emotional support and reassurance to the patient and family
  - Maintain a calm manner during patient interactions
  - Discuss plan of care with the patient and decide reasonable goals together
  - Notify the patient and family of changes in the plan of care
  - Identify barriers to care and compliance
  - Promote skin care and integrity
  - Cleanse the wound and apply appropriate dressing per injury staging (hydrocolloid or foam dressing preferred), advice from a wound expert is needed for more advanced staged injury. Consider a dressing that creates a warm, moist, wound healing environment (stages 2, 3, 4)
  - Avoid application of heating devices directly (bed warmers, heating pads) on the skin surface or near the pressure injury
  - Provide light clothing and bed linen
  - **Educational topics (as applicable to the patient):**
    - General information regarding the patient's pressure injury and differential diagnosis considerations
    - Procedure and intervention explanation and justification
    - Explanation regarding referrals and specialist who may see them for this issue
    - Pain scale and pain goals
    - Proper positioning and turning schedule
    - Peri-care and proper hygiene
    - Skin care
    - Dressing changes

- Safety needs and fall risk
- Handwashing and infection control measures
- High-protein diet
- Increased fluid intake
- Increased physical activity
- Blood glucose measurement techniques, frequency, and goals
- Signs and symptoms of skin infection
- Pressure injury prevention
- Dehydration prevention

ISBARR Recommendation Considerations

- Medication
  - Add PRN and/or scheduled pain medication
- IV fluid needs if oral intake is poor, there are signs of dehydration, and the patient is NPO or hypotensive
- Labs
  - Albumin
  - Wound culture
- Safety
  - Activity-level changes
  - Fall risk protocol
- Monitoring needs
  - Blood sugars including frequency and parameters to call the provider (if applicable)
  - Daily weights
  - Dressing change frequency
  - Skin assessment frequency
- Supportive cares
  - Compression stockings or SCDs
  - Specialty mattress, chair cushion, elbow and heel pads
- Change diet to
  - High protein
  - Push oral fluids

- Referrals
  - Dietician
  - General surgeon
  - Wound care specialist/nurse
- Ask if the provider wants anything else done
- Read back orders; ask that they enter all orders into the electronic medical record

ISBARR Template	
I **Introduction**	**Introduce Yourself and the Patient** • "Hello, Dr. Mortensen, this is Lisa Brown. I am the nurse for Daisy Garcia in Room 207. She is your patient that was admitted today for pneumonia. I know you have not been in to see her yet."
S **Situation**	**Sign/Symptom You Are Concerned About** • "I am calling because while doing an admission assessment, I noticed a 2-cm × 3-cm stage 2 pressure injury on her sacrum. It is moist, red, and warm. I do not see any other signs of infection." **Associated Signs/Symptoms** • "She is complaining of pain in the area."
B **Background**	**Vitals** • "Her blood pressure is 146/90, heart rate is 70, respirations are 14, and temperature is 100.1." **Exam** • "Besides her pressure injury, she has crackles in her right posterior lower lobe and a productive cough. I also noticed she has a thin body habitus and muscle atrophy in her bilateral lower extremities." **Past Medical History** • "She does have a history of CVA and is typically bedbound or in a chair. She is up with a Hoyer lift and doesn't move well on her own in bed." **Labs and Medications** • "Her albumin level on admission was low at 3.2."

ISBARR Template	
A **Assessment**	**Assessment** • "I am concerned about the progression of her pressure injury due to her immobility and signs of malnutrition."
R **Recommendations** **R** **Read Back**	**Nurse's Recommendations, Interventions, and Read Back** • "I have put her on a turning schedule of every two hours and put a foam dressing on the area. Would you consider a referral for wound care nurse and a dietician? I would also recommend a rotating air mattress. Would you like anything else done at this time?" • "Thank you, Dr. Mortensen. I will put in referrals for the wound nurse, dietician, and a rotating air mattress. I will make sure nursing is doing skin checks every eight hours."

Disclaimer: This dialogue is factitious and any resemblance to actual persons, living or dead, or actual events is purely coincidental.

In order to avoid order discrepancies, it is recommended that all orders be entered by the provider in the electronic medical record.

Select Differential Diagnosis Presentations

Arterial Ulcer

Overview: poor arterial blood flow leads to ischemic ulcers (typically) in the lower extremities

Patient may complain of: extremity ulceration, pain, numbness/tingling, and swelling

Objective findings: ulcer with well-defined wound margins; extremity will feel cool with weak pulses, sluggish capillary refill, atypical hair growth, and shiny, pale, taut skin

PMH considerations/risk factors: hx of PVD, obesity, peripheral neuropathy, diabetes, renal failure, HTN, trauma to the extremity, nicotine use, older age

Diagnostics: clinical diagnosis; arterial doppler and ABI may be considered initially

Cellulitis

Overview: bacterial infection of the skin

Patient may complain of: fever, chills, localized skin erythema, swelling, and pain; symptoms are progressive in nature

Objective findings: fever, localized skin erythema, swelling, warmth, tenderness, drainage, open wound(s)

PMH considerations/risk factors: hx of diabetes, PVD, (lymph) edema, preexisting skin condition, obesity, immunosuppression, trauma to the area, IV drug use, older age

Diagnostics: clinical diagnosis; CBC and wound culture may be considered

Venous Ulcer

Overview: poor venous circulation in the lower extremities leads to edema and breakdown of the skin

Patient may complain of: discoloration, swelling, and skin changes in the lower extremities

Objective findings: ulcer with ill-defined borders, typically shallow and painless; edema, surrounding skin may be red/brown/purple with "sock-like" appearance

PMH considerations/risk factors: hx of PVD, varicose veins, heart failure, diabetes, DVT, pregnancy, obesity, nicotine

Diagnostics: clinical diagnosis; venous doppler and ABI may be considered initially

References

American Medical Directors Association. (2010). *Know-it-all before you call: Data collection system.* Columbia, MD: Author.

Anders, T. (2017). Management of a patient with a coccyx ulcer in a nursing home. *Wounds UK, 13,* 54–58.

Armstrong, D., & Meyr, A. J. (2017). Basic principles of wound management. In K. A. Collins (Ed.), *UpToDate.* Retrieved from https://www.uptodate.com/contents/basic-principles-of-wound-management

Barbard, J. A. (2016). Increasing the accuracy of pressure ulcer classification using a pressure ulcer guidance tool. *Wounds UK, 12*(4), 52–57.

Berlowitz, D. (2017a). Clinical staging and management of pressure-induced skin and soft tissue injury. In K. A. Collins (Ed.), *UpToDate*. Retrieved from https://www.uptodate.com/contents/clinical-staging-and-management-of-pressure-induced-skin-and-soft-tissue-injury

Berlowitz, D. (2017b). Epidemiology, pathogenesis, and risk assessment of pressure ulcers. In K. A. Collins (Ed.), *UpToDate*. Retrieved from https://www.uptodate.com/contents/epidemiology-pathogenesis-and-risk-assessment-of-pressure-induced-skin-and-soft-tissue-injury

Berlowitz, D. (2018). Prevention of pressure-induced skin and soft tissue injury. In K. A. Collins (Ed.), *UpToDate*. Retrieved from https://www.uptodate.com/contents/prevention-of-pressure-induced-skin-and-soft-tissue-injury

Chapman, S. (2017). Preventing and treating pressure ulcers: Evidence review. *Community Wound Care, 22*(3), 37–40.

Chen, H. L., Caom Y. J., Zhang, W., Wang, J., & Huai, B. S. (2017). Braden scale (ALB) for assessing pressure ulcer risk in hospital patients: A validity and reliability study. *Applied Nursing Research, 33*, 169–174.

Ellis, M. (2016). Understanding the latest guidance on pressure ulcer prevention. *Journal of Community Nursing, 30*(4), 29–36.

Fletcher, J. (2017). An overview of pressure ulcer risk assessment tools. *Wounds UK, 13*(1), 18–26.

Gillespie, B. M., Chaboyer, W. P., McInnes, E., Kent, B., Whitty, J. A., & Thalib, L. (2014). Repositioning for pressure ulcer prevention in adults. *Cochrane Database of Systematic Reviews*, (4), 1–45. doi: 10.1002/14651858.CD009958.pub2

Gould, L., Stuntz, M., Giovannelli, M., Ahmad, A., Aslam, R., Mullen-Fortino, M., . . . Gordillo, G. M. (2016). Wound health society 2015 update on guidelines for pressure ulcers. *Wound Repair and Regeneration, 24*, 145–162.

Jarvis, C. (2015). *Physical examination & health assessment*. St. Louis, MO: Elsevier.

Lee, T. T., Lin, K. C., Mills, M. E., & Kuo, Y. H. (2012). Factors related to the prevention and management of pressure ulcers. *Computers, Informatics, Nursing, 30*(9), 489–495.

Moore, Z. E., & Cowman, S. (2015). Repositioning for treating pressure ulcers. *Cochrane Database of Systematic Reviews*, (1), 1–19. doi: 10.1002/14651858.CD006898.pub4

National Institute for Health and Care Excellence. (2014). *Pressure ulcers: Prevention and management of pressure ulcers in primary and secondary care.* Retrieved from https://www.ncbi.nlm.nih.gov/pubmedhealth/PMH0068960/

National Pressure Ulcer Advisory Panel, European Pressure Ulcer Advisory Panel and Pan Pacific Pressure Injury Alliance. (2014). *Prevention and treatment of pressure ulcers: Quick reference guide.* Retrieved from https://www.npuap.org/wp-content/uploads/2014/08/Updated-10-16-14-Quick-Reference-Guide-DIGITAL-NPUAP-EPUAP-PPPIA-16Oct2014.pdf

Papadakis, M. A., & McPhee, S. J. (2017). *Current medical diagnosis and treatment* (56th ed.). New York, NY: McGraw-Hill.

Qaseem, A., Humphrey, L. L., Forciea, M. A., Starkey, M., & Denberg, T. D. (2015). Treatment of pressure ulcers: A clinical practice guideline from the American college of physicians. *Annals of Internal Medicine, 162,* 370–379.

Registered Nurses' Association of Ontario. (2016). *Assessment and management of pressure injuries for the interprofessional team.* Retrieved from http://rnao.ca/sites/rnao-ca/files/Pressure_Injuries_BPG.pdf

Seller, R. H., & Symons, A. B. (2012). *Differential diagnosis of common complaints* (6th ed.). Philadelphia, PA: Elsevier.

Smith, B., Totten, A., Hickam, D. H., Fu, R., Wasson, N., Rahman, B., . . . Saha, S. (2013). Pressure ulcer treatment strategies. *Annals of Internal Medicine, 159*(1), 39–50.

Tayyib, N., & Coyer, F. (2016). Effectiveness of pressure ulcer prevention strategies for adult patients in intensive care units: A systematic review. *Worldviews on Evidence-Based Nursing, 13*(6), 432–444.

Tleyjeh, I., Berlowitz, D., & Baddour, L. M. (2018). Infectious complications of pressure ulcers. In A. Bloom (Ed.), *UpToDate.* Retrieved from https://www.uptodate.com/contents/infectious-complications-of-pressure-ulcers

Warner, J., Raible, M. A., Hajduk, G., & Collavo, J. (2017). Best practice for pressure ulcer prevention in the burn center. *Critical Care Nursing Quarterly, 40*(1), 41–48.

Wound, Ostomy and Continence Nurses Society. (2017). 2016 guideline for prevention and management of pressure ulcers (injuries). *Journal of Wound, Ostomy, and Continence Nursing, 44*(3), 241–246.

CHAPTER 28

Seizures

A seizure is caused by excessive neuronal firing in the brain. There are two broad categories of seizures: partial and generalized. Generalized seizures propagate throughout the entire brain, causing a loss of consciousness. Tonic-clonic seizures (formerly known as grand mal seizures) are the most common type of generalized seizures, and they characteristically cause generalized muscle stiffening (tonic) and rhythmic jerking (clonic). Partial seizures originate in one region of the brain which may or may not cause a change in consciousness. Some common behaviors during partial seizures include aphasia, hallucinations, aggression, head nodding, eye blinking, dysarthria, pelvic thrusting, crying, laughing, paralysis, nausea, vomiting, and palpitations.

In an acute care setting, it may be more common for the nurse to witness a provoked seizure that is caused by an underlying insult to the brain, such as a CVA, head trauma, withdrawal, infection, or electrolyte abnormalities. If the seizure is unprovoked and there has been no known insult to the brain, epilepsy is the most common cause. Epilepsy is defined by two or more unprovoked seizures occurring more than 24 hours apart. It can be confused with syncope, movement disorders, and psychogenic non-epileptic seizures. Determining the cause, type of seizure, risk of recurrence, and treatment is done by a neurologist.

Typically, seizures last less than 5 minutes. If the seizure is prolonged, the patient is at risk for status epilepticus, which is seizure activity lasting more than 30 minutes, either continuously, or having two or more seizures without full recovery in between. It is imperative that the nurse recognizes the patient's risk for status epilepticus because it has a mortality rate of almost 30% in adults.

After a seizure occurs, the patient will experience a postictal state that can last from seconds to several days. It is the nurse's priority to maintain the patient's airway and safety during the seizure, time the seizure, collect an accurate description of precipitating and postictal symptoms, and administer medication to help prevent seizure recurrence.

Differential Diagnosis Considerations

Common: benzodiazepine withdrawal, CVA/TIA, epilepsy, fever, hyperglycemia, hypoglycemia, hypokalemia, hypoxia, increased ICP, intracranial hemorrhage, TBI, uremia, withdrawal from alcohol

Consider: arrhythmia, AV malformation, BPPV, brain tumor, delirium, eclampsia, encephalitis, hypernatremia, hyperthyroidism, hypocalcemia, hypomagnesemia, hyponatremia, medication induced, meningitis, narcolepsy, panic attack, porphyrin, psychogenic non-epileptic seizures, sleep apnea, syncope

Questions to Ask the Patient/ Family/Witness/Yourself

- Was the seizure witnessed? By who?
- When did it start? How long did it last? (Exact timing is preferred.)
- Can you (the witness) describe the seizure (shaking, jerking, stiffness, staring, change in consciousness)?
- What were you/they doing before the seizure started?
- Did anything trigger the seizure (alcohol, emotion, lack of sleep, psychological stress, menstrual cycles, flashing light)?
- Have you/they had any recent: illness/infection? cranial surgery? trauma to your/their head?
- Have you/they taken any new prescribed or over-the-counter medications? Have there been any recent changes to your/their current medication?
- Do you/they drink alcohol? How many drinks per day/week? What kind and amount of alcohol do you/they drink? When was your/their last drink? (if applicable)

- Do you/they have a history of drug use? What types and how much? Do you/they use on a daily basis? When was your/their last use? (if applicable)

If the patient has a history of a seizure disorder

- When was your/their last seizure? How often do they happen?
- Can you tell when you/they are going to have a seizure (aura)?
- Do you/they take medication for your/their seizures as prescribed? Have you/they missed any doses? If so, how often do you/they miss doses per week?

Associated and Postictal Signs/Symptoms: PAIN: pain anywhere; GENERAL: fatigue, fever, chills, weakness; EENT: vision changes; CARDIOVASCULAR: chest pain/tightness, palpitations; GASTRO-INTESTINAL: nausea, vomiting; GENITOURINARY: incontinence; NEUROLOGICAL: dizziness, headache, numbness/tingling, (pre) syncope, tremors; PSYCHOLOGICAL: confusion, hallucinations, memory changes, sleeping issues, feelings of impending doom

Recommended Assessments

- Vital signs
- Temperature
- I/O
- Pain scale (if applicable)
  - Tolerable pain level
- General
  - Level of consciousness and orientation
  - Inspect: signs of acute distress, acute illness, affect, restlessness
  - Speech changes
  - GCS
- Skin
  - Inspect: cyanosis, diaphoresis, pallor
- Eyes
  - Inspect: nystagmus, ptosis, pupillary response

- Mouth
  - Inspect: tongue swelling or signs of biting
- Head/face/neck
  - Inspect: ROM of neck, signs of trauma
  - Palpate: swelling, tenderness
- Cardiovascular
  - Auscultate: heart sounds, rate, rhythm
- Respiratory
  - Inspect: respiratory effort, depth, pattern, use of accessory muscles
  - Auscultate: lung sounds
- Musculoskeletal
  - Palpate: muscle tone
- Neurological
  - Inspect: facial droop, tremors
  - Palpate: extremity strength, sensation
  - Cranial nerve exam
- Extremities
  - Inspect: IV site

Past Medical History Considerations

- Allergies

Puts the patient at risk for differential considerations

- Alcohol abuse/use
- Bleeding/clotting disorders
- CKD
- Diabetes
- Drug abuse/use
- Pregnancy

Chronic conditions associated with higher risk of seizures or can mimic seizure activity

- Alzheimer's disease/dementia
- Anxiety

- Arrhythmias (various)
- BPPV
- Brain malignancy
- CVA/TIA
- Depression
- Epilepsy
- Migraines
- Narcolepsy
- SLE
- Sleep apnea
- Syncope
- TBI
- Thyroid disease

Medication Evaluation

Associated with seizures and/or lowering the seizure threshold

- Albuterol
- Amphetamines
- Anesthetics
- Antiarrhythmics
- Anticancer drugs
- Anticholinergics
- Anticonvulsants
- Antiemetics
- Antihistamines
- Antimicrobials
- Antiparkinson agents
- Antipsychotics
- Benzodiazepine withdrawal
- Beta blockers
- Cholinesterase inhibitors
- Flumazenil
- MAO inhibitors
- Montelukast
- Muscle relaxants

- NSAIDs
- Opioids
- Phosphodiesterase-5 inhibitors
- Pseudoephedrine
- SNRIs
- SSRIs
- Theophylline
- Tricyclic antidepressants

Used to treat seizures/epilepsy

- Carbamazepine
- Clobazam
- Ethosuximide
- Felbamate
- Gabapentin
- Lacosamide
- Lamotrigine
- Levetiracetam
- Oxcarbazepine
- Phenobarbital
- Phenytoin
- Pregabalin
- Topiramate
- Valproate
- Zonisamide

Lab Evaluation and Trends

- Bedside capillary glucose trends
- BMP/CMP
- Seizure medication range/concentration

Nursing Intervention Considerations

- Call for help or rapid response/code team if vital signs are unstable or there are signs of urgent distress

- Maintain a patent airway
  - Apply oxygen if hypoxic
  - Suction as needed
  - Provide oral care throughout the day (q2–4hrs)
  - Never force anything into the patient's mouth during seizure activity
  - Call respiratory therapy for signs of respiratory distress
- Verify patent IV if IVF or IV medication treatment is anticipated
  - Flush according to facility protocol; watch for swelling, erythema, pain, and other signs of infiltration
- Blood sugar if hypo- or hyperglycemia is suspected
- Medications (if ordered or protocol allows)
  - PRN benzodiazepine if the patient has established seizure disorder diagnosis and discussion with the provider has taken place
  - If hypoglycemic and has altered mental status or is unable to swallow, give 1mg IV/IM/SQ glucagon, and/or 25–50mL IV 50% dextrose, or follow your facility's hypoglycemia protocol (goal is >100)
- Diet
  - If hypoglycemic, alert, and can swallow, give a fast-acting carbohydrate like a glucose tablet, 4oz of fruit juice, 8oz of milk, 4oz of non-diet soda, hard candy, or teaspoon of honey/sugar. Repeat until sugar is normalized (goal is >100)
- Activity
  - Keep the patient in bed until discussion with the provider
- Positioning
  - Side lying position if there is a decrease in LOC or the patient is vomiting
  - Avoid restraining the patient during seizure activity
  - Reposition every 2–4 hours or establish an individualized turning schedule
- Monitor
  - Stay with the patient until stable
  - Seizure time

- Pain levels
- Vital signs and trends
- Oxygen saturation/pulse oximetry
- Temperature trends
- Blood sugar trends (if applicable)
- Telemetry/cardiac monitor
- Orientation status changes, GCS
- Agitation levels
- Neurological exam
- Postictal injuries
- Skin assessment every 8–24 hours or more frequently if the patient is incontinent
- Signs of decreased cardiac output such as weak pulses, cool skin, altered mental status, hypotension, oliguria, and mottling
- Signs of respiratory distress such as cyanosis, tachypnea, hypoxia, use of accessory muscles, diaphoresis, and adventitious lung sounds
- Signs and symptoms of increased ICP such as worsening headache, nausea, vomiting, hypertension, bradypnea, altered mental status, vision changes, fixed or sluggish pupillary response, and GCS changes
- Safety
  - Perform a fall risk assessment and implement the appropriate strategies
  - Place bed rail padding
  - Initiate frequent checks or 1:1 care if needed
- Environment
  - Provide a calm, quiet environment and reduce stimulation
  - Maintain a well-lit environment
  - Utilize ways to reorient the patient with clocks, calendars, frequent family/friend interaction, and personal items from home

- Maintain a comfortable room temperature
- Utilize a fan (if appropriate)
- Supportive care
  - Maintain effective communication between yourself, patient, and family
  - Provide emotional support and reassurance to the patient and family
  - Maintain a calm manner during patient interactions
  - Discuss plan of care with the patient and decide reasonable goals together
  - Notify the patient and family of changes in the plan of care
  - Refrain from correcting or arguing with the patient during periods of confusion and reorient the patient as needed
  - Identify barriers to care and compliance
  - Provide light clothing and bed linen
  - Promote skin care and integrity
- **Educational topics (as applicable to the patient):**
  - General information regarding the patient's seizure and differential diagnosis considerations
  - Procedure and intervention explanation and justification
  - Explanation regarding referrals and specialist who may see them for this issue
  - New medication education including reason, side effects, and administration needs
  - Medication compliance
  - Medication changes
  - Laboratory monitoring needs
  - Oxygen therapy and maintenance
  - Relaxation techniques and breathing exercises
  - Trigger avoidance
  - Telemetry
  - Proper positioning and turning schedule

- Skin care
- Peri-care and proper hygiene
- Ketogenic diet
- Blood glucose measurement techniques and frequency
- Alcohol and/or drug cessation and support
- Home safety modifications and injury prevention
- Safety needs and fall risk
- 1:1 care
- Sleep hygiene
- Stimulus control
- Seizure calendar
- Stress reduction and management
- Driving restrictions
- When to notify the nurse or provider
- Signs and symptoms of hyper- and hypoglycemia
- Dehydration prevention
- Pressure injury prevention

ISBARR Recommendation Considerations

- Ask the provider to come assess the patient STAT if they are unstable or seizure activity is prolonged
- Transfer to the ICU if hemodynamically unstable, advanced medication management is required, or closer monitoring is needed
- Medication
  - Hold oral medications if the patient is unable to tolerate or NPO
  - Discuss changing medication routes with the provider (and pharmacy) if the patient is NPO
  - Discontinue/change suspected causative medication
  - Add anticonvulsant
  - Add PRN and/or scheduled benzodiazepine

- IV fluid needs if oral intake is poor, there are signs of dehydration, and the patient is NPO or hypotensive
- EEG
- ECG (recommended for first-time seizure)
- Imaging
  - Head CT scan/MRI
- Labs (depending on the suspected cause)
  - BMP/CMP
  - CBC
  - Magnesium
  - Seizure medication range/concentration
  - Toxicology screening
  - TSH
- Safety
  - 1:1 monitoring (if applicable)
  - Activity level changes
  - Bed rail padding
  - Fall risk protocol
- Monitoring needs
  - Blood sugars including frequency and parameters to call the provider (if applicable)
  - Continuous O_2 monitoring
  - Telemetry/continuous cardiac monitoring
  - Vital signs including frequency and parameters to call the provider
- Change diet to
  - Ketogenic
- Protocols
  - CIWA-Ar if alcohol withdrawal is suspected
- Referrals
  - Neurology
- Ask if the provider wants anything else done
- Read back orders; ask that they enter all orders into the electronic medical record

ISBARR Template	
I **Introduction**	**Introduce Yourself and the Patient** • "Hello, Dr. Schultz. This is Jen Simonson. I am the nurse for your patient Janet Carroll in Room 505."
S **Situation**	**Sign/Symptom You Are Concerned About** • "Ms. Carroll started having a generalized tonic-clonic seizure at 1030. The beginning of the seizure was witnessed by her husband. I was called into the room and the seizure lasted for roughly 90 seconds. She is now in a postictal state." **Associated Signs/Symptoms** • "She has been very fatigued since the seizure, but prior to her seizure her husband says she seemed more irritable and sweaty but did not have any headache, neck pain, or nausea complaints. She did not have incontinence during the seizure."
B **Background**	**Vitals** • "Vitals are stable. Blood pressure is 110/85, respiratory rate is 12, heart rate is 70, and temperature is 97.5." **Exam** • "She opens her eyes to her name but remains fatigued and sleepy. She responds to commands but mumbles when asked questions. She has no one-sided weakness or facial droop. I did notice she has signs of lateral tongue biting." **Past Medical History** • "She has a history of daily alcohol use. Her husband says she drinks six to eight beers a day but has not had any alcohol in over 24 hours. He also tells me that she has had seizures with alcohol withdrawal in the past, but I did not see anything about that in her past medical history. It sounds like it hasn't happened in a few years."

ISBARR Template	
	Labs and Medications
	• "She is not on any anticonvulsants. CMP and CBC were normal this morning."
A **Assessment**	**Assessment**
	• "I am concerned that her seizure is related to alcohol withdrawal."
R **Recommendations** **R** **Read Back**	**Nurse's Recommendations, Interventions, and Read Back**
	• "I have placed padding on her bed rails. Did you want to initiate the CIWA protocol? Do you want lorazepam or a different benzodiazepine ordered as needed? Do you want anything else like labs, EEG, or imaging done at this time? I would ask that you come assess her as soon as possible."
	• "Thank you, Dr. Schultz. I would like to read those orders back to you. You would like me to initiate fall risk and CIWA protocol. I will also put in for a STAT CT of the head, CBC, CMP, and toxicology screen. I will let the patient and her husband know you are coming to evaluate her as soon as possible."

Disclaimer: This dialogue is factitious and any resemblance to actual persons, living or dead, or actual events is purely coincidental.

In order to avoid order discrepancies, it is recommended that all orders be entered by the provider in the electronic medical record.

Select Differential Diagnosis Presentations

Arrhythmia

Overview: any irregular heart rhythm

Patient may complain of: fatigue, generalized weakness, (pre) syncope, palpitations, chest pain, dyspnea, dizziness, seizures, anxiety

Objective findings: signs of acute distress, lethargy, irritability, diaphoresis, irregular heart rhythm, bradycardia/tachycardia, murmur, hypertension/hypotension, tachypnea, seizures

PMH considerations/risk factors: hx of arrhythmia, CAD, HTN, heart failure, MI, cardiac valve disorders, diabetes, previous CV surgery, substance abuse, increased psychological stress, nicotine use, family hx of heart disease

Diagnostics: BMP/CMP, CBC, TSH, ECG, ECHO, Holter monitor/loop recorder/event recorder

Benign Paroxysmal Positional Vertigo

Overview: abnormal calcium debris within the inner ear causing obstruction of fluid movement, leading to acute dizziness

Patient may complain of: nausea, vomiting, dizziness with head position changes, balance disturbances; symptoms have a short duration

Objective findings: nystagmus, positive Dix–Hallpike maneuver, gait instability

PMH considerations/risk factors: hx of BPPV, orthostatic hypotension, recent head injury or ear infection, female gender

Diagnostics: clinical diagnosis; workup to rule out more emergent causes may be indicated

Cerebral Vascular Accident

Overview: partial or complete obstruction of blood flow to the brain due to ischemia or hemorrhage causing brain tissue death

Patient may complain of: vision changes, nausea, vomiting, dysphagia, headache, dizziness, seizures, insomnia, difficulty with memory, speaking, focusing, and understanding; unilateral paralysis of the face, arms, and legs

Objective findings: signs of acute distress, altered mental status, ptosis, dysarthria, hypertension, carotid bruit(s), facial droop, seizures, unilateral weakness and sensation disturbances, immobility, gait disturbances

PMH considerations/risk factors: hx of HTN, CAD, heart failure, hyperlipidemia, arrhythmia, cardiac valve disease, diabetes, obesity, nicotine use, substance abuse, family hx of heart disease

Diagnostics: head CT/MRI

Hypernatremia

Overview: elevated serum sodium

Patient may complain of: thirst, muscle spasms and cramps, tremors, seizures, anxiety; patient is typically asymptomatic unless severe

Objective findings: irritability, altered mental status, decreased skin turgor, dry mucous membranes, tachycardia, hypotension, bradypnea, decreased reflexes, seizures; exam is typically unremarkable unless severe

PMH considerations: hx of AKI, Cushing's syndrome, GI loss, burn injury, diabetes, diuretic use

Diagnostics: serum Na

Hyperthyroidism

Overview: overactive thyroid gland

Patient may complain of: anxiety, heat intolerance, fatigue, generalized weakness, palpitations, diarrhea, nausea, vomiting, weight loss, muscle cramps, tremors, seizures, insomnia

Objective findings: lethargy, irritability, diaphoresis, hair thinning, exophthalmos, goiter, tachycardia, hypertension, tremors, seizures

PMH considerations/risk factors: hx of Grave's disease, thyroiditis, pregnancy, thyroid cancer, family hx of thyroid dysfunction, female gender, older age

Diagnostics: TSH, T3, T4, thyroid US, radioactive iodine uptake scan

Hypocalcemia

Overview: low serum calcium

Patient may complain of: fatigue, diarrhea, muscle cramps, paresthesias, seizures, anxiety; patient is typically asymptomatic unless severe

Objective findings: lethargy, altered mental status, irritability, positive Trousseau's and Chvostek's sign, prolonged QT interval, hypotension, bradycardia, tachypnea, hyperactive bowel sounds, hyperactive reflexes, seizures; exam is typically unremarkable unless severe

PMH considerations/risk factors: hx of cancer, immobility, malnutrition, hypoparathyroidism, alcohol abuse/use, vitamin D deficiency

Diagnostics: serum Ca, ECG

Hypokalemia

Overview: low serum potassium

Patient may complain of: fatigue, palpitations, nausea, vomiting, constipation, muscle weakness and cramping, seizures, anxiety; patient is typically asymptomatic unless severe

Objective findings: lethargy, irritability, altered mental status, wide QRS, arrhythmia, bradypnea, hypoactive bowel sounds, decreased reflexes, seizures; exam is typically unremarkable unless severe

PMH considerations/risk factors: hx of CKD, diabetes, diarrhea, alcohol abuse/use, eating disorders, NPO status, diuretic use

Diagnostics: serum K, ECG

Hypomagnesemia

Overview: low serum magnesium

Patient may complain of: fatigue, generalized weakness, nausea, vomiting, constipation, confusion, paresthesias, tremors, seizures; patient is typically asymptomatic unless severe

Objective findings: altered mental status, lethargy, bradycardia, hypotension, wide QRS, peaked T waves, prolonged PR interval, arrhythmia, bradypnea, hypoactive bowel sounds, hyperactive reflexes, tremors, seizures; exam is typically unremarkable unless severe

PMH considerations/risk factors: hx of diarrhea, burn injury, alcohol abuse/use, malnutrition, DKA, pancreatitis

Diagnostics: serum Mg, ECG

Hyponatremia

Overview: low serum sodium

Patient may complain of: fatigue, thirst, nausea, vomiting, anorexia, muscle cramps and weakness, seizures, headache; patient is typically asymptomatic unless severe

Objective findings: altered mental status, lethargy, irritability, tachycardia, weak pulses, bradypnea, decreased reflexes, seizures; exam is typically unremarkable unless severe

PMH considerations/risk factors: recent GI loss, hx of CKD, heart failure, diuretic use, SIADH, dehydration

Diagnostics: serum Na

Increased Intracranial Pressure

Overview: rise in pressure within the cranial cavity

Patient may complain of: vision changes, nausea, vomiting, headache, confusion, seizures

Objective findings: signs of acute distress, altered mental status, GCS changes, sluggish/fixed pupillary response, hypertension, bradycardia, bradypnea

PMH considerations/risk factors: hx of TBI, CVA, CNS infections, hydrocephalus, cancer, seizures, HTN

Diagnostics: ICP monitoring, head CT/MRI

Meningitis

Overview: inflammation and infection of the meninges surrounding the brain and spinal cord

Patient may complain of: chills, fever, fatigue, photophobia, neck pain, anorexia, nausea, vomiting, headache, confusion, dizziness, seizures

Objective findings: signs of acute distress/illness, lethargy, fever, irritability, altered mental status, petechial rash, nuchal rigidity (positive Brudzinski, Kernig sign), seizures, signs of increased ICP

PMH considerations/risk factors: hx of TBI, immunosuppression, pregnancy, close quarter living situations, recent travel outside of the United States, alcohol abuse, older/younger age

Diagnostics: CBC, lumbar puncture, head CT

Transient Ischemic Attack

Overview: transient obstruction of blood flow to the brain mimicking a CVA

Patient may complain of: vision changes, nausea, vomiting, dysphagia, headache, dizziness, seizures, difficulty with memory, speaking, focusing, and understanding; unilateral paralysis of face, arms, and legs; signs and symptoms are transient in nature

Objective findings: signs of acute distress, altered mental status, ptosis, dysarthria, hypertension, carotid bruit(s), facial droop, seizures, unilateral weakness and sensation disturbances, immobility, gait disturbances; may not have abnormal exam findings due to transient nature of the issue

PMH considerations/risk factors: hx of HTN, CAD, heart failure, hyperlipidemia, arrhythmia, cardiac valve disease, diabetes, obesity, nicotine use, substance abuse, family hx of heart disease

Diagnostics: head CT/MRI

Withdrawal (Alcohol)

Overview: rapid or abrupt decrease in alcohol intake causing physical and psychological disturbances

Patient may complain of: fever, chills, palpitations, anorexia, nausea, vomiting, diarrhea, seizures, headache, alcohol craving, insomnia, anxiety

Objective findings: signs of acute distress, fever, irritability, altered mental status, diaphoresis, tachycardia, hypertension, hepatomegaly, ascites, seizures, tremors, hallucinations/delirium

PMH considerations: hx of alcohol abuse, longer cessation (>48 hrs) since last drink, other substance abuse

Diagnostics: toxicology screen; workup to rule out more emergent causes may be indicated

References

American Academy of Neurology. (n.d.). *Treatments for refractory epilepsy.* Retrieved from http://tools.aan.com/professionals/practice/pdfs/clinician_ep_treatment_e.pdf

American Medical Directors Association. (2010). *Know-it-all before you call: Data collection system.* Columbia, MD: Author.

Atkinson, M., Hari, K., Schaefer, K., & Shah, A. (2012). Improving safety outcomes in the epilepsy monitoring unit. *Seizure, 21,* 124–127.

Bradley, P. M., Lindsay, B., & Fleeman, N. (2016). Care delivery and self-management strategies for adults with epilepsy. *Cochrane Database of Systematic Reviews,* (2), 1–82. doi: 10.1002/14651858.CD006244.pub3

Choi, H., & Mendiratta, A. (2017a). Seizure and epilepsy in older adults: Etiology, clinical presentation, and diagnosis. In A. F. Eichler (Ed.), *UpToDate.* Retrieved from https://www.uptodate.com/contents/seizures -and-epilepsy-in-older-adults-etiology-clinical-presentation-and-diagnosis

Choi, H., & Mendiratta, A. (2017b). Treatment of seizures and epilepsy in older adults. In A. F. Eichler (Ed.), *UpToDate.* Retrieved from https:// www.uptodate.com/contents/treatment-of-seizures-and-epilepsy-in-older -adults

Desai, S. P. (2009). *Clinician's guide to laboratory medicine* (3rd ed.). Houston, TX: MD2B.

Fisher, R. S., Cross, J. H., D'Souza, C., French, J. A., Haut, S. R., Higurashi, N., . . . Zuberi, S. M. (2017). Instruction manual for the ILAE 2017 operational classification of seizure types. *Epilepsia, 58*(4), 531–542.

Gavvala, J. R., & Schuele, S. U. (2016). New-onset seizure in adults and adolescents: A review. *JAMA, 316*(24), 2657–2668.

Gilad, R. (2012). Management of seizures following a stroke: What are the options? *Drugs Aging, 29*(7), 533–538.

Glauser, T., Shinnar, S., Gloss, D., Alldredge, B., Arya, R., Bainbridge, J., . . . Treiman, D. M. (2016). American epilepsy society guideline: Evidence-based guideline: Treatment of convulsive status epilepticus in children and adults: Report of the guideline committee of the American epilepsy society. *Epilepsy Currents, 16*(1), 48–61.

Gulanick, M., & Myers, J. L. (2017). *Nursing care plans: Diagnosis, interventions, & outcomes* (9th ed.). St. Louis, MO: Elsevier.

Hale, A., & Hovey, M. J. (2014). *Fluid, electrolyte and acid-base imbalances.* Philadelphia, PA: F.A. Davis Company.

Hitchings, A. W. (2016). Drugs that lower the seizure threshold. *Adverse Drug Reaction Bulletin, 298*(1), 1151–1154. doi:10.1097/FAD .0000000000000016

Jarvis, C. (2015). *Physical examination & health assessment.* St. Louis, MO: Elsevier.

Karceski, S. (2017). Initial treatment of epilepsy in adults. In A. F. Eichler (Ed.), *UpToDate.* Retrieved from https://www.uptodate.com/contents /initial-treatment-of-epilepsy-in-adults

Korff, C. M., & Wirrell, E. (2017). ILAE classification of seizures and epilepsy. In A. F. Eichler (Ed.), *UpToDate*. Retrieved from https://www.uptodate.com/contents/ilae-classification-of-seizures-and-epilepsy

Krumholz, A., Wiebe, S., Gronseth, G. S., Shinnar, S., Levisohn, P., Ting, T., . . . French, J. A. (2015). Evidence-based guideline: Management of an unprovoked first seizure in adults. *Neurology, 84*, 1705–1713.

Kulhari, A., Strbian, D., & Sundararajan, S. (2014). Early onset seizures in stroke. *Stroke, 45*, 249–251.

LeBlond, R. F., Brown, D. D., Suneja, M., & Szot, J. F. (2015). *DeGowin's diagnostic examination* (10th ed.). New York, NY: McGraw-Hill.

McCance, K. L., Huether, S. E., Brashers, V. L., & Rote, N. S. (2014). *Pathophysiology: The biologic basis for disease in adults and children* (7th ed.). St. Louis, MO: Elsevier.

Munchie, H. L., Yasinian, Y., & Oge, L. (2013). Outpatient management of alcohol withdrawal syndrome. *American Family Physician, 88*(9), 589–595.

Papadakis, M. A., & McPhee, S. J. (2017). *Current medical diagnosis and treatment* (56th ed.). New York, NY: McGraw-Hill.

Raftery, A. T., Lim, E., & Ostor, A. J. (2014). *Differential diagnosis* (4th ed.). London: Elsevier.

Schachter, S. C. (2018a). Evaluation and management of the first seizure in adults. In A. F. Eichler (Ed.), *UpToDate*. Retrieved from https://www.uptodate.com/contents/evaluation-and-management-of-the-first-seizure-in-adults

Schachter, S. C. (2018b). Overview of the management of epilepsy in adults. In A. F. Eichler (Ed.), *UpToDate*. Retrieved from https://www.uptodate.com/contents/overview-of-the-management-of-epilepsy-in-adults

Seller, R. H., & Symons, A. B. (2012). *Differential diagnosis of common complaints* (6th ed.). Philadelphia, PA: Elsevier.

Smith, G., Wagner, J. L., & Edwards, J. C. (2015). Epilepsy update, part 2: Nursing care and evidence-based treatment. *American Journal of Nursing, 115*(6), 34–44.

Uphold, C. R., & Graham, M. V. (2013). *Clinical guidelines in family practice* (5th ed.). Gainesville, FL: Barmarrae Books.

Wilden, J. A., & Cohen-Gadol, A. A. (2012). Evaluation of first nonfebrile seizure. *American Family Physician, 86*(4), 334–340.

Ycaza-Gutierrez, M. C., Wilson, L., & Altman, M. (2015). Beside nurse-driven protocol for management of alcohol/polysubstance abuse withdrawal. *Critical Care Nurse, 35*(6), 73–76.

CHAPTER 29

Tachycardia

The basic definition of tachycardia is a heart rate greater than
100 beats per minute. Tachycardia can lead to decreased cardiac
output, reduced coronary blood flow, and increased myocardial
oxygen consumption. It can occur due to an abnormality or dysfunction in the heart's normal conduction pathway, or can be a
response to an underlying pathological issue. If a patient's tachycardia is sustained, an ECG should be performed immediately,
followed by continuous cardiac monitoring, because most cases
will require intervention such as medication, IV fluids, cardioversion, ablation, or emergency defibrillation. If the patient is hemodynamically unstable, a rapid response or code team is required.
It is the nurse's priority to maintain the patient's airway, breathing and circulation, call the proper support team if the patient is
unstable, help determine the heart rhythm, and actively participate in their stabilization. In this chapter, nursing intervention
considerations and plan of care recommendations should reflect
whatever the suspected cause is.

Differential Diagnosis Considerations

Narrow QRS complex and regular: atrial tachycardia, AVNRT,
AVRT, junctional tachycardia, PSVT, sinus tachycardia

Narrow QRS complex and irregular: atrial fibrillation,
atrial flutter, multifocal atrial tachycardia, sinus arrhythmia

Wide QRS complex and regular: SVT, ventricular tachycardia

Wide QRS complex and irregular: PVCs, Torsades de
pointes, ventricular fibrillation

Underlying pathologic considerations: AAA rupture,
anemia, anxiety, dehydration, DKA, ectopic pregnancy,
exercise, fever, heart failure, hyperkalemia, hypernatremia, hyperthyroidism, hypoglycemia, hypokalemia, hypomagnesemia, hyponatremia, hypotension, hypoxia, IBD,

infectious process, intestinal obstruction, medication induced, medication withdrawal, MI, ovarian cyst rupture, pacemaker malfunction, pain, pancreatitis, PE, pericarditis, pheochromocytoma, pneumothorax, POTS, sepsis, shock, sickle cell crisis, stable angina, stimulants (amphetamines, caffeine, cocaine, nicotine), unstable angina, withdrawal from alcohol/drugs

Questions to Ask the Patient/Family/Witness/Yourself

- Do you feel like your heart is racing?
- When did the tachycardia/fast heart rate start? Did it start gradually or suddenly?
- What were you doing before/when the tachycardia/fast heart rate started?
- Is it constant or does it come and go? If intermittent, how long does it last? How often is it happening per hour/day?
- What makes the tachycardia/fast heart rate better (bearing down, certain positions, medication, rest)?
- Does anything trigger the tachycardia/fast heart rate or make it worse (activity, anxiety, certain positions, caffeine, lack of sleep, medication)?
- Have you had any recent: CV/thoracic surgery? illness/infection? psychological trauma/stress? vigorous exercise?
- Have you taken any new prescribed or over-the-counter medications? Have there been any recent changes to your current medication?
- Do you have a history of a tachycardia/fast heart rate? If so, what has been done or used to treat it?
- How is your appetite? Are you able to keep down food and/or fluids? (if applicable)
- How much fluid are you drinking on a daily basis? (if applicable)
- When was your last menstrual period? (if applicable)
- Do you have a family history of fast heart rates or abnormal heart rhythms?

- Do you drink caffeine? How many drinks in a day? When was the last time you had any?
- Do you smoke? How much (ppd)? How long have you been smoking? (if applicable)
- Do you drink alcohol? How many drinks per day/week? What kind and amount of alcohol do you drink? When was your last drink? (if applicable)
- Do you have a history of drug use? What types and how much? Do you use on a daily basis? When was your last use? (if applicable)

If the patient has a history of HTN
- What medications do you take for your blood pressure?
- Have you been using your blood pressure medications as prescribed? If missing doses, how often do you miss doses per day/week?

Associated Signs/Symptoms: PAIN: pain anywhere; GENERAL: chills, fatigue, fever, weakness; EENT: vision changes; CARDIOVASCULAR: chest pain/tightness, palpitations, PND, orthopnea; RESPIRATORY: dyspnea, painful breathing/coughing; GASTROINTESTINAL: nausea, diarrhea, signs of GI bleeding, vomiting; NEUROLOGICAL: dizziness, headaches, (pre)syncope; PSYCHOLOGICAL: anxiety, confusion, feelings of impending doom

Recommended Assessments
- Vital signs
  - Orthostatic blood pressure (if applicable)
- Temperature
- Weight
- I/O
- Pain scale (if applicable)
  - Tolerable pain level
- General
  - Level of consciousness and orientation

- Inspect: signs of acute distress, acute illness, affect, restlessness
  - Difficulty speaking due to breathlessness
- Skin
  - Inspect: cyanosis, diaphoresis, dryness, mottling, pallor
  - Palpate: temperature, turgor
- Head/face/neck
  - Inspect: JVD, tracheal deviation
  - Auscultate: carotid bruits
- Mouth
  - Inspect: mucous membrane moisture level
- Cardiovascular
  - Auscultate: heart sounds, rate, rhythm
  - Palpate: heaves, thrills
- Respiratory
  - Inspect: chest asymmetry, respiratory effort, depth, pattern, use of accessory muscles
  - Auscultate: lung sounds
- Gastrointestinal
  - Inspect: distention
  - Auscultate: bowel sounds, bruits
  - Palpate: guarding, (rebound) tenderness
- Extremities
  - Inspect: IV site
  - Palpate: capillary refill, edema, pulses, temperature

Note: Other examinations may be necessary depending on the underlying cause.

Past Medical History Considerations

- Allergies

Puts the patient at risk for differential considerations

- Alcohol use/abuse
- CAD
- CKD

- COPD
- CV/thoracic surgery
- Diabetes
- Drug use/abuse
- HTN
- Immobilization
- Nicotine use
- Ovarian cysts
- Pacemaker/ICD
- Sickle cell anemia

Reoccurrence/exacerbation should be considered

- Arrhythmias (various)
- MI
- PE

Chronic conditions that can cause tachycardia

- Anemia
- Anxiety
- Arrhythmias (various)
- Cardiac valve disorders
- Chronic pain
- Congenital heart defect(s)
- Heart failure
- POTS
- Thyroid disease

Medication Evaluation

Most common causative/exacerbating medication

- Antiarrhythmics
- Anticholinergics
- Antihistamines
- Antimicrobials
- Antipsychotics
- Atropine

- Beta blocker withdrawal
- Bronchodilators
- Decongestants
- Diuretics
- Levothyroxine
- Opioids
- PPIs
- SSRIs
- Tricyclic antidepressants
- Vasodilators

Used to treat tachyarrhythmias

- Adenosine
- Amiodarone
- Beta blockers
- Digoxin
- Diltiazem
- Dofetilide
- Flecainide
- Ivabradine
- Verapamil

Lab Evaluation and Trends

- Bedside capillary glucose trends
- BMP/CMP
- Cardiac enzymes
- CBC

Nursing Intervention Considerations

- Call for help or rapid response/code if vital signs are unstable or there are signs of urgent distress. If defibrillation is required for ventricular tachycardia or ventricular fibrillation, cardiac arrest protocol should be followed
- Maintain a patent airway
  - Apply oxygen if hypoxic

- Encourage slow relaxed deep breathing if hyperventilating
- Call respiratory therapy for signs of respiratory distress
- Verify patent IV if IVF or IV medication treatment is anticipated
  - Flush according to facility protocol; watch for swelling, erythema, pain, and other signs of infiltration
  - Large bore IV is preferred
- ECG STAT
- Blood sugar if hypoglycemia is suspected
- Medications (if ordered or protocol allows)
  - Hold suspected causative medication until discussion with the provider
  - If hypoglycemic and has altered mental status or unable to swallow, give 1mg IV/IM/SQ glucagon, and/or 25–50mL IV 50% dextrose, or follow your facility's hypoglycemia protocol (goal is >100)
- Diet
  - NPO if procedure or surgery is anticipated
  - Push fluids if there are no contraindications (>2,000mL/day)
  - Avoid caffeine
  - Encourage heart healthy, low-sodium food choices
  - If hypoglycemic, alert, and can swallow, give a fast-acting carbohydrate like a glucose tablet, 4oz of fruit juice, 8oz of milk, 4oz of non-diet soda, hard candy, or teaspoon of honey/sugar. Repeat until sugar is normalized (goal is >100)
- Activity
  - Keep the patient in bed until discussion with the provider
- Positioning
  - Supine position while performing vagal maneuvers
  - Lay supine with feet elevated if the patient is hypotensive
  - HOB raised to comfort for respiratory distress
  - Reposition every 2–4 hours or establish an individualized turning schedule

- Monitor
  - Stay with the patient until stable
  - Pain levels
  - Vital signs and trends
  - Oxygen saturation/pulse oximetry
  - Temperature trends
  - I/O
  - Telemetry/cardiac monitor
  - Blood sugar trends (if applicable)
  - Weight trends
  - Orientation status changes
  - Agitation levels
  - Peripheral pulses
  - Skin assessment every 8–24 hours
  - Signs of decreased cardiac output such as weak pulses, cool skin, altered mental status, hypotension, oliguria, and mottling
  - Signs of respiratory distress such as cyanosis, tachypnea, hypoxia, use of accessory muscles, diaphoresis, and adventitious lung sounds
  - Signs and symptoms of sepsis such as fever, chills, hypotension, altered mental status, hypoxia, cool clammy skin, dyspnea, oliguria, tachycardia, and tachypnea
  - Signs of dehydration such as lethargy, decreased skin turgor, dry mucous membranes, tachycardia, and (orthostatic) hypotension
  - Signs and symptoms of blood loss such as fatigue, dizziness, dyspnea, melena, hematochezia, hematemesis, hematuria, epistaxis, pallor, ecchymosis, altered mental status, hypotension, tachycardia, tachypnea, and hemoptysis
- Safety
  - Perform a fall risk assessment and implement the appropriate strategies
- Environment
  - Provide a calm, quiet environment and reduce stimulation

- Maintain a well lit environment
- Provide distractions
- Avoid bothersome odors in the room
- Maintain a comfortable room temperature
- Offer aromatherapy and/or music therapy (if appropriate)
- Utilize a fan (if appropriate)
- Supportive care
  - Maintain effective communication between yourself, patient, and family
  - Provide emotional support and reassurance to the patient and family
  - Maintain a calm manner during patient interactions
  - Discuss plan of care with the patient and decide reasonable goals together
  - Notify the patient and family of changes in the plan of care
  - Identify barriers to care and compliance
  - Reorient the patient as needed
  - Promote skin care and integrity
  - Provide light clothing and bed linen
  - Encourage vagal maneuvers (if appropriate)
  - Offer back rubs, warmed blankets, warm drinks, and new bed linens (if appropriate)
- **Educational topics (as applicable to the patient):**
  - General information regarding the patient's tachycardia and differential diagnosis considerations
  - Procedure and intervention explanation and justification
  - Explanation regarding referrals and specialist who may see them for this issue
  - New medication education including reason, side effects, and administration needs
  - Medication compliance
  - Medication changes
  - Pain scale and pain goals

- Relaxation techniques and breathing exercises
- Oxygen therapy and maintenance
- Trigger avoidance
- Telemetry
- Energy conservation techniques: placing items within reach, sitting to do tasks, taking breaks in between activities, sliding rather than lifting, pushing rather than pulling
- Vagal maneuvers
- Cardioversion and ablation
- Proper positioning and turning schedule
- Skin care
- Safety needs and fall risk
- Caffeine restriction
- NPO diet, DASH diet
- Increased fluid intake
- Smoking cessation
- Alcohol and/or drug cessation and support
- Stress reduction and management
- When to notify the nurse or provider
- Signs and symptoms of hypoglycemia
- Signs and symptoms of cardiac emergencies
- Signs and symptoms of respiratory emergencies
- Signs and symptoms of abnormal bleeding
- Dehydration prevention
- Pressure injury prevention

ISBARR Recommendation Considerations

- Ask the provider to come assess the patient STAT if they are symptomatic or unstable
- Transfer to the ICU if hemodynamically unstable, advanced medication management is required or closer monitoring is needed

- Medication
  - Hold oral medications if the patient is unable to tolerate or NPO
  - Discuss changing medication routes with the provider (and pharmacy) if the patient is NPO
  - Discontinue/change suspected causative medication
  - Add PRN and/or scheduled medication for anxiety or irritability
  - Add PRN and/or scheduled pain medication
- IV fluid needs if oral intake is poor, there are signs of dehydration, and the patient is NPO or hypotensive
- ECG if repeat testing is needed
- Imaging (depending on the suspected cause)
  - Chest X-ray
- Labs (depending on the suspected cause)
  - ABG
  - Blood culture
  - BMP/CMP
  - BNP
  - Cardiac enzymes
  - CBC
  - D-dimer
  - Magnesium
  - Toxicology screen
  - TSH
- Safety
  - Activity-level changes
  - Fall risk protocol
- Monitoring needs
  - Blood sugars including frequency and parameters to call the provider (if applicable)
  - Continuous O_2 monitoring
  - Telemetry/continuous cardiac monitoring
  - Strict I/O

- Daily weights
  - Vital signs including frequency and parameters to call the provider
- Supportive care
  - Compression stockings or SCDs
- Change diet to (depending on the suspected cause)
  - NPO
  - Caffeine restriction
  - DASH, low sodium
  - Push oral fluids
- Protocols
  - CIWA-Ar if alcohol withdrawal is suspected
- Referrals
  - Cardiology or Electrophysiology
- Ask if the provider wants anything else done
- Read back orders; ask that they enter all orders into the electronic medical record

ISBARR Template	
I **Introduction**	**Introduce Yourself and the Patient** • "Hello, Dr. Seefeldt, this is Mckenzie Saunders. I am the nurse for your patient Anne Caskey in Room 101 who was just admitted for complaints of chest pain with an unknown etiology. I know you have not been in to see her yet."
S **Situation**	**Sign/Symptom You Are Concerned About** • "I am calling because she developed constant tachycardia five minutes ago. Heart rates are between 130–150." **Associated Signs/Symptoms** • "Mrs. Caskey is feeling anxious and having constant palpitations but is denying chest pain at this time."

Tachycardia

ISBARR Template	
B **Background**	**Vitals** • "Blood pressure is stable at 158/89. Respirations are 22 and she is afebrile with a temperature of 97.4." **Exam** • "She appears anxious, is mildly diaphoretic, but has no new murmur and lungs are clear." **Past Medical History** • "She has a history of hypertension but no history of atrial fibrillation or other arrhythmias." **Labs and Medications** • "She took her lisinopril this morning and is not on any other medications for her blood pressure. The CMP and troponin from the ED were both normal."
A **Assessment**	**Assessment** • "I was concerned about an arrhythmia."
R **Recommendations** **R** **Read Back**	**Nurse's Recommendations, Interventions, and Read Back** • "I performed a 12-lead ECG. It appears that she is in rapid atrial fibrillation. I am keeping the patient in bed. Can you please come assess the patient as soon as possible? Would you like the patient on telemetry? Did you want any labs? What else would you like done before you come to see her?" • "Thank you, Dr. Seefeldt. I will place the patient on telemetry while you make your way down to see her. I will also call pharmacy to prep a diltiazem drip."

Disclaimer: This dialogue is factitious and any resemblance to actual persons, living or dead, or actual events is purely coincidental.

In order to avoid order discrepancies, it is recommended that all orders be entered by the provider in the electronic medical record.

Select Differential Diagnosis Presentations

Abdominal Aortic Aneurysm Rupture

Overview: abnormal dilation of the abdominal aorta leads to vessel rupture

Patient may complain of: severe abdominal/back pain, palpitations, nausea, vomiting, dizziness

Objective findings: signs of acute distress, altered mental status, diaphoresis, tachycardia, hypotension, pulsating abdominal mass, abdominal bruit

PMH considerations/risk factors: hx of CAD, HTN, heart failure, diabetes, connective tissue disorders, trauma to the abdomen, nicotine use, family hx of AAA, male gender, older age

Diagnostics: abdominal US/CT/MRI

Angina (Stable)

Overview: chest pain caused by a decrease in myocardial oxygen supply that is improved with rest

Patient may complain of: fatigue, chest pain/tightness/heaviness that is worse with activity, better with rest or NTG, radiation of the pain to the left arm/neck/jaw, palpitations, dyspnea, activity intolerance, nausea, dyspepsia, dizziness, feelings of impending doom, anxiety; symptoms have a short duration

Objective findings: signs of acute distress, lethargy, diaphoresis, hypertension, tachycardia, murmur, weak pulses, sluggish capillary refill, tachypnea

PMH considerations/risk factors: hx of angina, CAD, HTN, heart failure, hyperlipidemia, diabetes, cardiac valve disorders, obesity, increased psychological stress, nicotine use, family hx of heart disease

Diagnostics: cardiac enzymes, ECG, stress test, coronary angiography

Angina (Unstable)

Overview: chest pain caused by a decrease in myocardial oxygen supply that is not improved with rest

Patient may complain of: fatigue, chest pain/tightness/heaviness that is worse with activity, not improved with rest or NTG, radiation of the pain to the left arm/neck/jaw, palpitations, dyspnea, activity intolerance, nausea, dyspepsia, dizziness, feelings of impending doom, anxiety; symptoms have a longer duration than stable angina

Objective findings: signs of acute distress, lethargy, diaphoresis, hypertension, tachycardia, murmur, weak pulses, sluggish capillary refill, tachypnea

PMH considerations/risk factors: hx of angina, CAD, HTN, heart failure, hyperlipidemia, diabetes, cardiac valve disorders, obesity, increased psychological stress, nicotine use, family hx of heart disease

Diagnostics: cardiac enzymes, ECG, stress test, coronary angiography

Anxiety

Overview: psychiatric disorder that can cause intense fear and worry

Patient may complain of: fatigue, chest pain, palpitations, dyspnea, nausea, vomiting, abdominal pain, constipation/diarrhea, paresthesias, tremors, dizziness, headache, insomnia, mind racing, feelings of impending doom

Objective findings: signs of acute distress, irritability, inability to focus, diaphoresis, tachycardia, hypertension, tachypnea, muscle tension

PMH considerations/risk factors: hx of anxiety, depression, PTSD, insomnia, substance abuse, physical abuse, recent physical or emotional trauma, family hx of psychiatric diseases

Diagnostics: clinical diagnosis; workup to rule out more emergent causes may be indicated

Arrhythmia

Overview: any irregular heart rhythm

Patient may complain of: fatigue, generalized weakness, (pre) syncope, palpitations, chest pain, dyspnea, dizziness, anxiety

Objective findings: signs of acute distress, lethargy, irritability, diaphoresis, irregular heart rhythm, bradycardia/tachycardia, murmur, hypertension/hypotension, tachypnea, seizures

PMH considerations/risk factors: hx of arrhythmia, CAD, HTN, heart failure, MI, cardiac valve disorders, diabetes, previous CV surgery, substance abuse, increased psychological stress, nicotine use, family hx of heart disease

Diagnostics: BMP/CMP, CBC, TSH, ECG, ECHO, Holter monitor/loop recorder/event recorder

Dehydration

Overview: abnormal loss of extracellular fluid volume

Patient may complain of: fatigue, thirst, dry mouth, palpitations, constipation, oliguria, muscle cramps, dizziness, headache

Objective findings: fever, altered mental status, lethargy, irritability, decreased skin turgor, generalized skin dryness, dry mucous membranes, (orthostatic) hypotension, tachycardia, oliguria

PMH considerations/risk factors: hx of liver or renal disease/failure, recent vomiting and/or diarrhea, GI bleeding, polyuria, diuretic use, burn injury, or intense physical activity

Diagnostics: BMP/CMP, CBC, urine Na, I/O

Heart Failure

Overview: broad term to describe pumping malfunction of the heart

Patient may complain of: fatigue, activity intolerance, chest pain, palpitations, dyspnea, orthopnea, PND, coughing, sputum production, weight gain/loss, anorexia, nausea, nocturia, insomnia

Objective findings: signs of acute distress, lethargy, diaphoresis, cyanosis, JVD, bradycardia/tachycardia, hypertension/hypotension, displaced PMI, murmur, gallop, weak pulses, sluggish capillary refill, digital clubbing, edema, breathlessness, tachypnea, cough, adventitious lung sounds, sputum, hepatomegaly, ascites

PMH considerations/risk factors: hx of heart failure, HTN, CAD, cardiac valve disorders, MI, diabetes, arrhythmias, hyper/hypothyroidism, obesity, nicotine use, substance abuse, family hx of heart disease

Diagnostics: BNP, BMP/CMP, TSH, ECG, I/O, chest X-ray, ECHO, cardiac catheterization

Hyperkalemia

Overview: elevated serum potassium

Patient may complain of: fatigue, palpitations, diarrhea, nausea, vomiting, dyspepsia, muscle weakness and cramps, paresthesias; patient is typically asymptomatic unless severe

Objective findings: lethargy, hypotension, peaked T waves, arrhythmia, weak pulses, hyperactive bowel sounds; exam is typically unremarkable unless severe

PMH considerations/risk factors: hx of arrhythmia, CKD, AKI, Addison's disease, diabetes, burn injury, recent surgery

Diagnostics: serum K, ECG

Hypernatremia

Overview: elevated serum sodium

Patient may complain of: thirst, muscle spasms and cramps, tremors, seizures, anxiety; patient is typically asymptomatic unless severe

Objective findings: irritability, altered mental status, decreased skin turgor, dry mucous membranes, tachycardia, hypotension, bradypnea, decreased reflexes; exam is typically unremarkable unless severe

PMH considerations: hx of AKI, Cushing's syndrome, GI loss, burn injury, diabetes, diuretic use

Diagnostics: serum Na

Hyperthyroidism

Overview: overactive thyroid gland

Patient may complain of: anxiety, heat intolerance, fatigue, generalized weakness, palpitations, diarrhea, nausea, vomiting, weight loss, muscle cramps, tremors, seizures, insomnia

Objective findings: lethargy, irritability, diaphoresis, hair thinning, exophthalmos, goiter, tachycardia, hypertension, tremors, seizures

PMH considerations/risk factors: hx of Grave's disease, thyroiditis, pregnancy, thyroid cancer, family hx of thyroid dysfunction, female gender, older age

Diagnostics: TSH, T3, T4, thyroid US, radioactive iodine uptake scan

Hypokalemia

Overview: low serum potassium

Patient may complain of: fatigue, palpitations, nausea, vomiting, constipation, muscle weakness and cramping, seizures, anxiety; patient is typically asymptomatic unless severe

Objective findings: lethargy, irritability, altered mental status, wide QRS, arrhythmia, bradypnea, hypoactive bowel sounds, decreased reflexes; exam is typically unremarkable unless severe

PMH considerations/risk factors: hx of CKD, diabetes, diarrhea, alcohol abuse/use, eating disorders, NPO status, diuretic use

Diagnostics: serum K, ECG

Hyponatremia

Overview: low serum sodium

Patient may complain of: fatigue, thirst, nausea, vomiting, anorexia, muscle cramps and weakness, seizures, headache; patient is typically asymptomatic unless severe

Objective findings: altered mental status, lethargy, irritability, tachycardia, weak pulses, bradypnea, decreased reflexes; exam is typically unremarkable unless severe

PMH considerations/risk factors: recent GI loss, hx of CKD, heart failure, diuretic use, SIADH, dehydration

Diagnostics: serum Na

Myocardial Infarction

Overview: decreased or no blood flow through the coronary arteries causing cardiac muscle death

Patient may complain of: fatigue, chest pain not improved with rest, radiation of the pain to the left arm/neck/jaw, palpitations, dyspnea, activity intolerance, abdominal pain, nausea, dizziness, anxiety, feelings of impending doom; symptoms have longer duration than stable angina

Objective findings: signs of acute distress, lethargy, irritability, altered mental status, diaphoresis, cool clammy skin, hypertension/hypotension, tachycardia/bradycardia, arrhythmia, murmur, ST elevations, pathologic Q waves, weak pulses, sluggish capillary refill, tachypnea

PMH considerations/risk factors: hx of MI, CAD, HTN, heart failure, hyperlipidemia, diabetes, cardiac valve disorders, sedentary lifestyle, NSAID use, nicotine use, substance abuse, family hx of heart disease, older age

Diagnostics: cardiac enzymes, ECG, stress test, coronary angiography

Pneumothorax

Overview: abnormal air or fluid in the pleural cavity causing lung collapse

Patient may complain of: sudden onset of chest pain, palpitations, dyspnea, coughing, anxiety, feelings of impending doom

Objective findings: signs of acute distress, tachycardia, hypotension, tachypnea, diminished/absent unilateral breath sounds, uneven chest excursion, tracheal deviation, hypoxia, cough

PMH considerations/risk factors: hx of Marfan syndrome, COPD, cystic fibrosis, asthma, TB, trauma to the chest/back, thin

body habitus, recent thoracentesis or pulmonary biopsy, family hx of pneumothorax, nicotine use, male gender
Diagnostics: chest X-ray

Pulmonary Embolism

Overview: a blood clot in the pulmonary vasculature

Patient may complain of: chills, fever, chest pain, pain with deep breaths, palpitations, activity intolerance, dyspnea, coughing, hemoptysis, abdominal pain, dizziness

Objective findings: signs of acute distress, fever, pallor, cyanosis, diaphoresis, tachycardia, S3/S4 heart sounds, hypotension, tachypnea, hypoxia, cough, signs of DVT

PMH considerations/risk factors: hx of DVT, PE or CVA, bleeding/clotting disorder, cancer, pregnancy, HRT/birth control use, IV drug use, recent surgery, immobility, nicotine use

Diagnostics: D-dimer, chest CT, V/Q scan, chest X-ray

Sepsis

Overview: severe inflammatory response due to an infection causing organ dysfunction

Patient may complain of: chills, fever, fatigue, generalized weakness, palpitations, (pre)syncope, dyspnea, oliguria; symptoms of whatever infection is suspected (i.e., appendicitis, diverticulitis, cholecystitis, pneumonia, cellulitis, meningitis, UTI)

Objective findings: signs of acute distress/illness, lethargy, fever, altered mental status, cyanosis, cool clammy skin or warm to the touch, tachycardia, hypotension, tachypnea, hypoxia, oliguria; signs of whatever infection is suspected

PMH considerations/risk factors: hx of immunosuppression, diabetes, cancer, recent infection or hospitalization, older/younger age

Diagnostics: blood culture, lactate, CBC, BMP/CMP, PT/INR; workup may also relate to whatever infection is suspected

Withdrawal (Alcohol)

Overview: rapid or abrupt decrease in alcohol intake causing physical and psychological disturbances

Patient may complain of: fever, chills, palpitations, anorexia, nausea, vomiting, diarrhea, seizures, headache, alcohol craving, insomnia, anxiety

Objective findings: signs of acute distress, fever, irritability, altered mental status, diaphoresis, tachycardia, hypertension, hepatomegaly, ascites, seizures, tremors, hallucinations/delirium

PMH considerations: hx of alcohol abuse, longer cessation (>48 hrs) since last drink, other substance abuse

Diagnostics: toxicology screen; workup to rule out more emergent causes may be indicated

Withdrawal (Opioids)

Overview: rapid or abrupt decrease in opioid intake causing physical and psychological disturbances

Patient may complain of: fever, body aches, nasal congestion, nasal drainage, anorexia, abdominal cramping, diarrhea, nausea, vomiting, tremors, opioid craving, anxiety, insomnia

Objective findings: signs of acute distress, fever, irritability, altered mental status, diaphoresis, piloerection, frequent yawning, pupil dilatation, rhinorrhea, hypertension, tachycardia, hyperactive bowel sounds

PMH considerations/risk factors: hx of daily opioid use, chronic pain, other substance abuse

Diagnostics: toxicology screen; workup to rule out more emergent causes may be indicated

References

Al-Khatib, S. M., Arshad, A., Balk, E. M., Das, S. R., Hsu, J. C., Joglar, J. A., & Page, R. L. (2015). Risk stratification for arrhythmic events in patients with asymptomatic pre-excitation: A systematic review for the 2015 ACC/AHA/HRS guideline for the management of adult patients with supraventricular tachycardia. *Circulation, 133*(14), 575–586.

Al-Khatib, S. M., & Page, R. L. (2016). Acute treatment of patients with supraventricular tachycardia. *JAMA Cardiology, 1*(4), 483–485.

Al-Zaiti, S. S., & Magdic, K. S. (2016). Paroxysmal supraventricular tachycardia: Pathophysiology, diagnosis, and management. *Critical Care Nursing Clinics of North America, 28*(3), 309–316.

American Medical Directors Association. (2010). *Know-it-all before you call: Data collection system.* Columbia, MD: Author.

Baldzizhar, A., Manuylova, E., Marchenko, R., Kryvalap, Y., & Carey, M. G. (2016). Ventricular tachycardias: Characteristics and management. *Critical Care Nursing Clinics of North America, 28*(3), 317–329.

Busmer, L. (2011). Postural orthostatic tachycardia syndrome. *Primary Health Care, 21*(9), 16–20.

Cantillon, D. J., Loy, M., Burkle, A., Pengel, S., Brosovich, D., Hamilton, A., … Lindsay, B. D. (2016). Association between off-site central monitoring using standardized cardiac telemetry and clinical outcomes among non-critically ill patients. *JAMA, 316*(5), 519–524.

Colucci, R. A., Silver, M. J., & Shubrook, J. (2010). Common types of supraventricular tachycardia: Diagnosis and management. *American Family Physician, 82*(8), 942–952.

Desai, S. P. (2009). *Clinician's guide to laboratory medicine* (3rd ed.). Houston, TX: MD2B.

Ganz, L. I. (2016). Clinical manifestations, diagnosis, and evaluation of narrow QRS complex tachycardias. In B. C. Downey (Ed.), *UpToDate.* Retrieved from https://www.uptodate.com/contents/clinical-manifestations-diagnosis-and-evaluation-of-narrow-qrs-complex-tachycardias

Ganz, L. I. (2018). Wide QRS complex tachycardias: Approach to management. In B. C. Downey (Ed.), *UpToDate.* Retrieved from https://www.uptodate.com/contents/wide-qrs-complex-tachycardias-approach-to-management

Hale, A., & Hovey, M. J. (2014). *Fluid, electrolyte and acid-base imbalances.* Philadelphia, PA: F.A. Davis Company.

Heidenreich, P. A., Solis, P., Estes, N. A., Fonarow, G. C., Jurgens, C. Y., Marine, J. E., … McNamara, R. L. (2016). 2016 ACC/AHA clinical performance and quality measures for adults with atrial fibrillation or atrial flutter. *Journal of the American College of Cardiology, 68*(5), 525–568.

Helton, M. R. (2015). Diagnosis and management of common types of supraventricular tachycardia. *American Family Physician, 92*(9), 793–802.

Homound, M. (2018). Sinus tachycardia: Evaluation and management. In B. C. Downey (Ed.), *UpToDate.* Retrieved from https://www.uptodate.com/contents/sinus-tachycardia-evaluation-and-management

January, C. T., Wann, S., Alpert, J. S., Calkins, H., Cleveland, J. C., Cigarroa, J. E., … Halperin, J. (2014). 2014 AHA/HRS guideline for the management of patients with atrial fibrillation: A report of the American college of cardiology/American heart association task force on practice guidelines and the heart rhythm society. *Circulation, 130*(23), 199–267.

Jarvis, C. (2015). *Physical examination & health assessment.* St. Louis, MO: Elsevier.

Kaufmann, H., & Freeman, R. (2015). Postural tachycardia syndrome. In J. L. Wilterdink (Ed.), *UpToDate.* Retrieved from https://www.uptodate.com/contents/postural-tachycardia-syndrome

LeBlond, R. F., Brown, D. D., Suneja, M., & Szot, J. F. (2015). *DeGowin's diagnostic examination* (10th ed.). New York, NY: McGraw-Hill.

McCance, K. L., Huether, S. E., Brashers, V. L., & Rote, N. S. (2014). *Pathophysiology: The biologic basis for disease in adults and children* (7th ed.). St. Louis, MO: Elsevier.

Page, R. L., Joglar, J. A., Caldwell, M. A., Calkins, H., Conti, J. B., Deal, B. J., … Al-Khatib, S. M. (2016). 2015 ACC/AHA/HRS guideline for the management of adult patients with supraventricular tachycardia. *Journal of the American College of Cardiology, 67*(13), 27–115.

Payne, L., Zeigler, V. L., & Gillette, P. C. (2011). Acute cardiac arrhythmias following surgery for congenital heart disease: Mechanisms, diagnostic tools, and management. *Critical Care Nursing Clinics of North America, 23,* 255–272.

Papadakis, M. A., & McPhee, S. J. (2017). *Current medical diagnosis and treatment* (56th ed.). New York, NY: McGraw-Hill.

Peyrol, M., & Levy, S. (2016). Clinical presentation of inappropriate sinus tachycardia and differential diagnosis. *Journal of Interventional Cardiac Electrophysiology, 46,* 33–41.

Priori, S. G., Blomstrom-Lundqvist, C., Mazzanti, A., Blom, N., Borggrefe, M., Camm, J., . . . Veldhuisen, D. J. (2015). 2015 ESC guidelines for the management of patients with ventricular arrhythmias and the prevention of sudden cardiac death. *European Heart Journal, 36,* 2793–2867.

Prutkin, J. M. (2016). Overview of the acute management of tachyarrhythmias. In B. C. Downey (Ed.), *UpToDate.* Retrieved from https://0-www.uptodate.com.libus.csd.mu.edu/contents/overview-of-the-acute-management-of-tachyarrhythmias?source=search_result&search=tachycardia&selectedTitle=2~150

Raftery, A. T., Lim, E., & Ostor, A. J. (2014). *Differential diagnosis* (4th ed.). London: Elsevier.

Raj, S., & Sheldon, R. (2016). Management of postural tachycardia syndrome, inappropriate sinus tachycardia and vasovagal syncope. *Arrhythmia and Electrophysiology Review, 5*(2), 122–129.

Seller, R. H., & Symons, A. B. (2012). *Differential diagnosis of common complaints* (6th ed.). Philadelphia, PA: Elsevier.

Swift, J. (2013). Assessment and treatment of patient with acute tachyarrhythmia. *Nursing Standard, 28*(5), 50–59.

Uphold, C. R., & Graham, M. V. (2013). *Clinical guidelines in family practice* (5th ed.). Gainesville, FL: Barmarrae Books.

CHAPTER 30

Urinary Retention

Urinary retention is the patient's inability to pass urine or completely empty their bladder. It can be caused by inflammation, obstruction, infection, neurological diseases, and medication. Men are more commonly affected than women. If left untreated, urinary retention can lead to renal failure. The volume of urine associated with retention is defined as >500mL.

Acute retention usually presents with abdominal pain and bladder distention, while chronic retention is typically painless. The main priority of the nurse is to measure the patient's urine output, performed most accurately via catheterization. Catheterization is also the gold standard treatment for acute urinary retention. Other priorities include distinguishing retention from oliguria, which is urine production of <0.5mL/kg/day, and anuria, which is urine production of <50mL/day. Oliguria and anuria are usually associated with acute kidney injury or chronic kidney disease and are not topics covered in this chapter.

Differential Diagnosis Considerations

Common: BPH, constipation, medication induced, perineal trauma, post-surgical state, pyelonephritis, urethritis, urolithiasis, UTI

Consider: AKI, balanitis, CKD, CVA, cystocele, detrusor sphincter, diabetic neuropathy, dyssynergia, Fowler's syndrome, GU malignancy, Guillain-Barré syndrome, herpes zoster, MS, Parkinson's disease, pelvic organ prolapse, post-partum complication, prostatitis, spinal cord injury, urethral stricture, vulvovaginitis

Questions to Ask the Patient/ Family/Witness/Yourself

- When did the urinary difficulty start? Are you able to urinate at all?

- When was the last time you urinated?
- Is it difficult to start the stream?
- Do you feel like you empty your bladder completely?
- What color is your urine (yellow, amber, red, pink, cola colored)?
- Have you seen any blood in your urine?
- Do you have any pain when you urinate?
- How much fluid are you drinking on a daily basis?
- Do you have a history of difficulty emptying your bladder/urination? If so, what has been done or used to treat it?
- Have you had any recent: radiation therapy? surgery? trauma to the abdomen or pelvis?
- Have you had any recent invasive interventions such as spinal anesthesia or a urinary catheter?
- Have you taken any new prescribed or over-the-counter medications? Have there been any recent changes to your current medication?

Associated Signs/Symptoms: PAIN: pain anywhere; GENERAL: chills, fatigue, fever, weakness; CARDIOVASCULAR: edema; GASTROINTESTINAL: bloating, constipation, LBM, nausea, vomiting; GENITOURINARY: bladder fullness, incontinence, nocturia, penile/vaginal discharge, urinary urgency; PSYCHOLOGICAL: anxiety, confusion

Recommended Assessments

- Vital signs
- Temperature
- I/O
- Pain scale (if applicable)
  - Tolerable pain level
- General
  - Level of consciousness and orientation
  - Inspect: signs of acute distress, acute illness, affect, restlessness
- Skin
  - Inspect: dryness, ecchymosis, vesicular rash
  - Palpate: turgor

- Gastrointestinal
  - Inspect: distention
  - Auscultate: bowel sounds
  - Palpate: masses, hernias, organomegaly, (rebound) tenderness
- Genitourinary
  - Inspect: cystocele, external drainage, erythema, swelling, lesions, uterine prolapse
  - Palpate: bladder distention, CVAT
- Extremities
  - Inspect: IV site (if applicable)
  - Palpate: capillary refill, edema, pulses

Past Medical History Considerations

Puts the patient at risk for differential considerations

- CKD
- Diabetes
- Immobilization
- Incontinence
- Radiation therapy to the abdomen/pelvis

Reoccurrence/exacerbation should be considered

- Prostatitis
- Urolithiasis
- UTI

Chronic conditions that can cause urinary retention

- BPH
- Constipation
- CVA/TIA
- Cystocele
- GU malignancy
- Guillain-Barré syndrome
- MS

- Neuropathy
- Parkinson's disease
- Spinal cord injury

Medication Evaluation

Most common causative/exacerbating medication

- Antiarrhythmics
- Anticholinergics
- Antihistamines
- Antiparkinson agents
- Antipsychotics
- HRT
- Hydralazine
- Muscle relaxers
- Nifedipine
- NSAIDs
- Opioids
- Sympathomimetic agents
- Tricyclic antidepressants

Lab Evaluation and Trends

- BMP/CMP

Nursing Intervention Considerations

- Verify patent IV if IVF or IV medication treatment is antici-
  pated
  - Flush according to facility protocol; watch for
    swelling, erythema, pain, and other signs of
    infiltration
- Bladder scan/PVR
- Medications (if ordered or protocol allows)
  - Hold suspected causative medication until discussion
    with the provider

- Diet
  - Avoid bladder irritants such as soda, coffee, tea, and chocolate
  - Avoid foods that can discolor urine, such as beetroot, blackberries, blueberries, rhubarb, fava beans, and foods with artificial coloring
  - Offer warm fluids before elimination attempts
- Activity
  - Encourage activity and ambulation if safety permits
- Collect
  - Urine sample (if able)
- Monitor
  - Pain levels
  - Vital signs and trends
  - Temperature trends
  - I/O
  - Orientation status changes
  - Agitation levels
  - Skin assessment every 8–24 hours or more frequently if incontinent
  - Signs of dehydration such as lethargy, decreased skin turgor, dry mucous membranes, tachycardia, and (orthostatic) hypotension
  - Signs and symptoms of GU infection such as fever, chills, dysuria, hematuria, increased urinary frequency and urgency, fatigue, altered mental status, and back/flank pain
  - Catheter patency and kinking
  - PVR
  - Urine output color, frequency, and volume
- Environment
  - Provide a calm, quiet environment and reduce stimulation
  - Remove distractions during elimination attempts
  - Provide privacy and "Do Not Disturb" notice on the patient's door during elimination if safety permits

- Supportive care
  - Maintain effective communication between yourself, patient, and family
  - Provide emotional support and reassurance to the patient and family
  - Maintain a calm manner during patient interactions
  - Discuss plan of care with the patient and decide reasonable goals together
  - Notify the patient and family of changes in the plan of care
  - Identify barriers to care and compliance
  - Promote skin care and integrity
  - Encourage frequent attempts to void
  - **Educational topics (as applicable to the patient):**
    - General information regarding the patient's urinary retention and differential diagnosis considerations
    - Procedure and intervention explanation and justification
    - Explanation regarding referrals and specialist who may see them for this issue
    - Medication changes
    - Pain scale and pain goals
    - Relaxation techniques and breathing exercises
    - Bladder scanning/PVR
    - Catheter care and irrigation
    - Strict I/O
    - Peri-care and proper hygiene
    - Skin care
    - Handwashing and infection control measures
    - Avoidance of bladder irritants
    - Avoidance of food/fluid that can discolor the urine
    - Increased physical activity
    - When to notify the nurse or provider
    - Signs and symptoms of GU infection
    - Dehydration prevention
    - Pressure injury prevention

ISBARR Recommendation

Considerations

- Medication
  - Discontinue/change suspected causative medication
- IV fluid needs if oral intake is poor, there are signs of dehydration, and the patient is NPO or hypotensive
- Bladder scan/PVR if a rescan is needed
- Bladder irrigation
- Foley catheter or straight catheter insertion
- Imaging (depending on the suspected cause):
  - Abdominal CT scan, bladder US (if unavailable on unit)
- Labs
  - BMP/CMP
  - Urinalysis
  - Urine culture
- Safety
  - Activity-level changes
- Monitoring needs
  - Daily weights
  - Strict I/O
- Referrals
  - Urology
- Ask if the provider wants anything else done
- Read back orders; ask that they enter all orders into the electronic medical record

ISBARR Template	
I **Introduction**	**Introduce Yourself and the Patient** • "Hello, Dr. Amidon. This is AJ Tindall. I am the nurse for your patient Adam Schlicht in Room 109. He returned to me from PACU after his cholecystectomy about eight hours ago."

ISBARR Template	
S **Situation**	**Sign/Symptom You Are Concerned About** • "Mr. Schlicht has not been able to urinate since getting to the floor and has tried multiple times over the past few hours." **Associated Signs/Symptoms** • "He is otherwise asymptomatic besides 4/10 abdominal pain surrounding his sutures." **Vitals** • "Vitals are stable. BP is 112/80, heart rate is 70, and temperature is 98.8." **Exam** • "His bladder is palpable and mildly distended with no tenderness. Bowel sounds are heard throughout."
B **Background**	**Past Medical History** • "The Foley catheter was removed in PACU. He does not have a history of any urinary difficulties." **Labs and Medications** • N/A in this patient scenario
A **Assessment**	**Assessment** • "I am concerned about urinary retention relating to his surgery and possible irritation from the Foley."
R **Recommendations** **R** **Read Back**	**Nurse's Recommendations, Interventions, and Read Back** • "I performed a bladder scan. He has 550cc in his bladder. Would you like me to use a straight catheter intervention? Would you like anything else done at this time?" • "Thank you, Dr. Amidon. I would like to read those orders back to you. You would like the patient to be straight cathed X 1. Measure post-void residual, then notify you if patient is still unable to urinate in two to three hours. Is all that correct?"

Disclaimer: This dialogue is factitious and any resemblance to actual persons, living or dead, or actual events is purely coincidental.
In order to avoid order discrepancies, it is recommended that all orders be entered by the provider in the electronic medical record.

Select Differential Diagnosis Presentations

Benign Prostatic Hyperplasia

Overview: enlargement of the prostate due to hyperplasia

Patient may complain of: urinary hesitancy, diminished stream force, urinary retention, increased urinary frequency, nocturia, incontinence, hematuria

Objective findings: enlarged prostate with digital rectal exam, bladder distention

PMH considerations/risk factors: hx of BPH, prostatitis, urinary retention, prostate cancer, diabetes, obesity, recent UTI or trauma to pelvis/genitals, older age

Diagnostics: PSA, urinalysis and urine culture, biopsy, PVR

Parkinson's Disease

Overview: progressive movement disorder of the central nervous system

Patient may complain of: fatigue, generalized weakness, vision changes, dysphagia, constipation, urinary retention, gait instability, joint rigidity, tremors, confusion, hallucinations, insomnia; symptoms are progressive in nature

Objective findings: altered mental status, lethargy, flat affect, dysarthria, (orthostatic) hypotension, bradykinesia, generalized muscle and joint rigidity, postural instability, resting tremor, psychosis

PMH considerations/risk factors: hx of Parkinson's disease, trauma to the head, family hx of Parkinson's disease, male gender, older age

Diagnostics: clinical diagnosis; head MRI may be ordered initially

Pyelonephritis

Overview: bacterial infection of the kidney

Patient may complain of: fever; chills; nausea; vomiting; abdominal/back/flank pain; increased urinary frequency, retention, and urgency; dysuria; hematuria; urine odor; confusion (elderly)

Objective findings: signs of acute distress/illness, altered mental status (elderly), fever, tachycardia, CVAT, abdominal tenderness, bladder distention

PMH considerations: hx of frequent UTIs, diabetes, urolithiasis, urinary retention, immunosuppression, pregnancy, poor fluid intake, immobility, recent catheter use or GU surgery, female gender

Diagnostics: CBC, urinalysis, urine culture, renal US

Renal Disease/Failure

Overview: broad term to describe damage and malfunction of the kidneys

Patient may complain of: fatigue, itching, dyspnea, anorexia, nausea, vomiting, oliguria, confusion

Objective findings: lethargy, altered mental status, arrhythmia, edema, pericardial rub, hypertension/hypotension, adventitious lung sounds, oliguria or anuria; exam is typically unremarkable unless severe

PMH considerations/risk factors: hx of CKD, diabetes, HTN, CAD, sepsis, BPH, burn injury, heart failure, dehydration, GI/blood loss, NSAID use, ACE inhibitor use, diuretic use, older age

Diagnostics: BMP/CMP, anion gap, urinalysis, renal US

Urolithiasis

Overview: calculi that form in the urinary tract

Patient may complain of: severe flank/back pain, may radiate to the abdomen, nausea, vomiting, urinary urgency and retention, increased urinary frequency, dysuria, hematuria

Objective findings: signs of acute distress/illness, irritability, fidgeting, CVAT, abdominal tenderness

PMH considerations/risk factors: hx of urolithiasis, short bowel syndrome, malnutrition, diabetes, gout, obesity, dehydration, bariatric surgery, family hx of urolithiasis, female gender

Diagnostics: urinalysis, KUB, renal US

Urinary Tract Infection

Overview: broad term for infection of the urinary tract including the urethra, bladder, ureters, and kidneys

Patient may complain of: fever; chills; abdominal/back/flank/pelvic pain; nausea; vomiting; dysuria; increased urinary frequency, retention, and urgency; hematuria; incontinence; urine odor; confusion (elderly)

Objective findings: fever, altered mental status (elderly), pelvic tenderness, bladder distention; exam is typically unremarkable

PMH considerations/risk factors: hx of frequent UTIs, diabetes, interstitial cystitis, urinary retention, immunosuppression, dehydration, pregnancy, incontinence, recent catheter use, GU surgery or sexual activity, immobility, female gender

Diagnostics: urinalysis/urine dipstick, urine culture

References

Addison, B., & Harvey, M. (2013). Herpes zoster-induced acute urinary retention. *Emergency Medicine Australasia, 25*(3), 279–281. doi:10.1111/1742-6723.12079

American Medical Directors Association. (2010). *Know-it-all before you call: Data collection system.* Columbia, MD: Author.

Barrisford, G. W., & Steele, G. (2018). Acute urinary retention. In H. Libman (Ed.), *UpToDate.* Retrieved from https://www.uptodate.com/contents/acute-urinary-retention

Buchko, B. L., & Robinson, L. E. (2012). An evidence-based approach to decrease early post-operative urinary retention following urogynecologic surgery. *Urological Nursing, 32*(5), 260–264. Retrieved from http://www.medscape.com/viewarticle/773058_5

Desai, S. P. (2009). *Clinician's guide to laboratory medicine* (3rd ed.). Houston, TX: MD2B.

Fatehi, P., & Hsu, C. (2017). Evaluation of acute kidney injury among hospitalized adult patients. In A. Sheidan (Ed.), *UpToDate.* Retrieved from https://www.uptodate.com/contents/evaluation-of-acute-kidney-injury-among-hospitalized-adult-patients

Fatehi, P., & Hsu, C. (2018). Diagnostic approach to adult patients with subacute kidney injury in an outpatient setting. In A. M. Sheridan

(Ed.), *UpToDate*. Retrieved from https://www.uptodate.com/contents /diagnostic-approach-to-adult-patients-with-subacute-kidney-injury -in-an-outpatient-setting

Gardner, J., Mooney, J., & Forester, A. (2013). HEAL: A strategy for advanced practitioner assessment of reduced urine output in hospital inpatients. *Journal of Clinical Nursing, 23*, 1562–1572.

Gulanick, M., & Myers, J. L. (2017). *Nursing care plans: Diagnosis, interventions, & outcomes* (9th ed.). St. Louis, MO: Elsevier.

Hale, A., & Hovey, M. J. (2014). *Fluid, electrolyte and acid-base imbalances*. Philadelphia, PA: F.A. Davis Company.

Jarvis, C. (2015). *Physical examination & health assessment*. St. Louis, MO: Elsevier.

Johansson, R. M., Malmvall, B. E., Andersson-Gare, B., Larsson, B., Erlandsson, I., Sund- Levander, M., . . . Christensson, L. (2013). Guidelines for preventing urinary retention and bladder damage during hospital care. *Journal of Clinical Nursing, 22*(3), 347–355.

LeBlond, R. F., Brown, D. D., Suneja, M., & Szot, J. F. (2015). *DeGowin's diagnostic examination* (10th ed.). New York, NY: McGraw-Hill.

Liangos, O., & Jaber, B. (2018). Kidney and patient outcomes after acute kidney injury in adults. In A. Sheridan (Ed.), *UpToDate*. Retrieved from https://www.uptodate.com/contents/kidney -and-patient-outcomes-after-acute-kidney-injury-in-adults

McCance, K. L., Huether, S. E., Brashers, V. L., & Rote, N. S. (2014). *Pathophysiology: The biologic basis for disease in adults and children* (7th ed.). St. Louis, MO: Elsevier.

Mody, L., & Juthani-Mehta, M. (2014). Urinary tract infections in older women: A clinical review. *JAMA, 311*(8), 844–854. doi:10.1001/ jama.2014.303

National Institute of Health. (2014). Urinary retention. *NIH Publications, 14*, 1–16.

Okusa, M. D., & Rosner, M. H. (2017). Overview of the management of acute kidney injury (acute renal failure). In A.M. Sheridan (Ed.), *UpToDate*. Retrieved from https://www.uptodate.com/contents/overview -of-the-management-of-acute-kidney-injury-in-adults

Papadakis, M. A., & McPhee, S. J. (2017). *Current medical diagnosis and treatment* (56th ed.). New York, NY: McGraw-Hill.

Raftery, A. T., Lim, E., & Ostor, A. J. (2014). *Differential diagnosis* (4th ed.). London: Elsevier.

Seller, R. H., & Symons, A. D. (2012). *Differential diagnosis of common complaints* (6th ed.). Philadelphia, PA: Elsevier.

Smith, M. D., Seth, J. H., Fowler, C. J., Miller, R. F., & Panicker, J. N. (2013). Urinary retention for the neurologist. *Practical Neurology, 13*(5), 288–291. doi:10.1136/practneurol-2012-000478

Stoffel, J., Lightner, D., Peterson, A., Sandhu, J., Suskind, A., & Wei, J. (2016). *Non-neurogenic chronic urinary retention: Consensus definition, management strategies, and future opportunities.* Retrieved from http://www.auanet.org/guidelines/chronic-urinary-retention

Uphold, C. R., & Graham, M. V. (2013). *Clinical guidelines in family practice* (5th ed.). Gainesville, FL: Barmarrae Books.

Abbreviations

Disclaimer: Please review your organization's approved abbreviation list and The Joint Commission's "Do Not Use" abbreviation list (https://www.jointcommission.org/facts_about _do_not_use_list/).

AAA: abdominal aortic aneurysm
ABCs: airway, breathing, circulation
ABD/abd: abdomen
ABG: arterial blood gas
ABI: ankle brachial index
ACE: angiotensin converting enzyme
ACS: acute coronary syndrome
ADLs: activities of daily living
AIDS: acquired immunodeficiency syndrome
AKI: acute kidney injury
ALS: amyotrophic lateral sclerosis
ALT: alanine transaminase
AM: morning
ARB: angiotensin II receptor blockers
ARDS: acute respiratory distress syndrome
ASA: aspirin
AST: aspartate transaminase
AV: atrioventricular
AVNRT: atrioventricular node re-entry tachycardia
AVRT: atrioventricular re-entry tachycardia
BID: twice a day
BMP: basic metabolic panel
BNP: brain natriuretic peptide
BP: blood pressure
BPH: benign prostatic hyperplasia
BPPV: benign paroxysmal positional vertigo

BRAT: banana, rice, applesauce, toast
BUN: blood urea nitrogen
Ca: calcium
CAD: coronary artery disease
CAM: Confusion Assessment Method
CANVAS: cerebellar ataxia neuropathy and vestibular areflexia
   syndrome
CBC: complete blood count
cc: cubic centimeter
CCB: calcium channel blocker
cm: centimeter
CHF: congestive heart failure
CIWA-Ar: Clinical Institute Withdrawal Assessment for Alcohol
   revised
CKD: chronic kidney disease
Cl: chloride
CMP: comprehensive metabolic panel
CMV: cytomegalovirus
CNA: certified nursing assistant
CNS: central nervous system
CO: carbon monoxide
COPD: chronic obstructive pulmonary disease
CRP: C-reactive protein
CSF: cerebrospinal fluid
CT: computed tomography
CV: cardiovascular
CVA: cerebrovascular accident
CVAT: costovertebral angle tenderness
D50: dextrose 50%
DASH: dietary approaches to stop hypertension
DBP: diastolic blood pressure
DDD: degenerative disc disease
DIC: disseminated intravascular coagulation
DJD: degenerative joint disease
DKA: diabetic ketoacidosis
dL: deciliter

DVT. deep vein thrombosis
ECG: electrocardiogram
ECHO: echocardiogram
EEG: electroencephalogram
EENT: eyes, ears, nose, throat
EMG: electromyography
ENT: ears, nose, throat
ER: emergency room
ESR: erythrocyte sedimentation rate
ETOH: alcohol
F: Fahrenheit
fL: femtoliter
g: gram
GCA: giant cell arteritis
GCS: Glasgow coma scale
GDH: glutamate dehydrogenase
GERD: gastroesophageal reflux disease
GFR: glomerular filtration rate
GI: gastrointestinal
gtt: drops
GU: genitourinary
GYN: gynecological
Hcg: human chorionic gonadotropin
HCO_3: bicarbonate
HCP: health care provider
Hct: hematocrit
Hgb: hemoglobin
HHS: hyperosmolar hyperglycemic state
HIDA scan: hepatobiliary scan
HIV: human immunodeficiency virus
HOB: head of bed
HPI: history of the present illness
hrs: hours
HRT: hormone replacement therapy
HSV: herpes simplex virus
HTN: hypertension

hx: history
IBD: inflammatory bowel disease
IBS: irritable bowel syndrome
ICD: implantable cardioverter defibrillator
ICP: intracranial pressure
ICS: inhaled corticosteroids
ICU: intensive care unit
IGF: insulin growth factor
IM: intramuscular
INR: international normalized ratio
I/O: intake/output
ISBARR: introduction, situation, background, assessment, recommendations, read back
IU: international units
IUD: intrauterine device
IV: intravenous
JVD: jugular vein distention
K: potassium
kg: kilogram
KUB: kidneys, ureters, and bladder X-ray
L: liter
LABA: long-acting beta agonist
LAMA: long-acting muscarinic antagonist
Lat: lateral
LBM: last bowel movement
lbs: pounds
LLQ: left lower quadrant
LMP: last menstrual period
LOC: level of consciousness
LUQ: left upper quadrant
LVAD: left ventricular assistive device
MAOI: monoamine oxidase inhibitor
max: maximum
mcg: microgram
MCV: mean corpuscular volume
MDI: meter dosed inhaler

mEq: milliequivalents
Mg: magnesium
mg: milligram
MI: myocardial infarction
mIU: milli-international units
mL: milliliter
mmHg: millimeter of mercury
mmol: millimole
MRI: magnetic resonance imaging
MS: multiple sclerosis
MSM: men who have sex with men
MVP: mitral valve prolapse
Na: sodium
N/A: not applicable
NC: nasal cannula
NG: nasogastric
ng: nanogram
NPO: nothing by mouth
NRB: non-rebreather mask
NSAID: non-steroidal anti-inflammatory drug
NTG: nitroglycerin
O_2: oxygen
ox: oximetry
oz: ounce
PA: posterior anterior
PACU: post-anesthesia care unit
PAD: peripheral arterial disease
pCO_2: carbon dioxide partial pressure
PCP: phencyclidine
PE: pulmonary embolism
PEF: peak expiratory flow
pg: picogram
pH: potential of hydrogen
PID: pelvic inflammatory disease
PMH: past medical history
PMI: point of maximum impulse

PND: paroxysmal nocturnal dyspnea

PO: oral

pO_2: partial pressure of oxygen

POTS: postural orthostatic tachycardia syndrome

ppd: pack per day

PPI: proton pump inhibitor

PRN: as needed

PSA: prostate specific antigen

PSVT: paroxysmal supraventricular tachycardia

PT: prothrombin time

PTSD: post-traumatic stress disorder

PTT: partial thromboplastin time

PTU: propylthiouracil

PUD: peptic ulcer disease

PVCs: pre-ventricular contractions

PVD: peripheral vascular disease

PVR: post-void residuals

q: every

QID: four times a day

RBC: red blood cell

RDW: red cell distribution width

RLQ: right lower quadrant

RN: registered nurse

ROM: range of motion

RR: respiratory rate

RSV: respiratory syncytial virus

RUQ: right upper quadrant

SA: sinoatrial

SABA: short-acting beta agonist

SAMA: short-acting muscarinic antagonist

SARS: severe acute respiratory syndrome

sat: saturation

SBP: systolic blood pressure

SCD: sequential compression device

SIADH: syndrome of inappropriate anti-diuretic hormone

SIBO: small intestinal bacterial overgrowth

SL: sublingual
SLE: systemic lupus erythematosus
SNRI: serotonin norepinephrine reuptake inhibitor
SOB: shortness of breath
SQ: subcutaneous
SSI: surgical site infection
SSRI: selective serotonin reuptake inhibitor
STAT: short turnaround time
STD: sexually transmitted disease
SVT: supraventricular tachycardia
TB: tuberculosis
TBI: traumatic brain injury
TEE: transesophageal echocardiography
THC: tetrahydrocannabinol
TIA: transient ischemic attack
TID: three times a day
TMJ: temporomandibular joint disorders
TSH: thyroid stimulating hormone
TZD: thiazolidinedione
U: units
UA: urinalysis
UACS: upper airway cough syndrome
URI: upper respiratory infection
US: ultrasound
UTI: urinary tract infection
V/Q scan: ventilation and perfusion scan
WBC: white blood cell

Labs

Albumin

Normal: 3.4–5.4g/dL

Albumin is produced by the liver and low levels can be indicative of liver disease, malnutrition, and malabsorption.

Amylase and Lipase

Normal: amylase 23–85U/L, lipase 0–160U/L

Amylase and lipase are digestive enzymes that are elevated when the pancreas is inflamed (pancreatitis).

Arterial Blood Gas

Normal: pH 7.35–7.45, pCO_2 35–45, HCO_3 22–28, pO_2 80–100, O_2 saturation 95–100%

Analyzing an ABG will determine if the patient is in an acidotic or alkalotic state, whether it is respiratory or metabolic in nature, and if there is compensation. Common situations where an ABG may be indicated include respiratory dysfunction, sepsis, shock, liver failure, kidney failure, excessive bodily fluid loss, and carbon monoxide poisoning.

Basic Metabolic Panel/Comprehensive Metabolic Panel

Normal BMP: BUN 7–20mg/dL, CO_2 20–29mmol/L, creatinine 0.8–1.2mg/dL, glucose 64–100mg/dL, chloride 96–106mmol/L, potassium 3.7–5.2mEq/L, sodium 136–144mEq/L, calcium 8.5–10.9mg/dL

Normal CMP (including all above tests): albumin 3.4–5.4g/dL, alkaline phosphatase 44–147IU/L, ALT 7–55IU/L, AST 10–48IU/L, total bilirubin 0.2–1.9mg/dL

A BMP includes measurements for kidney function, glucose, and electrolytes. A complete metabolic panel also includes liver function tests. They can be ordered for an extensive list of issues, but are most commonly used when there is concern for kidney dysfunction, liver dysfunction, dehydration, and electrolyte imbalances.

Brain Natriuretic Peptide

Normal: less than 100pg/mL

A BNP level aides in the diagnosis of CHF and heart failure exacerbation. Elevations occur in response to ventricular dilation and fluid overload.

Cardiac Enzymes

Normal: troponin less than 0.01ng/mL, CK 22–198U/L, myoglobin less than 90mcg/L

Cardiac enzymes include troponin, creatine kinase (CK), and myoglobin. They are used to detect myocardial ischemia or infarction. Some providers may only order a troponin level because it is more specific for cardiac injury.

Complete Blood Count

Normal: RBC 3.9–5.7 $\times$ 10^{12}/L, hemoglobin 12.0–17.5g/dL, hematocrit 34–50%, MCV 81–98fL, RDW 11.8–15.6%, WBC 3.5–10.5 $\times$ 10^9/L, platelets 150–450 $\times$ 10^9/L, neutrophils 1.7–7.0 $\times$ 10^9/L, lymphocytes 0.9–2.9 $\times$ 10^9/L, monocytes 0.3–0.9 $\times$ 10^9/L, eosinophils 0.1–0.5 $\times$ 10^9/L, basophils 0.0–0.3 $\times$ 10^9/L

A basic CBC includes measurements of WBCs, RBCs, hemoglobin, hematocrit, and platelets. When ordered with a differential, percentages of the various types of WBCs are given. A CBC can be ordered for an extensive list of issues, but is most commonly used for detecting anemia, as well as signs of inflammation, dehydration, and infection.

Culture (Sputum, Stool, Urine, Wound)

Normal: negative or no growth

A culture is used to detect and identify the specific type of virus, bacteria, parasite, or fungi causing an infection. It will take at least 3–4 days to analyze the specimen. Typically, the patient is treated empirically with broad spectrum antimicrobials until the exact pathogen is identified.

D-Dimer

Normal: less than 500ng/mL

A D-dimer is ordered when there is suspicion for thrombus formation. If the D-dimer is negative, a DVT or PE is unlikely. If levels are elevated, further investigation is necessary.

Digoxin Drug Level

Therapeutic: 0.5–2.0ng/mL

Digoxin is a medication used to treat certain heart conditions such as heart failure and arrhythmias. It has a small therapeutic window, and levels should be checked if toxicity is suspected. Symptoms of digoxin toxicity include headache, sensitivity to light, confusion, nausea, and palpitations.

Helicobacter pylori (Biopsy, Breath, Stool, Serum)

Normal: negative

Testing should strongly be considered in any patient with signs and symptoms of *Helicobacter pylori* infection, which include abdominal pain, bloating, nausea, anorexia, dyspepsia, and signs of GI bleeding. It is important to assess if the patient has had a previous *H. pylori* infection, recently used PPIs, certain antibiotics, and bismuth subsalicylate, because these can all affect the accuracy of the test.

Hemoglobin A1C

Normal: less than 5.7%
Prediabetes: 5.7–6.4%
Diabetes: equal to or greater than 6.5%

A hemoglobin A1C measures the patient's average blood glucose concentration over the past 3 months. An A1C greater than 7.0 indicates poorly controlled glucose levels.

Histamine

Normal: less than 1.0ng/mL

Plasma histamine levels may be considered if an anaphylaxis diagnosis is unclear. A caveat to this test is that levels peak shortly after symptoms begin and rapidly decline thereafter, making it hard to detect if samples are not drawn quickly.

Human Chorionic Gonadotropin

Not pregnant: less than 5.0mIU/mL

A serum or urine Hcg will be ordered if there is suspicion for pregnancy (including ectopic).

Lactate Dehydrogenase

Normal: 0.6–2.3mmol/L

Lactate or lactate dehydrogenase (LDH) is elevated in a wide variety of conditions that cause cellular injury and tissue damage. Levels are usually drawn when there is suspicion for sepsis and shock.

Magnesium

Normal: 1.7–2.3mg/dL

Magnesium levels are not typically drawn with a BMP and have to be ordered separately. A level may be considered if the patient has severe hypocalcemia or hypokalemia, kidney dysfunction, or signs of significant hyper/hypomagnesemia such as muscle weakness, seizures, confusion, or arrhythmias.

Occult Stool

Normal: negative

Occult stool testing, also known as a fecal occult blood test, is done to detect hidden blood in the patient's stool. If positive, additional testing with a colonoscopy is usually required to determine the source of the bleeding.

Prothrombin Time/International Normalized Ratio

Normal: PT 9.4–12.5, INR 0.9–1.1
Therapeutic INR: standard 2.0–3.0, high intensity 2.5–3.5

PT/INR is a measurement of how long it takes the patient's blood to coagulate. The higher the PT/INR level, the higher the patient's bleeding risk. It is most commonly used to manage the dosing of the anticoagulant Coumadin (warfarin). If the patient is not taking Coumadin, an elevation in the PT/INR could indicate liver disease, clotting disorders, or vitamin K deficiency.

Serum Seizure Drug Levels

Therapeutic: phenytoin 10–20mcg/mL, phenobarbital 10–40mcg/mL, valproate 5–25mcg/mL

Many of the seizure medications require close monitoring of their serum levels. Levels too low will have a non-therapeutic effect and the risk for seizures is higher, while elevated levels put the patient at risk for toxicity. Medications that are commonly monitored include phenytoin, phenobarbital, and valproate.

Thyroid Stimulating Hormone

Normal: 0.3–4.2mIU/L

TSH is used to screen for thyroid dysfunction and monitor thyroid function while on replacement therapy. Elevated levels indicate a hypoactive thyroid, while low levels indicate a hyperactive thyroid.

Toxicology Screening

Normal: negative

Toxicology screening via the urine or blood may be indicated if substance abuse is suspected. Typical screening includes the detection of alcohol, amphetamines, barbiturates, benzodiazepines, methadone, cocaine, opiates, PCP, and THC.

Tryptase

Normal: less than 11.5ng/mL

Tryptase is produced by mast cells and will be elevated 15 minutes after the onset of anaphylaxis. Levels may be considered if an anaphylaxis diagnosis is unclear.

Type and Cross Match

Normal: N/A

Type and cross match is used to determine the patient's blood type. It is important to perform this test pre-operatively or if the patient needs a blood transfusion.

Urinalysis

Normal: color pale yellow-amber, clarity clear-hazy, pH 4.5–8.0, specific gravity 1.005–1.040, glucose negative, ketones negative, nitrites negative, leukocyte esterase negative, bilirubin negative, urobilinogen negative, protein negative, RBCs negative, WBCs negative, casts negative, crystals negative, bacteria negative

A urinalysis is commonly ordered when there is concern for kidney dysfunction, GU infection, nephrolithiasis, and DKA.

References

Desai, S. P. (2009). *Clinician's guide to laboratory medicine* (3rd ed.). Houston, TX: MD2B.

Hale, A., & Hovey, M. J. (2014). *Fluid, electrolyte and acid-base imbalances.* Philadelphia, PA: F.A. Davis Company.

McCance, K. L., Huether, S. E., Brashers, V. L., & Rote, N. S. (2014). *Pathophysiology: The biologic basis for disease in adults and children* (7th ed.). St. Louis, MO: Elsevier.

Index

Index

Index

Index

Index

Index

Index

Index

Index

Index

Index

Index